ULTRASOUND OF THE PROSTATE

ULTRASOUND OF THE PROSTATE

Matthew D. Rifkin, M.D.
*Professor of Radiology and Urology
Jefferson Medical College
Thomas Jefferson University
Philadelphia, Pennsylvania*

Raven Press New York

To my wife, Susan—without her constant support, this work would not have been possible

Raven Press, 1185 Avenue of the Americas, New York, New York 10036

© 1988 by Raven Press, Ltd. All rights reserved. This book is protected by copyright. No part of it may be reproduced, stored in a retrieval system, or transmitted, in any form or by any means, electronical, mechanical, photocopying, or recording, or otherwise, without the prior written permission of the publisher.

Made in the United States of America

Library of Congress Cataloging-in-Publication Data

Rifkin, Matthew D.
  Ultrasound of the prostate.

  Bibliography: p.
  Includes index.
    1. Prostate—Diseases—Diagnosis. 2. Prostate—Imaging. 3. Diagnosis, Ultrasonic. I. Title.
  [DNLM: 1. Prostate—pathology. 2. Ultrasonic Diagnosis. WJ 750 R564u]
RC899.R54   1988   616.6′507543   87-45467
ISBN 0-88167-434-6

    The material contained in this volume was submitted as previously unpublished material, except in the instances in which credit has been given to the source from which some of the illustrative material was derived.
    Great care has been taken to maintain the accuracy of the information contained in the volume. However, neither Raven Press nor the author can be held responsible for errors or for any consequences arising from the use of the information contained herein.

9 8 7 6 5 4 3

Preface

Prostate ultrasound—in particular, the endorectal (also known as transrectal) approach—has become, during the past few years, an exciting field with important clinical implications. Although the technique of endorectal ultrasound was actually developed over 20 years ago, its use has become more widespread only during the past few years.

The clinical implications of the technique are immense. It has the potential of being a tool that may markedly decrease the mortality of a prevalent and, in many instances, lethal disease process. However, regardless of the excitement with this technique, there is much information that is yet to be known in terms of its efficacy.

This volume presents an overview of ultrasound imaging of the prostate. Because of the superiority of the endorectal approach, this approach will be emphasized.

Endorectal ultrasound is not necessarily a definitive procedure. There is still overlap in the presentation of different diseases. Although a great deal of knowledge has been gathered over the past few years, there is still much to be learned. While there may be some limitations to prostate ultrasound, its uses and clinical applications are extremely important. The strengths and weaknesses of prostate ultrasound will be discussed.

This book should interest all radiologists, urologists, and other physicians interested in imaging and diagnosis of the prostate. This volume deals with the basic and most elementary aspects of ultrasound and extends to the most advanced techniques and applications of the procedures. Clinicians, sonographers, and nurses, as well as other technologists and medical support personnel, should find this information timely and useful.

Matthew D. Rifkin

Acknowledgments

This book could not have been produced without the support of many individuals. In particular, I would like to thank Larry D. Kradle for photographic credits, Larry Waldroup for visual aids, Saundra Ehrlich for editorial assistance, and Mary M. Rogers of Raven Press for her continuous support. I would also like to thank Dr. Albert Goldstein for his excellent contribution (Chapter 3).

Finally, without the dedication, support, and long hours required (beyond the call of duty) of my secretary, JoAnn A. Gardner, the completion of this text would not have been possible.

Contents

1	Introduction	1
2	Embryology and Normal Anatomy	3
3	Physical Principles of Ultrasound Imaging *Albert Goldstein*	15
4	Scanning Techniques, Equipment, and Patient Preparation	31
5	Normal Sonographic Anatomy	51
6	Prostate and Seminal Vesicle Size Determination	93
7	Sonographic Approach to the Diagnosis of Prostatic Disease	101
8	Biopsy Techniques	113
9	Prostate Cancer: General Considerations	141
10	Prostate Cancer: Sonographic Characteristics	157
11	Percutaneous Use of Radiation Treatment and Treatment Planning	185
12	Benign Prostatic Hyperplasia	191
13	Inflammation of the Prostate and Seminal Vesicles	221
14	Infertility and Seminal Vesicle Disease	229
15	The Prostatic Urethra	241
16	Endorectal Prostatic Ultrasound: Clinical Indications and Clinical Implications	259
	References and Selected Bibliography	267
	Subject Index	285

1 // Introduction

The prostate, despite being a small organ in volume, has the ability to undergo extensive pathophysiologic changes. Although many of these changes are clinically asymptomatic and innocuous, some may be physically debilitating; others may even be life threatening. The prostate gland can be affected by benign neoplastic changes and inflammatory disease. More importantly, the prostate can also harbor malignant degeneration. Most men, during the course of aging, are affected by one or more of these processes, the most significant of which is prostate cancer. Cancer of the prostate is the second most frequently diagnosed cancer in the United States male population and is the third most frequent cause of cancer death (461).

Until recently, a diagnosis of prostatic pathology and cancer, in particular, was determined by clinical symptomatology, the physical examination, a variety of blood serum, and other laboratory examinations; occasionally, diagnosis was determined by diagnostic imaging studies which were of limited value.

Plain and contrast radiographs have had little benefit in evaluation of subtle intrinsic prostate pathology (2,104,274). The radiograph cannot define the prostate directly and only poorly indirectly, even with the administration of iodinated contrast material. A soft tissue mass may cause impression upon the fluid (urine or iodinated contrast) filled urinary bladder. Prostatic calculi may be defined, but the remainder of the soft tissue abnormalities within the prostate appear similar and not identifiable by routine radiography. Soft tissue masses (i.e., those from lymphadenopathy) may cause deviation of the bladder and/or ureters.

The radionuclide study has, in general, shown no usefulness in the evaluation of intrinsic prostatic disease (223,478). In early studies, technetium 99m phytate and technetium 99m antimony sulfacolloid were injected into the prostate gland, but the evaluation of intraprostatic abnormalities and periprostatic lymph nodes has had only limited, if any, success (145). Isotope studies have been utilized with great success to evaluate metastatic lesions, particularly to the bone and possibly within the liver.

Computed tomography (CT), which is able to demonstrate extension of pathology outside the gland, has not been successful in delineating intrinsic prostatic disease (97,98,103,114,159,251,271,481,514). Other than demonstrating the size of the prostate gland, and extension of malignancy, CT of prostatic disease is nonspecific; that is, there are no specific findings to differentiate between focal benign and malignant processes. Both processes will demonstrate homogeneous attenuation of the gland. Extension beyond the capsule of the prostate to stage prostatic carcinoma has only been positive with CT with very invasive lesions. Lymphadenopathy in the pelvic region and in the periprostatic bed is possible, but differentiation of normal-sized nodes with tumor infiltration is not possible from the normal lymph node.

With the recent innovations in magnetic resonance imaging (MRI), pathology within the internal structures of the prostate can now be identified, but this also has its limitations.

MRI is expensive, relatively immobile, requires a long examination time, and may not always be readily available. MRI has been able to demonstrate portions of the prostate. The peripheral zone is clearly delineated on T2 weighted images from the central and periurethral tissues. Tumors will frequently be clearly distinguished in the peripheral zone; however, there is great overlap between benign and malignant prostatic disease (54,196,277). Staging of known carcinomas has had relatively good success in distinguishing between capsular invasion and confined tumors. Further work must be undertaken to clearly identify the roles of MRI and the other complementary imaging modalities.

The introduction of ultrasound during the 1960s was a primary force in the evaluation of prostatic disease. The ability of this unique imaging modality to detect extensive internal derangement of the gland yielded important information, even with the earlier and less sophisticated equipment. The application of diagnostic ultrasound to the genitourinary system, particularly to the prostate, was immediate from the time of initial development.

Almost immediately following the initial production of conventional ultrasound imaging equipment, specialized machines and transducers were developed for endosonography. These instruments allowed placement of ultrasound transducers into various viscera (hollow structures) to allow, theoretically, better resolution of the internal organs. This technique was applied to the upper gastrointestinal system (i.e., endoesophageal and endogastric ultrasound), the bladder (i.e., endovesical, endo/transurethral), and the rectum (i.e., endorectal/transrectal ultrasound). The surrounding structures to the hollow structures could thus be identified.

In the late 1960s, with the early use of ultrasound, only crude images were possible. Equipment was developed slowly over the next few years, progressing from bistable to grayscale imaging. However, it is only in the past few years that increased attention has been given to these endosonographic techniques, particularly for diagnosis of prostatic disease. With these newer developments, endourethral and, in particular, endorectal equipment have become so sophisticated that very small lesions can now be clearly defined. These small areas of abnormality, although present on previous scans, could not be identified because of the technical considerations in the development of the equipment and lack of sophistication of the machines.

During the past two decades, special attention has also been given to the prostate with regard to anatomical considerations. New theories and increased knowledge of the prostate and its relationship to pathogenesis and treatment of various disease processes has occurred. This knowledge, in conjunction with the newer and more highly specialized ultrasound equipment, has allowed the development of this important imaging technique and its applications to the diagnosis, treatment, and follow-up of prostatic disease.

Because of these above considerations, while all aspects of prostatic ultrasound will be discussed, only the endorectal approach will be examined in detail. This is because of the major uses and information obtained that this study alone can provide. When indicated, the other techniques will be discussed. In other instances, only the endorectal study will be mentioned.

2 // *Embryology and Normal Anatomy*

Embryology 3
The Urinary Bladder
Sex Determination
Prostate
Vas Deferens
Seminal Vesicles
Ejaculatory Ducts
Normal Anatomy 5
Gross Anatomy
Histological Anatomic Considerations

Conventional anatomic orientation of the prostate and periprostatic tissues is quite different from the cross-sectional approaches. The former approach is generally taught in medical school; until recently, anatomy relating to axial, sagittal, and coronal imaging was reserved for radiologists. However, when imaging the prostate and periprostatic structures, particularly for sonographic evaluation, a clear understanding of anatomy in all planes is essential. It is also important to understand the embryological development of the prostatic and periprostatic tissues.

EMBRYOLOGY

The Urinary Bladder

The embryogenesis of the urogenital system involves a complex interaction of three developmental systems: the pronephros, the mesonephros, and either the mesonephric duct (in the male) or the paramesonephric duct (in the female). The pronephros, which appears early in embryological life, develops evaginations that grow segmentally in a dorsolateral and caudad projection and fuse to form the pronephric duct. This continues to grow in a caudad direction and then opens into the cloaca. After the pronephros stage of growth, the pronephric duct becomes the mesonephric or Wolffian duct.

The mesonephros develops into the mesonephric tubules, which subsequently become the nephrons. These tubules collectively are termed the *mesonephros* or *Wolffian body*. The permanent kidney develops from the metanephros, as the mesonephros atrophies and disappears.

The urinary bladder is formed from a combination of the cloaca and portions of the mesonephric ducts. The cloaca is divided by the urorectal septum into a ventral urogenital sinus and dorsal rectum. The urogenital sinus is further divided into three parts. These consist of: (i) an *anterior* or *vesicourethral portion* continuous above the allantois; the mesonephric ducts open into this area; (ii) an intermediate section called the *pelvic portion*; and (iii) the posteriorly placed *phallic segment*.

The mesonephric ducts are absorbed by the vesicourethral portion and become the area of the trigone of the bladder and portions of the prostatic urethra. The remainder of the vesicourethral portions develop into the body of the bladder and the remainder of the prostatic urethra. The apex or cephalad allantoic portion becomes elongated as it extends to the umbilicus. This then becomes a narrow channel and is termed the *urachus*. The male mesonephric or Wolffian duct continues to develop into the epididymis, the ductus deferens (vas deferens), and the ejaculatory duct.

Sex Determination

While genetic sexual determination is made at fertilization, gonadal sex is determined by the sex chromosome complex. Both genetically determined male and female embryos are identical in appearance prior to the 7th week of gestation. It is the presence of the Y chromosome which influences development of the testis and seminiferous tubules. The absence of this chromosome leads to ovarian development.

Prostate

The earliest cells of the prostate gland appear during the third month of fetal life. Just prior to the appearance of the prostatic buds, the bladder, which is already formed, tapers into what will become the prostatic urethra. Wolffian ducts open into the area that becomes the verumontanum. On either side of this area, called Müller's hillock, are two laterally placed depressions that will become the prostate. At approximately 12 weeks of fetal life, the appearance of the gland is noted by the development of five areas of solid epithelial tissue. These grow from the prostatic urethra and penetrate the surrounding mesenchymal area. Four weeks later, the buds have developed into tubules with lumina that elongate and multiply. These newly formed groups are called *lobes* (the fibromuscular stroma of the prostate develops in the newborn infant).

The male urethra has two portions: (i) the true urethra, which is situated superior to the openings of the Wolffian ducts, and (ii) the urogenital sinus. The prostatic urethra is composed of the true urethra and a small part of the urogenital sinus. The upper portion of the prostatic urethra will become the vesicle neck, and the lower portion unites with the membranous urethra.

Vas Deferens

Each of the vas deferens develops embryologically from the superior (cranial) end of the Wolffian duct. By the 12th week, the prostatic buds emerge from the urethra, and the vas deferens descends behind the developing bladder. During early embryological development, each of the vas deferens descend and become quite large, dwarfing the urethra in size. They remain large until the 16th week of fetal life, at which time they diminish rapidly in size.

Seminal Vesicles

The seminal vesicles are lateral outpouchings from the vas deferens which develop at approximately the 13th week of fetal life. They develop at the level of the internal vesical sphincter and grow posterolaterally, producing numerous short convoluted channels. By 30 weeks of fetal life, the seminal vesicles are situated posterior to the trigone and communicate with the vas deferens at the base of the prostate where the ejaculatory ducts form. As embryological development progresses, the openings of the ejaculatory ducts shrink in size and the seminal vesicles enlarge. At birth, the seminal vesicles are situated in their normal anatomical position, beneath the base of the bladder, at either side of the trigone.

Ejaculatory Ducts

The two, paired ejaculatory ducts develop from the caudad extension of the Wolffian ducts. They are a continuation of the vas deferens inferior to the seminal vesicles. The ejaculatory ducts, similar to the vas deferens, are relatively large through the 16th week of fetal life, and at that time they begin to shrink in size.

NORMAL ANATOMY

Gross Anatomy

The prostate is surrounded by a thin capsule that is indistinct from the surrounding fascial tissue. The capsule consists of dense fibrous tissue and smooth muscle which connects with the muscular layers of the prostatic urethra and cannot be separated from the prostate without tearing the glandular tissue. The normal postpubescent prostate weights approximately 20 g, although slightly larger glands are considered normal in the over-40-year-old male population (266). The average-sized normal prostate measures approximately 4 cm in maximum transverse diameter, 3 cm in anterior-posterior dimension, and 3.8 cm in cephalocaudad projection.

The prostate is situated immediately superior to the urogenital diaphragm (Fig. 2.1). It is separated from its anterior border, the symphysis pubis, and pubic bones by a collection of vessels (predominantly veins), fat, lymphatics, nerves, and fascial tissues, all termed the *anterior prostatic fat and fascia*. Laterally, the obturator internus (more pronounced superiorly) and levator ani (more pronounced inferiorly) muscles border the glands on either side (Figs. 2.2–2.6). These margins are separated from the prostate by an internal fascial layer. Posteriorly, areolar tissue and Denonvilliers' fascia separate the prostate from the rectum. The superior margin of the gland, the base of the prostate, abuts the inferior aspect of the urinary bladder, the base of the urinary bladder. The seminal vesicles are paired structures, situated on the posterior-superior aspect of the prostate, between the urinary bladder (situated anteriorly) and the rectum (situated posteriorly) (Figs. 2.1 and 2.5). The vas deferens are paired structures originating from the epididymis. They join the seminal vesicles medially (Fig. 2.7). Anterolaterally, there is a collection of veins (Santorini's plexus) bordering the gland, and laterally other venous plexi are present bilaterally.

The prostate is shaped like a flattened cone with its caudad margin, the tip (also known as the apex), providing an exit for the prostatic (also known as the posterior) urethra (Fig.

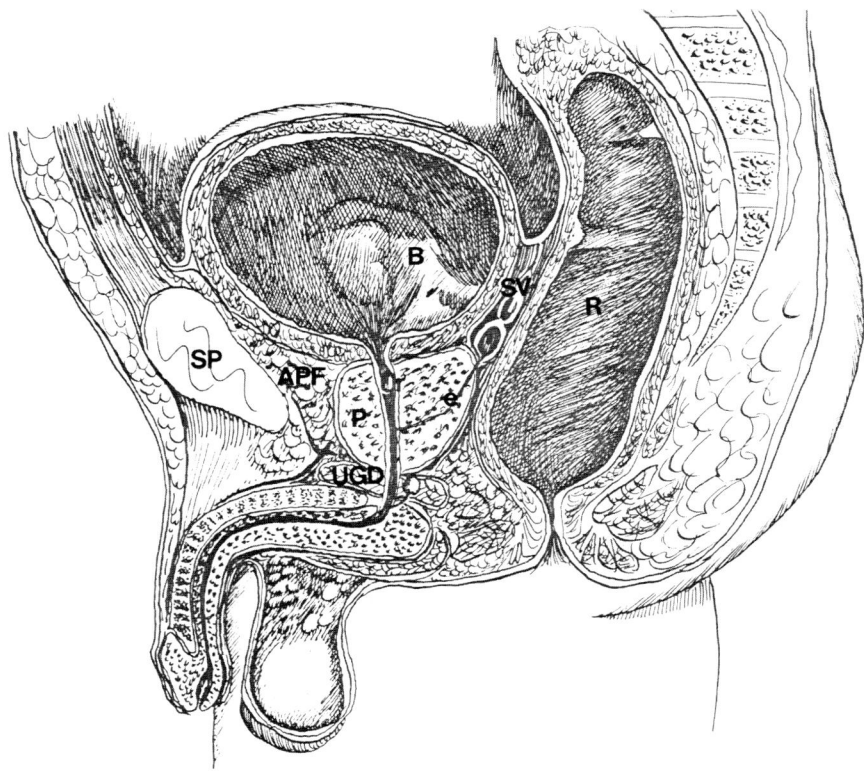

FIG. 2.1. Diagram of the male pelvis in a midline sagittally oriented section, demonstrating the position of the prostate in relation to its structures. (APF) Anterior prostatic fascia; (B) bladder; (e) ejaculatory duct; (P) prostate; (R) rectum; (SP) symphysis pubis; (SV) seminal vesicle; (UGD) urogenital diaphragm; (Ur) prostatic urethra.

2.8). The apex is angled downward and lies slightly anterior, abutting the superior fascia of the urogenital diaphragm. The anterior surface of the prostate is convex, small, and attached to the symphysis pubis and pubic bones by puboprostatic ligaments. The posterior surface which borders the rectum is broader, triangular, and flattened. The posterior surface of the prostate contains a midline depression known as the *median furrow* or *median sulcus*.

The prostatic urethra courses through the prostate from the bladder to the apex of the gland, where it exits and becomes the membranous urethra (Fig. 2.1). There are two bilaterally paired ejaculatory ducts which pass from the junction of the vas deferens and seminal vesicles and angle slightly anteriorly and inferiorly as they join the prostatic urethra at the verumontanum.

The internal sphincter is the area of the proximal prostatic-urethra and consists of the musculature that connects the bladder to the urethra. It consists of a complex or urethral musculature with incorporation of both collagen and elastic fibers.

The external (the voluntary) sphincter is composed of striated skeletal muscle and surrounds the membranous urethra at the level of the urogenital diaphragm.

The older anatomic description of the prostate (i.e., lobar anatomy) divides the prostate into five major lobes. These are: (i) the anterior lobe, which is situated between the anterior

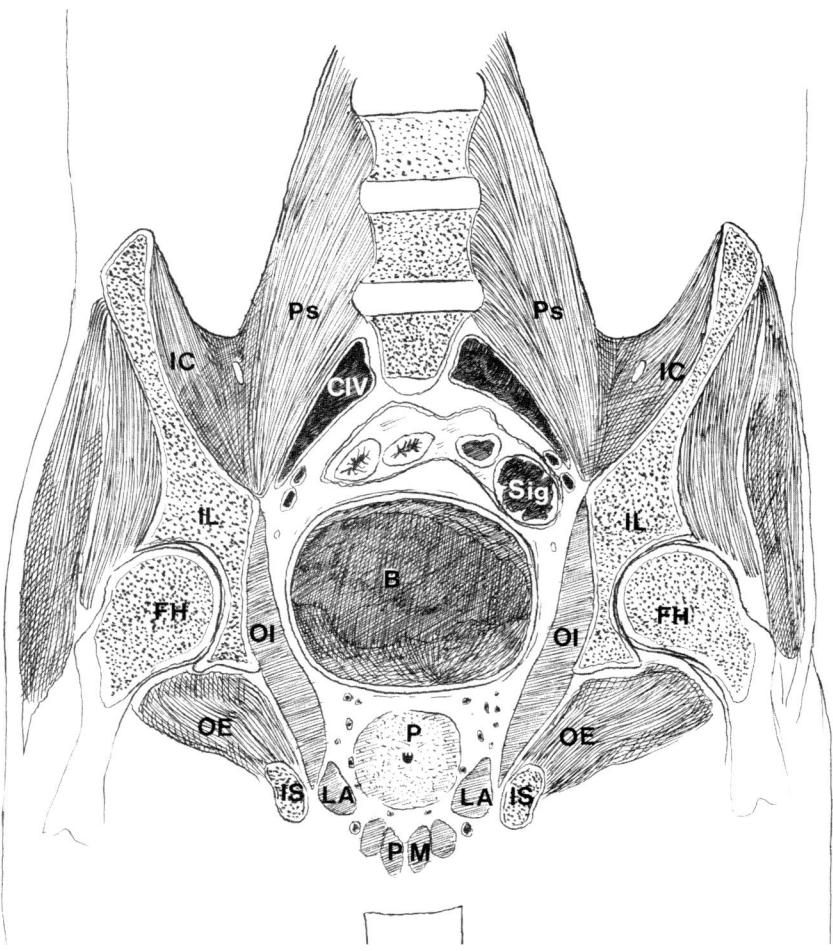

FIG. 2.2. Diagram of the male pelvis in coronal orientation, demonstrating the prostate and its adjacent structures. (B) Bladder; (CIV) common iliac vein; (FH) femoral head; (IC) iliacus muscle; (IL) ilium; (IS) ischium; (LA) levator ani muscle; (OI) obturator internus muscle; (OE) obturator externus muscle; (P) prostate; (PM) penile muscles; (Ps) psoas muscle; (Sig) sigmoid colon. (From reference 393.)

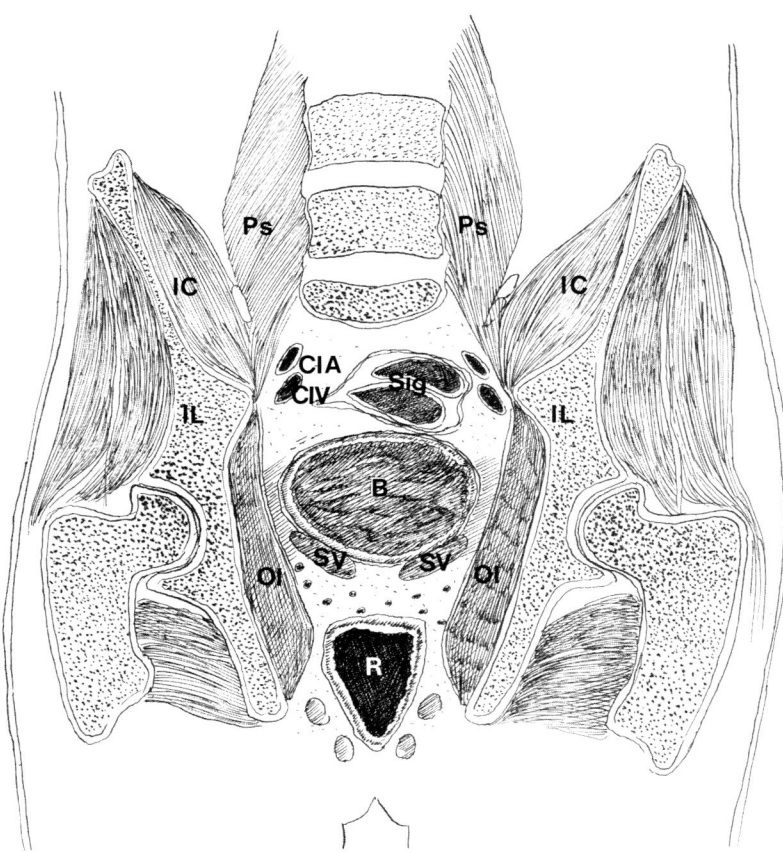

FIG. 2.3. Diagram of the male pelvis in coronal orientation, just posterior to the prostate at the level of the seminal vesicles, demonstrating normal anatomical structures. (B) Bladder; (CIA) common iliac artery; (CIV) common iliac vein; (IC) Iliacus muscle; (IL) ilium; (OI) obturator internus muscle; (Ps) psoas muscle; (R) rectum; (Sig) sigmoid colon; (SV) seminal vesicles. (From reference 393.)

margin of the prostate and the prostatic urethra; (ii) the median or middle lobe, which is delineated by the prostatic urethra anteriorly and the ejaculatory ducts posteriorly; (iii) the posterior lobe, which extends from its anterior margins, the ejaculatory ducts, to the posterior surface of the gland; and (iv and v) two lateral lobes, which are positioned relatively symmetrically. Contiguous with the posterior lobe, the lateral lobes angle toward the prostatic urethra and comprise the majority of the gland. Two minor accessory lobes, poorly defined in the adult, are (i) the subcervical lobe and (ii) the subtrigonal lobe.

Although this is a gross description of anatomy and is important for the surgeon in defining landmarks (i.e., position of possible benign nodule impingement), this is not an accurate anatomic description. Histologically, the prostate is a far more complex structure requiring a different type of description and evaluation.

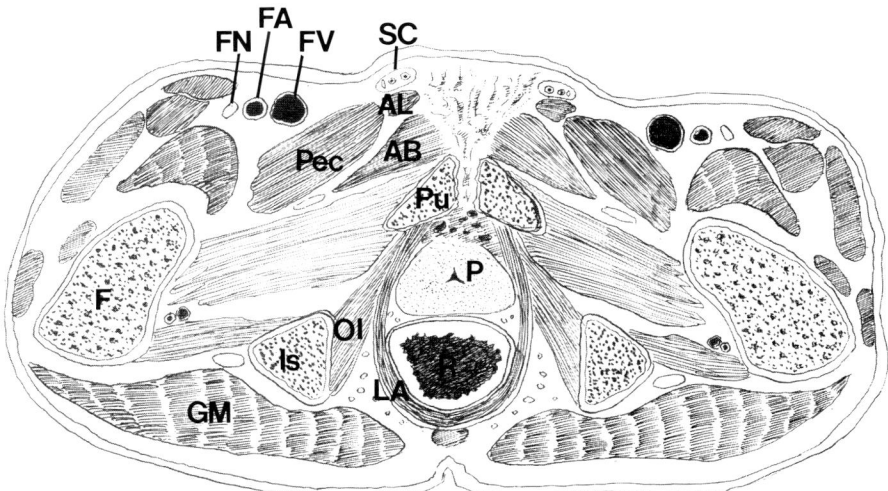

FIG. 2.4. Diagram of the male pelvis in axial orientation at the level of the base of the prostate, demonstrating the normal anatomical structures. (AB) Adductor brevis; (AL) adductor longus; (FA) femoral artery; (FN) femoral nerve; (FV) femoral vein; (GM) gluteus maximus muscle; (Is) ischium; (LA) levator ani muscle; (OI) obturator internus muscle; (P) prostate; (Pec) pectineus muscle; (Pu) pubic bone; (R) rectum; (SC) spermatic cord. (From reference 393.)

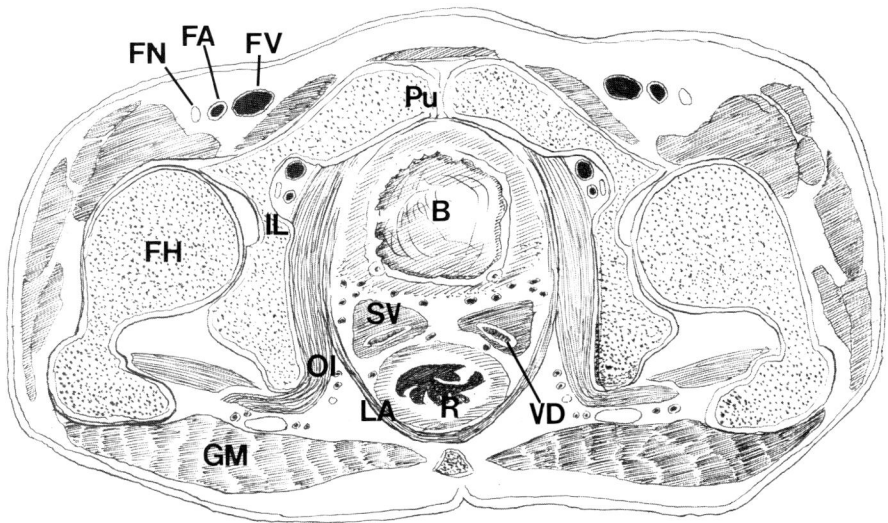

FIG. 2.5. Diagram of the male pelvis in axial orientation at the level of the seminal vesicle, demonstrating normal structures. (B) Bladder; (FA) femoral artery; (FH) femoral head; (FN) femoral nerve; (FV) femoral nerve; (GM) gluteus maximus muscle; (IL) ilium; (LA) levator ani muscles; (OI) obturator internus muscle; (Pu) pubic bones; (R) rectum; (SV) seminal vesicles; (VD) vas deferens. (From reference 393.)

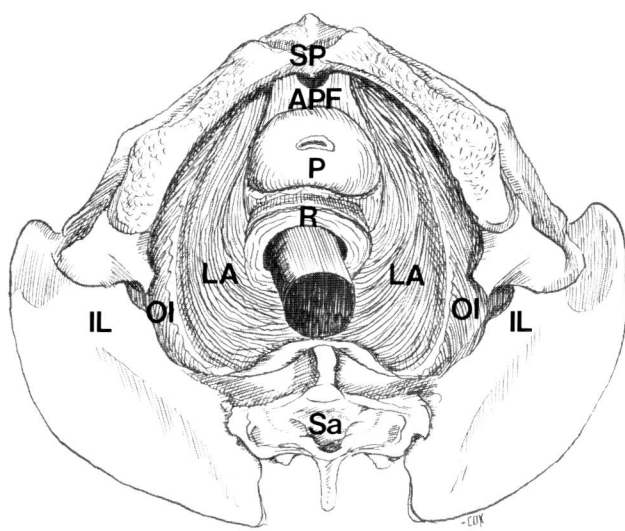

FIG. 2.6. Diagram of the normal male pelvis in an oblique axial orientation with a probe placed within the rectum, demonstrating the prostate and the surrounding normal structures. (APF) Anterior prostatic fat and fascia; (IL) iliac bone; (LA) levator ani muscle; (OI) obturator internus muscle; (P) prostate; (R) rectum; (Sa) sacrum; (SP) symphysis pubis. (From reference 393.)

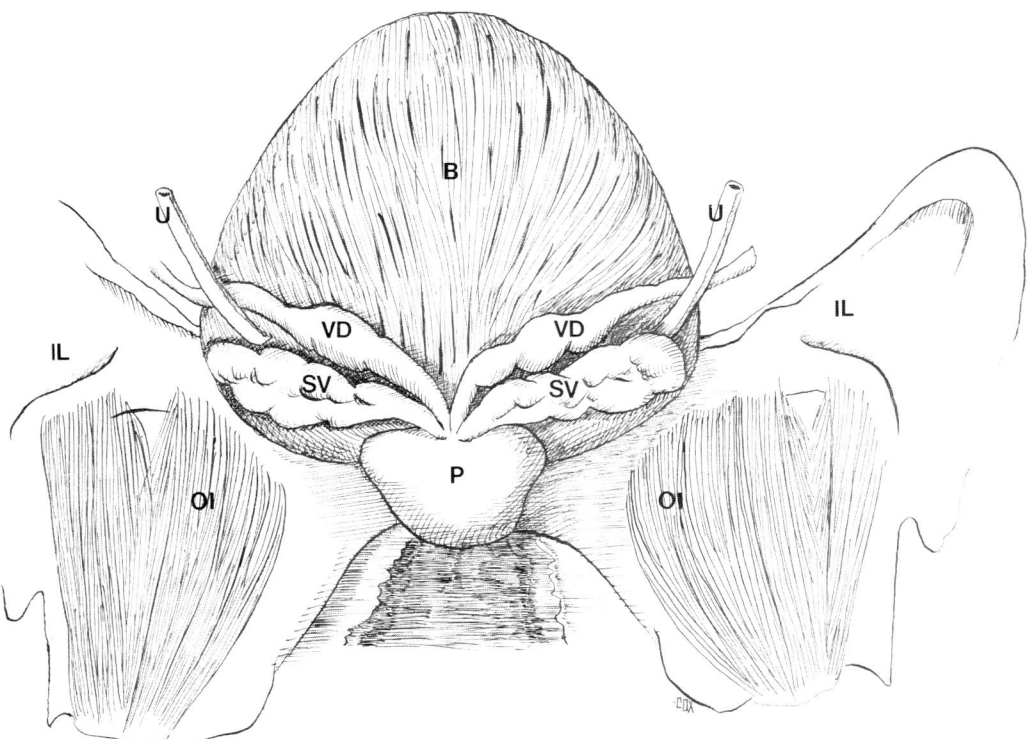

FIG. 2.7. Diagram of the normal male pelvis, demonstrating the orientation of the prostate, vas deferens, and seminal vesicles in relation to the urinary bladder and surrounding musculature. (B) Bladder; (IL) iliac bone; (OI) obturator internus muscle; (P) prostate; (SV) seminal vesicles; (U) ureter; (VD) vas deferens. (From reference 393.)

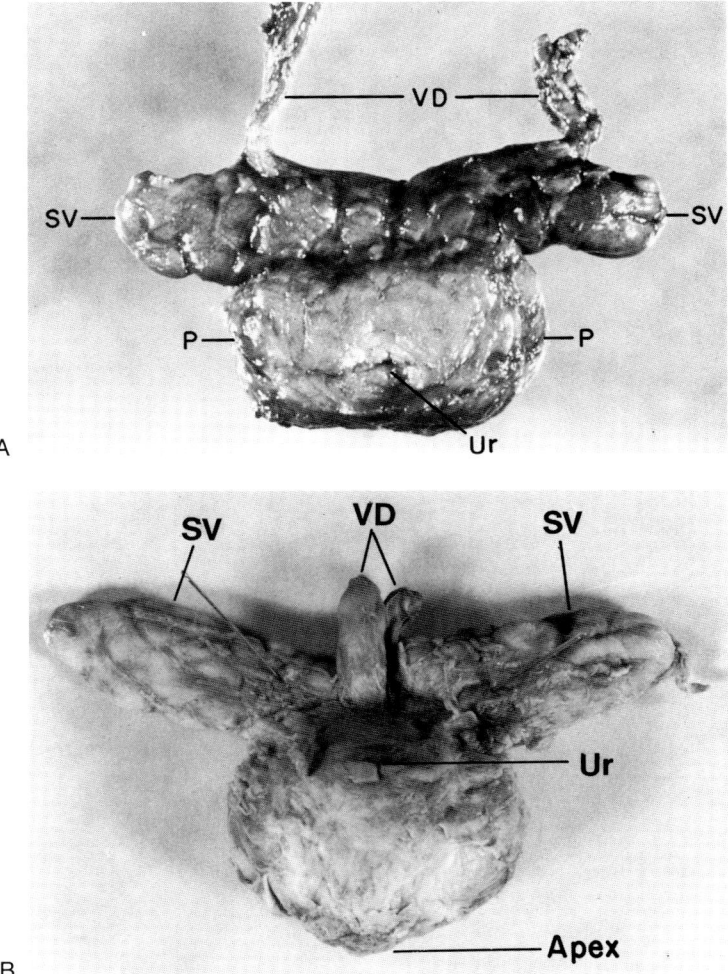

FIG. 2.8. Gross specimen of the prostate (**A**) prior to and (**B**) after formalin fixation, demonstrating the orientation of the vas deferens (VD) and seminal vesicles (SV) to the prostate (P) and the prostatic urethra (Ur).

Histological Anatomic Considerations

The more recent histologic studies have differentiated the prostate into two major areas, the prostatic glandular zones and the periurethral area (also poorly termed the central gland) (Figs. 2.9 and 2.10) (296–306).

The glandular prostate is separated into a peripheral and a central zone of acinar tissue. The peripheral zone encompasses 75%, and the central zone encompasses 25%, of the total volume of the prostatic acinar or glandular prostate (304).

Morphologically, these two zones are quite different. The ejaculatory ducts throughout their entire course in the prostate are surrounded by the central zone. The orifices of the central ducts surround the orifices of the ejaculatory ducts and radiate toward the verumon-

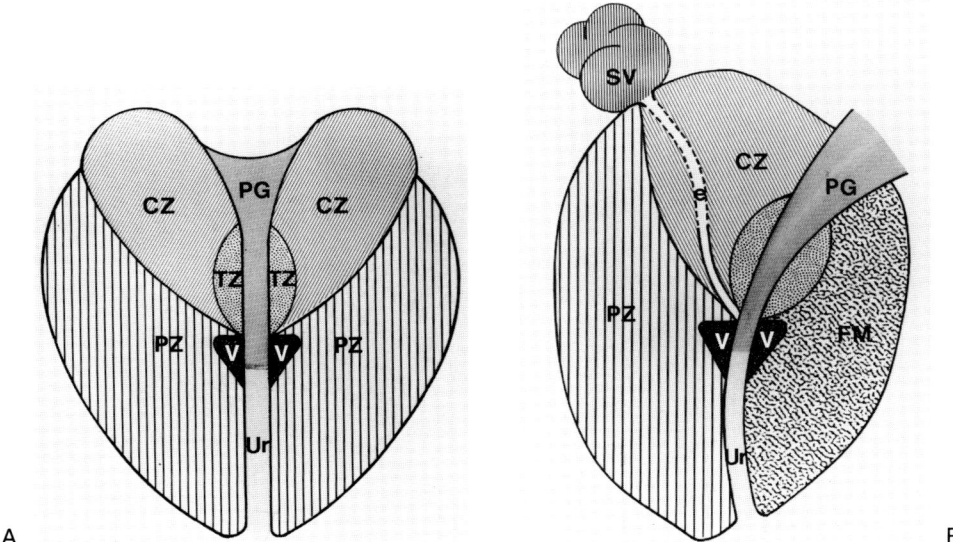

FIG. 2.9. Diagrams of the prostate in a curved coronal section (**A**) along the axis of the prostatic urethra and in a sagittally oriented view (**B**) with the rectum to the left and the anterior aspect of the prostate, the anterior fibromuscular stroma (FM), to the right. The position of the seminal vesicles (SV), the verumontanum (V), and the ejaculatory ducts (e) are shown. Additionally noted are the periurethral glandular zone (tissue) (PG), the prostatic urethra (Ur), and the transition (TZ), central (CZ), and peripheral zones (PZ).

tanum. The peripheral zone ductal system joins the urethra distinctly separate from those of the central zone. A double lateral line is formed which extends along the posterolateral aspects of the distal urethral segment from the area of the verumontanum toward the apex of the prostate.

The central zone is comprised of irregular, large acini. The acini of the peripheral zone are smaller and rounder with smooth walls and are more uniform in size. The muscular stroma is also different. The central zone's stroma is compactly arranged and longitudinally positioned. The musculature of the peripheral zone is more random and not as tightly interwoven. In the normal male, this difference is apparent, both histologically and visually; that is, in a normal individual, the zones are distinctly separate and different.

The periurethral (or central) glandular area is divided into the periurethral glandular tissue (or zone) and a transition zone. The periurethral glandular tissue has ducts that arise from the proximal aspect of the urethra and appears to be a continuation of the peripheral and transition zone ductal systems. Histologically, the periurethral glandular tissue resembles both the peripheral zone and the transition zone tissues. Small microscopic ducts and acini

FIG. 2.10. Diagrams of the prostate (**A**) showing sections from the seminal vesicles (**B**) and the prostate in sequential axial section from the base of the gland to the apex (**C–H**), demonstrating the orientation of the different tissues. (CZ) Central zone; (e) ejaculatory duct; (FM) fibromuscular stroma; (PG) periurethral glandular zone; (SV) seminal vesicles; (TZ) transition zone; (Ur) prostatic urethra; (V) verumontanum.

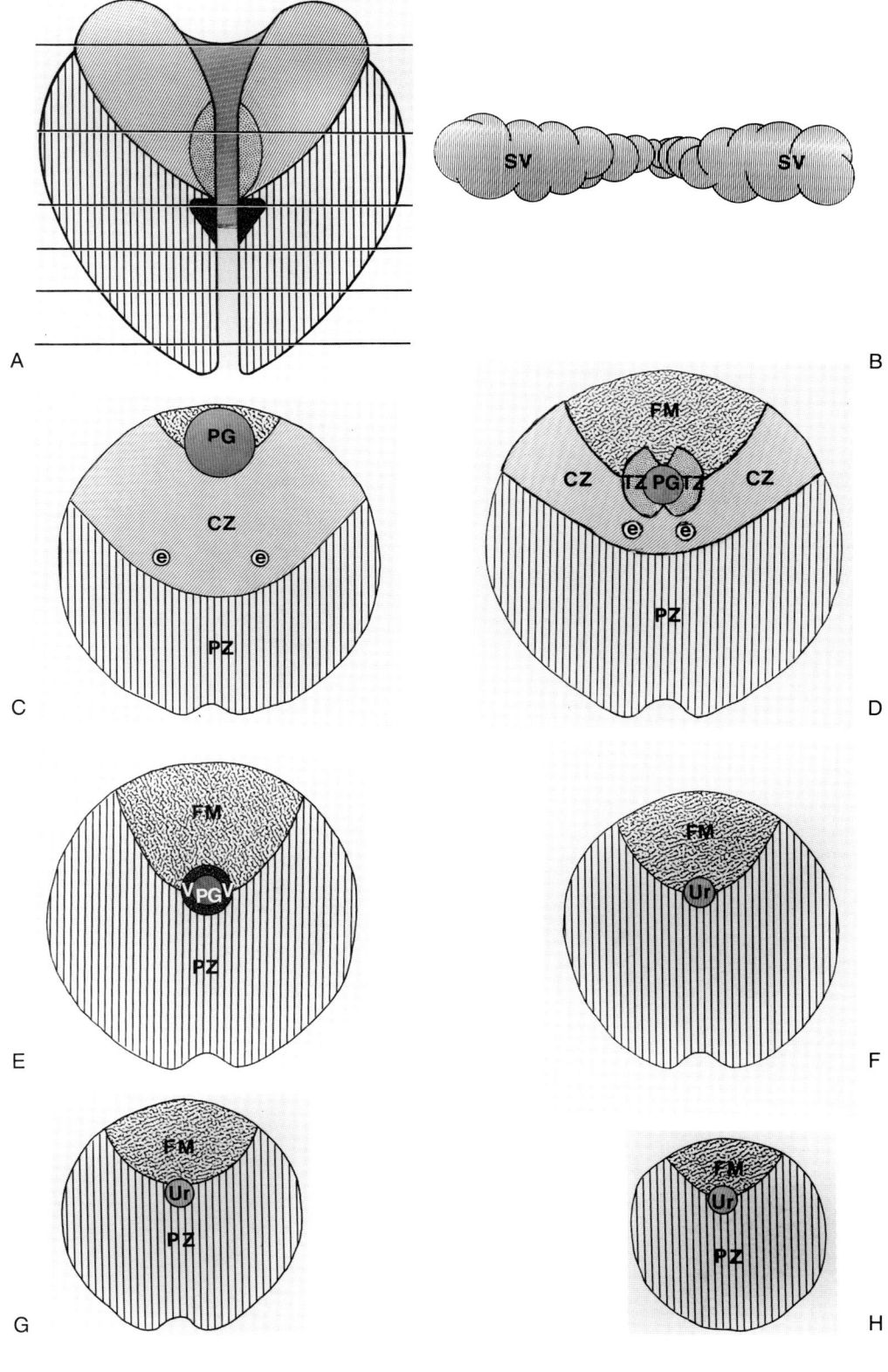

are seen situated in the longitudinal smooth muscle that surrounds the urethra. The periurethral glandular tissue courses from the bladder neck to the area of the verumontanum.

The transition zone represents approximately 5% of the glandular prostate. This area is a bilobed zone situated just lateral to the preprostatic sphincter and surrounds the proximal aspect of the urethra between the bladder neck and the verumontanum. The ductal system of the transition zone branches along the proximal aspect along the proximal urethral segment, and the ducts insert into the urethra just proximal to the verumontanum. Histologically, the glandular tissue of the transition zone appears identical to that of the peripheral zone. However, the borders of the transition zone appear to be anatomically distinct and separate from the peripheral zone.

A third area of prostatic tissue is the anterior fibromuscular stroma previously described as the anterior lobe. It is situated anterior to the urethra and is composed of smooth muscle that is continuous with the detrusor muscle fibers of the anterior bladder wall at the bladder neck. The fibromuscular stroma is thickest just distal to the verumontanum, where it is mainly comprised of fibrous tissue. It becomes narrower at the verumontanum and thins markedly as it reaches the apex of the prostate.

This type of differentiation of the various zones is important because of the pathologic processes that can be involved from each area. For example:

1. Prostatic carcinoma appears to originate mostly from the peripheral zone of the acinar or glandular prostate. A small number of cancers also arise from the transition and central zones (308).

2. Prostatitis can originate in any area of the prostate but usually presents initially in the peripheral zone (297).

3. Benign prostatic hyperplasia appears to originate in the transition zone predominantly, but it also develops, to a lesser degree, in the periurethral glandular zone (300,308).

4. The central zone (except for a small number of cancers) appears relatively immune to the development of various pathological processes, although it can be involved secondarily (308).

Despite the changes that appear to occur in each zone, nothing is definitive and, as previously noted, there is some overlap. However, an understanding of this newer anatomic terminology becomes essential in the utilization of sonography for evaluation of the prostate.

3 // Physical Principles of Ultrasound Imaging*

Ultrasound-Image Generation	16
Pulse-Echo Principle	
Equipment Design	
Real-Time Ultrasound	
Difficulties in Image Generation	19
Image Spatial Resolution	
Focus Characteristics	
Side Lobes	
Scan Plane Thickness	
Tissue Attenuation	
Fat	
Bones	
Air	
Other Difficulties	
Acoustic Windows	
New High-Quality Ultrasound Images	26
Small-Parts Scanners	
Endorectal Prostate Scanners	

Over the past 20 years, ultrasound imaging has developed into one of the most commonly used methods of obtaining diagnostic quality medical images in a safe, noninvasive manner. There are three reasons for this development. The first is that it permits the noninvasive visualization and identification of internal soft tissue structures. The second is that the results of clinical and animal bioeffects studies indicate that ultrasound radiation is posing little danger of biological effects to the operator, the patient, or even a fetus *in utero*. The third is that the relatively low cost and clinical effectiveness of ultrasound imaging make it a preferred imaging modality in today's cost-effective medical-imaging marketplace. To fully appreciate and utilize the diagnostic medical information presented in ultrasound images, those using the technique should have some knowledge of the operational principles of ultrasound equipment and the acoustic information contained in the images. This chapter contains a correct, but highly simplified, description of ultrasound image generation. The reader interested in a more complete understanding should consult refs. 157, 214, 243, 290, 334, and 375.

---

*This chapter has been written by Albert Goldstein, Ph.D., Associate Professor, Departments of Ob/Gyn and Radiology, Wayne State University School of Medicine, Detroit, Michigan 48201.

ULTRASOUND-IMAGE GENERATION

Sound waves which travel in air are similar to medical ultrasound radiation. Both are mechanical pressure waves with alternating regions of high and low pressure requiring a medium in which to propagate (sound waves will not propagate in a vacuum). The acoustic velocity of sound waves depends on the propagation medium. In air, the velocity is approximately 333 m/sec. In soft tissues, the average acoustic velocity is 1,540 m/sec. The frequency of a sound wave is the number of cycles (repetitions) of high pressure (or low pressure) that a listener receives per second. The audible range of frequencies of the human ear is approximately 20 to 16,000 Hz (hertz, or cycles per second). The sound waves used in medical imaging have much higher frequencies in the 3- to 15-MHz range (millions of cycles per second), and that is why the term ultrasound is used to describe them.

Pulse-Echo Principle

The pulse-echo ranging principle of radar and sonar is used to produce ultrasound images. Since the acoustic velocity in a medium is known and the time of travel from a transmitter to a receiver can be measured, the distance between the transmitter and receiver may be calculated using the following relation: distance = acoustic velocity × time of travel. In ultrasound imaging equipment, the transducer performs both the acoustic transmission and reception. The transducer is placed on the skin surface, and a short ultrasound wave (pulse) is transmitted into the body. As the ultrasound pulse traverses the soft tissues in the body, some of the ultrasound energy (echo) is reflected back toward the transducer. The equipment measures two quantities for each received echo: (i) the time delay between the transmission pulse and the reception of the echo and (ii) the amplitude (strength) of the received echo.

Each transmitted ultrasound pulse produces a series of echoes from internal reflectors along the pulse path through the body, with the earliest echoes coming from close internal reflectors and the later echoes coming from correspondingly distant reflectors. The exact anatomical location of each reflector may be calculated from the known direction of the ultrasound beam in the body and the measured time of arrival of its echo. Since the acoustic velocity of most soft tissues is within 3% of the average soft tissue value (1,540 m/sec), there is only minimum spatial distortion in the image if the equipment assumes that all soft tissue has this average acoustic velocity. The narrow ultrasound beam is slowly scanned across the body, whereas the transducer is repetitively fired to obtain a two-dimensional image containing many transducer lines of sight. Each line in the image represents a separate pulsing of the transducer and the subsequent reception of echoes along the transducer beam direction. The resulting image is that of the scanned cross-sectional anatomy. The transducer beam always cuts a planar cross section (transverse, longitudinal, or oblique to the long body axis) or scan plane so that the two-dimensional ultrasound image will represent a planar two-dimensional patient cross section.

In ultrasound gray-scale images, shades of gray are used to represent the echo amplitudes at the anatomic site of interest. The gray-scale image can be either white on black or black on white. In a white on black image, the background (echo absence) is black and the succeedingly lighter shades of gray represent higher echo amplitudes. The darker shades of gray represent higher amplitude echoes in a black on white image. On most equipment, the viewer has the choice of which type of gray-scale image to display.

There are two types of echoes displayed in gray-scale images, namely, specular and diffuse. Specular echoes are from large mirror-like reflectors (interfaces) in the body (e.g., liver capsule, kidney capsule, diaphragm, fat layers). They are high in amplitude but difficult to present in the image because they bounce off of the interface much like light reflecting from a mirror, and only when the transducer beam is perpendicular to the interface will the echo be captured (transmitted back toward the transducer) in the image. The specular echoes are important in the ultrasound image because they help locate the boundaries of the large organ masses.

Diffuse echoes arising from internal organ parenchyma are much different from specular echoes. Since they are caused by small, weak reflectors, they have low amplitudes but scatter equally in all directions so that they will always be captured by the transducer and presented in the gray-scale ultrasound image. It has been demonstrated clinically that the diffuse echo amplitudes contain vital diagnostic information. Because of the different salt-and-pepper appearance of the diffuse gray-scale echo patterns from each soft tissue structure, it is the diffuse echoes, not the specular ones, which generally show the size, shape, and location of internal organs. Focal disease usually occurs in the images as small isolated regions of echo amplitudes that are either higher in amplitude (hyperechoic) or lower in amplitude (hypoechoic) than the surrounding normal tissue. Diffuse disease usually occurs in the image as a region where the salt-and-pepper pattern of the internal diffuse echoes differs from the tissue's normal salt-and-pepper appearance. The ability of the ultrasound-imaging equipment to properly capture and display the diffuse echoes' gray-scale appearance is of paramount importance in the diagnostic information content of the resultant ultrasound images.

Equipment Design

Piezoelectric transducers make possible pulse-echo ultrasound imaging. A transducer is a device that transforms energy from one form into another (the electrical energy from the wall plug is converted into sound waves by the transducer). Inside the transducer, the active element is a thin piezoelectric disk. Electric voltages cause slight changes in thickness of the piezoelectric disk as a result of the piezoelectric (pressure-electric) effect. The transducer is pressed against the patient's skin surface, and the high-frequency changes in disk thickness cause the disk front surface to repetitively push against the patient's skin, thus generating an ultrasound pulse that propagates inward. Returning echoes enter the transducer, and their acoustic pressures produce (again, by the piezoelectric effect) voltages across the thickness of the disk whose magnitudes are proportional to their amplitudes.

In order for the ultrasound pulse to leave the transducer and enter the patient (and return as an echo), the transducer must be acoustically coupled to the patient. Although this sounds rather complicated, it is really quite simple to understand. A partial reflection occurs at each interface that an ultrasound pulse traverses. The reflection magnitude depends on the differences in acoustic properties between the two media forming the interface. If the patient's skin surface is dry, then no matter how hard one presses, there will always be a thin layer of air between the transducer's front surface and the patient's skin. Since the acoustic properties of air are quite dissimilar to those of plastic (the transducer front surface) and skin, there will be a very strong reflection (and thus very little transmission) at both the plastic-air and air-skin interfaces. Acoustic coupling simply means replacing the thin layer of air with a layer of gel whose acoustic properties are much more similar to those of plastic and skin than to those of air. This is the reason all patients to be scanned ultrasonically have their skin surfaces covered by a coupling gel. This type of scanning is called *contact scanning* because the transducer is held in contact with the gel-covered skin. There is another type of scanning, called *immersion scanning*, where a liquid bath (usually water) is used to couple the ultrasound energy between the transducer and the patient. Breast and ophthalmological ultrasound scans are commonly performed using the immersion technique. In automated breast scanning, the breasts are usually immersed in a large water tank containing the transducers and their mechanical drives. In ophthalmological scans, a small bath of water is formed over the eye socket, and the transducer is immersed in the bath to ultrasonically view the eye interior.

Real-Time Ultrasound

The first ultrasound contact scanners used a single-element piezoelectric disk transducer which an operator moved over the patient's skin surface. The image took 5 to 20 sec to be produced, and it presented a static view of the internal patient cross section. These scanners are now known as *static scanners* and have the advantage of large fields of view demonstrating the total cross-sectional skin surface. It was relatively easy for the viewer to identify the precise anatomical location of the scan plane obtained independently by the operator.

Modern ultrasound imaging equipment has more complex transducers which are capable of acquiring 15 to 30 images (frames) a second. With these high frame rates, internal patient anatomy is presented in real time, and tissue may be studied temporally as well as spatially. Advantages of real-time ultrasound include rapid and complete survey capability, reduced examination time, and less required operator scanning skill. There is a trade-off between spatial and temporal resolution because the output pulse repetition frequency (prf) of the transducer is limited by the requirement that the echoes from the furthest depths in the image must be received before the transducer can be pulsed again for the next image line. Depending on the depth of the imaged field of view, there is a maximum number of image lines that may be acquired each second. The number of lines per second equals the lines per frame multiplied by the frames per second. The equipment designer must now decide how many lines to place in each frame and how many frames to present each second. When one is increased, the other must be decreased to keep their numerical product constant, so a compromise between spatial and temporal resolution must be made. If the equipment has a large number of lines per frame, the image spatial detail will be quite fine, but the ability to follow tissue temporal motion will be limited. If the equipment has a higher image frame rate, the temporal resolution will be good, but the spatial resolution in each frame must be reduced. Typically, in real-time abdominal scanners, the frame rate is 15 frames/sec and there are 256 lines/frame leading to adequate spatial resolution. In real-time cardiac scanners, where visualization of the valve motion is of prime importance, the frame rate is 30 frames/sec and there are 128 lines/frame. (The high tissue-blood contrast in a cardiac image lessens the spatial resolution requirements.)

In order to acquire the ultrasound images automatically and repetitively, several different types of real-time transducers have been developed. The simplest is the *mechanical sector scanner*, in which a single-element transducer is mechanically oscillated back and forth (Fig. 3.1). The resulting field of view is sector-shaped, with a limited field of view for anterior tissue and a widening field of view for more posterior tissue. Some mechanical sector scanners

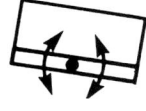
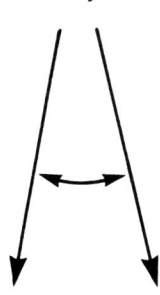

FIG. 3.1. Real-time mechanical sector transducer. A single-element transducer (with an attached backing layer) oscillates back and forth around an axis through the element. The oscillating beam direction defines a sector-shaped field of view in the patient.

have a single-element transducer that continuously rotates in a circle and only fires and receives when its beam direction is inside of the sector field of view.

Another type of real-time transducer is mechanically simpler but much more complex electronically. The *sector* (or *phased*) *array* is a multielement linear array of small single elements arranged linearly (Fig. 3.2). When the elements are all pulsed simultaneously, the beam leaves the multielement transducer perpendicular to its face. Conversely, if the multielement transducer is fired with a small time delay between the sequential pulsing of adjacent elements, the beam will leave the transducer at an angle (depending on the magnitude of the time delay) to its central ray. A similar set of time delays is applied to the returning echo signals, and this multielement transducer can effectively steer its beam in both transmission and reception defining a sector-shaped field of view. Actually, a more complex set of time delays is used when firing this multielement transducer to focus its beam pattern in both transmission and reception. The advantage of the sector field of view is that only a limited contact area is required on the patient's skin, with various anterior acoustic obstructions being avoided.

The third type of real-time transducer, called the *line* (or *linear*) *array*, is again a multielement linear array of single elements (Fig. 3.3). It is much longer than the sector array; also, for each image line, only a small number of adjacent elements are fired. Beam steering is not used because the element groups are fired sequentially along the array so that the image field of view will be rectangular. The rectangular field of view requires a large contact area on the patient's skin surface but gives a superior presentation of anterior soft tissue in the image. A group of elements is fired for each image line so that it forms a large effective aperture with a more collimated beam pattern than that from a single element. Its beam pattern can also be focused (in transmission and reception) using small time delays between the individual elements in the group.

DIFFICULTIES IN IMAGE GENERATION

Gray-scale ultrasound image generation has been discussed above. In clinical images, soft tissue structures are visible and two-dimensional cross-sectional anatomy is acquired in a manner which permits localization of internal soft tissue structures in preparation for surgical procedures. However, there are certain soft tissue characteristics, as well as certain equipment limitations, which affect the spatial resolution and gray-scale integrity in the image. Im-

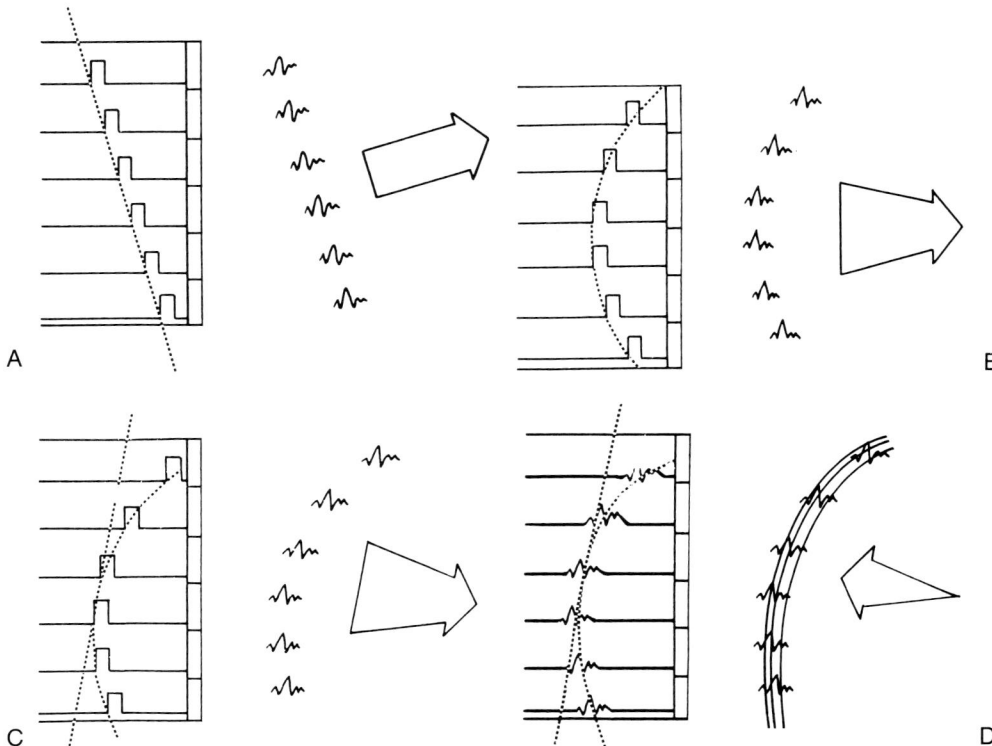

FIG. 3.2. Real-time sector array transducer. This multielement linear array of small piezoelectric elements steers and focuses the ultrasound beam by the use of electronically controlled time delays between the firings of the individual elements. **A:** Diagram demonstrating (for a six-element linear array) beam steering. At the left of the line of elements, the square waves on the electrical cables to the elements represent the driving electrical pulses (which shock the elements into producing ultrasound pulses) at an instant of time before firing. At the right of the elements, the short waveforms in the medium represent the individual element acoustic pulses at an instant after firing. The constant time difference between element firings has produced a composite "steered" ultrasound plane wave which is propagating at an angle to the central ray of the transducer. **B:** In a similar fashion, the use of time delays to produce a composite curved ultrasound wave in the medium which will focus at a predetermined depth is demonstrated. **C:** Diagram demonstrating that in actual practice a combination of "steering" and "focusing" time delays are used to produce the series of focused ultrasound beams which interrogate the entire sector-shaped field of view. Since the pulse-echo principle is used in ultrasound image generation, part **D** demonstrates that in reception, the same time delays (as used in transmission) must be applied to the received individual element signals to focus the multielement array in reception.

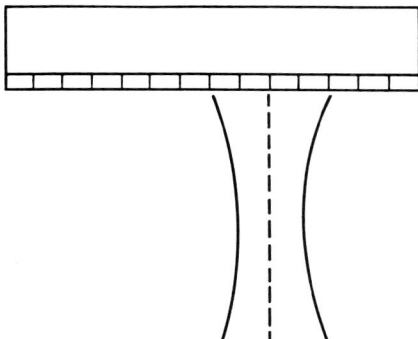

FIG. 3.3. Real-time linear-array transducer. This multielement linear array of elements is much longer than a sector array; and for each image line, only a small group of elements is sequentially fired along the array (without beam steering). In the case shown, four elements transmit and receive (with focusing time delays) to produce the focused ultrasound beams which define a rectangular image field of view.

provements in equipment design are continually sought to counter these limitations for inclusion of more spatial or echo amplitude detail in the images.

Image Spatial Resolution

Image spatial resolution refers to the amount of spatial detail present in the image. One factor in spatial resolution is the number of lines (transducer firings) in each frame. The closer together the image lines are, the more tissue detail that can be presented in the image (Fig. 3.4). The other important factor is the amount of blurring inherent in the imaging of small tissue details (point reflectors). The blurring arises because the ultrasound pulse that is transmitted into the soft tissue has finite dimensions both axial and lateral to the beam

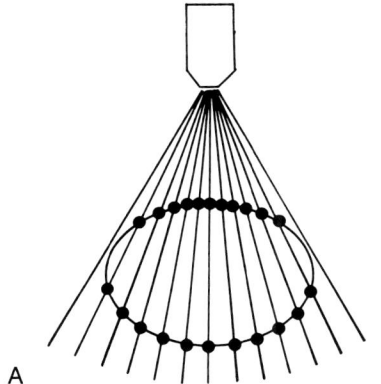
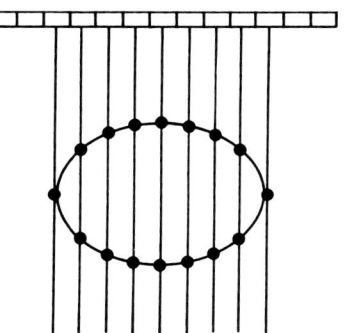

FIG. 3.4. Multielement array line density. The spatial density of the lines in an ultrasound image frame is an important parameter affecting image detail (spatial resolution). **A:** Diagram demonstrating the line density of a sector array scanning a fetal head. The fetal skull is shown in ellipsoidal cross section, with dots representing the imaged skull echoes using equipment with minimum spatial blur. Since the lines all emanate from the center of the array, the line density and image detail reduce with depth in the image. **B:** Diagram demonstrating the line density of a line array scanning the same fetal head. Since there is no beam steering, the line density and image detail are constant with depth.

assumption and the gray-scale image presents a true representation of the scanned patient cross section. However, some transducers do not send out all of their ultrasound energy straight ahead. Because of design or fabrication difficulties, the transducer may send out a small portion of its ultrasound energy at an angle to the transducer line of sight. Then, any reflectors in the path of this extra side-lobe radiation can send back echoes which will be picked up and incorrectly interpreted as being due to reflectors located along the transducer line of sight (main lobe). Usually, the amount of ultrasound energy contained in side lobes is so small that their contribution to the gray-scale ultrasound image is negligible. However, if the side lobe is unusually strong or there are very strong reflectors in its path and the main lobe is receiving little or no echo signal, then it is possible for the side-lobe echoes to be presented in the image. The most common imaging situation for this side-lobe fill-in would be when the transducer beam is aimed at an anechoic portion of the patient cross section such as a liquid-filled cyst, a full urinary bladder, amnionic fluid, or a region of an acoustic shadow in the image.

Multielement array transducers are particularly susceptible to side-lobe effects. Beam steering a multielement linear array increases the strength of its side lobes. Generally, the larger the beam steering angle, the greater the amount of ultrasound energy in the side lobe. Thus, sector (phased) array transducers are the most susceptible to side-lobe fill-in in their images. The fill-in will usually occur at the largest beam-steering angles, which means at the edges of the sector image field of view.

Scan Plane Thickness

The two-dimensional gray-scale patient image is usually interpreted as representing a thin cross section (thin scan plane) in the patient. The actual thickness of the scan plane is a very important transducer parameter because too wide a scan plane will degrade the image as a result of both partial volume effects and loss of spatial resolution. Partial volume effects refer to the fact that the image shades of gray represent the sum of the echo signals received from a given image depth (from the sampling volume). If the scan plane is too thick, the image shades of gray can be influenced by tissue at the edges of the thick scan plane. Spatial resolution refers to the ability to accurately image small objects (such as focal lesions) in the patient. A small focal lesion has small dimensions both in the scan plane and out of the scan plane. If the scan plane is wider than the small lesion, then (a) the edges of the lesion will be blurred in the image and (b) partial volume effects may obscure visualization of the lesion when it has low contrast with the background tissue (which is usually the case).

Tissue Attenuation

The received echo amplitude depends upon the reflectivity of the soft tissue reflectors and the attenuation of the overlying tissue (between the transducer and the internal reflector). Tissue attenuation refers to the reduction in amplitude of ultrasound pulses (or echoes) as they propagate through tissue as a result of the tissue's acoustic scattering and absorption characteristics. An unfortunate characteristic of the tissue attenuation of ultrasound is that it increases with increasing ultrasound frequency. The best image detail can be obtained at higher ultrasound frequencies; however, as a result of tissue attenuation, the higher-frequency ultrasound echoes from large image depths can have amplitudes too weak to be detected by the equipment. Thus, the selection of the ultrasound frequency to use in a clinical scan is always a compromise between image detail and tissue penetration. The general rule is to use the highest available frequency that will penetrate to the depths of interest. When imaging large fields of view, higher frequencies cannot be used because of their limited tissue penetration, and image detail suffers. One way to increase the penetration of ultrasound waves in tissue would be to increase the output power of the equipment. This is possible to some extent on available equipment, but the output power is limited to a level that has been deemed safe by bioeffects studies. Another way to increase the penetration of higher frequencies is to make the equipment amplifier more sensitive to very low amplitude echoes. Equipment designers are always striving to develop amplifiers with increased sensitivity. As new amplifiers are developed, the higher frequencies can be used more effectively in general ultrasound scanning.

Fat

Body fat has an acoustic velocity that is much less (6%) than the average value for soft tissue. This leads to two important consequences in ultrasound imaging. The first is due to the phenomenon of refraction. Refraction simply refers to the bending (change of direction) of the ultrasound path as the pulse crosses an interface formed by two soft tissue types with different acoustic velocities. With obliquely incident ultrasound, large planar interfaces can cause a change of direction of the transmission pulse and returning echoes which will "fool" the scanner (which is programmed to expect only straight-line propagation) into misregistering the reflector positions in the ultrasound image. This image spatial distortion is usually slight because in most scanning situations, the transducer beam direction is fairly close to being perpendicular to refracting interfaces such as the subcutaneous fat–soft-tissue interface, which is generally parallel to the skin contours. Internal fat layers, such as those surrounding the kidneys, can cause reflector position misregistration when the beam is incident obliquely to this fat layer and its two soft tissue interfaces.

The second consequence of fat–soft-tissue refraction occurs in obese individuals who have fat globules distributed throughout their soft tissue masses. The fat globules act like a small acoustic lens unfocusing and scattering the ultrasound beam. Because of their large numbers and their relatively high reflection coefficients, the fat globules substantially add to the tissue attenuation. This causes the well-known clinical observation that obese individuals produce poor ultrasound images with more limited penetration and reduced tissue detail.

Bones

Bones have acoustic properties that are very different from most soft tissues. The acoustic velocity of skull bone is between two and three times higher than the soft tissue average, and its attenuation of ultrasound is also considerably higher. Because of the resulting severe refraction and attenuation, the skull bone surrounding the brain effectively shields this important organ from diagnostic ultrasound imaging. Fetuses, neonates, and young infants have skull bones that have not yet sufficiently ossified to prevent ultrasound imaging of the brain. In a similar fashion, the vertebral bodies prevent ultrasound scans of the enclosed spinal cord. The ribs also cause difficulties in ultrasound images. Because of their acoustic attenuation, they reduce the amplitude of echoes received from posterior reflectors. Because of their high acoustic velocity, they act like acoustic lenses, distorting the beam focal properties and reducing the amplitude of the posterior echoes. As a result of ultrasound energy being trapped and reverberating between the two highly reflecting rib–soft-tissue interfaces, a ladder of posterior image artifacts known as *reverberation artifacts* are produced which also obscures the visualization of posterior soft tissue information.

Air

Air pockets, such as trapped gas in the upper and lower intestines, also block the passage of ultrasound waves. In this case it is the large acoustic mismatch at the air–soft-tissue boundaries which cause almost complete reflection of the transmitted ultrasonic pulse, preventing it from penetrating through the gas pocket and into the posterior soft tissue. Thus, air pockets cause "reflection" acoustic shadows in ultrasound images (as opposed to "attenuation" acoustic shadows caused by highly attenuating tissues).

Other Difficulties

Scar tissue and body hair may also affect the penetration of the ultrasound waves. In both cases they present an attenuating and scattering layer between the transducer and the patient which causes a reduction in penetration and image detail.

Acoustic Windows

In contact scanning, the clinical solution to the imaging problems caused by some of the above-mentioned difficulties is to find appropriate acoustic windows for each imaging situation. Acoustic windows are regions on or adjacent to the patient's skin surface which readily transmit ultrasound waves and quite effectively serve as conduits to the posterior soft-tissue structures below. The filled urinary bladder serves as an acoustic window for the ultrasonic imaging of the female reproductive organs and the first-trimester fetus. Amnionic fluid is an acoustic window for *in utero* fetal scans. The highest-quality ultrasonic brain scans of neonates and newborn infants will result when the fontanel is used as an acoustic window. In cardiac imaging, the deleterious effects of the ribs can be avoided if the small transducer front face is placed in an intercostal space. Clearly, the identification of an appropriate acoustic window can be a vital factor in difficult imaging situations.

NEW HIGH-QUALITY ULTRASOUND IMAGES

Small-Parts Scanners

These new scanners have been specifically designed to produce images of limited depths into the body. High-quality thyroid, breast, testes, and peripheral vascular scans may be effectively obtained using small-parts scanners. By limiting the depth of penetration of the image field of view, several important advantages are realized. The first is that the limited tissue depth reduces the attenuation of overlying tissue (and fat) so that higher ultrasound frequencies (with superior spatial resolution capabilities) can be used. Second, the image line density is higher in small-parts images, which also increases their imaged tissue detail.

The increased line density is due to two factors: (i) Since the image is a magnified one, the image lines per frame cover a smaller field of view so the line density per patient dimension is higher; and (ii) because of the decreased image depth, the real-time scanner can be pulsed more rapidly (it does not have to wait as long for the echoes from the furthest image depths to arrive), leading to a higher number of lines per frame. And third, small-diameter transducers with long focal zones at the required focal lengths (image depths) can be used in small-parts scanners because their beams are not as strongly focused as compared with larger-diameter transducers (which would have shorter focal zones at these depths). However, only soft-tissue areas adjacent to the skin surface can be effectively scanned with this new contact scan equipment. Because of their proximity to the skin, the internal, external, and common carotid arteries may be quite effectively imaged using a small-parts scanner.

Endorectal Prostate Scanners

Detailed high-quality images of deep-lying organs such as the prostate are not attainable with contact scanning because the overlying tissue restricts the maximum values of both the ultrasound frequency and number of image lines acquired per second (which are the two important parameters governing image spatial resolution). One way to solve this proximity problem and get the transducer closer is to insert the transducer into the body through a natural orifice, the rectum, and maneuver it close to the prostate. Then the resulting ultrasound images will have all of the benefits associated with small-parts scanning, higher spatial resolution, and greater tissue detail. The small diameter necessary for the short-focal-length, high-frequency transducers also makes them more readily insertible in the rectum. Depending on the imaging situation, either small line arrays or sector scanners are utilized.

The transducer is mounted on a long, thin probe which is covered with a condom and inserted into the rectum. When the probe is in position, the condom is filled with water. In effect, an immersion scan situation exists, with the water in the condom providing the acoustic coupling between the transducer and the patient's internal anatomy. The liquid-filled condom also pushes aside any fecal matter or air bubbles in the rectum, providing a shadow-free acoustic window to the prostate. Two scan-plane orientations are used. Transaxial scan planes are oriented perpendicular to the rectum axis. They may be acquired using a single-element mechanical sector transducer or a sector array. In either case, a sector field of view is provided, with the sector angle sufficiently wide to include the entire prostate in the image field of view. Sagittal scan planes are oriented parallel to the rectum's longitudinal axis. They may be acquired using sector or line arrays. Recently, a number of manufacturers have developed biplane transrectal prostate probes containing two different transducers so that both scan planes may be conveniently acquired without the necessity of changing probes during the examination. Proper positioning of the probe in the dilated, liquid-filled rectum is important for optimal visualization of the prostate's peripheral zone, where most primary cancerous lesions develop. The effect of shifting the focal zone in the image by using the water in the condom as a standoff is shown in Figs. 3.7 and 3.8. These figures were acquired using a phantom (PIRTO Phantom, Model 419, RMI, Inc., Middleton, WI, 53562) specifically designed to demonstrate the transducer focus over the image field of view. It consists of an anechoic gel into which is placed a uniform dispersion of small-point scatters. The images of the point reflectors are small and well defined at the image depths of the focal zone. Outside of the focal zone, the point reflector images are blurred, indicating a lack of image detail (or transducer focus at these depths). The probe positioning demonstrated in

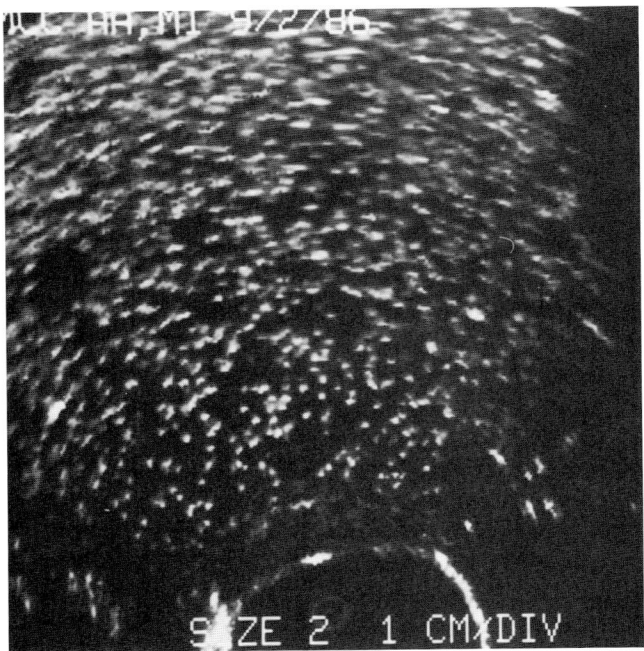

FIG. 3.7. Probe close to rectal wall. Image from a transducer focus phantom [PIRTO Phantom, Model 419, RMI, Inc., Middleton, WI] shows the transducer's 2–4-cm focal zone to be located roughly 1 cm from the rectal wall. The position of the probe in the dilated condom is shown by the small circle.

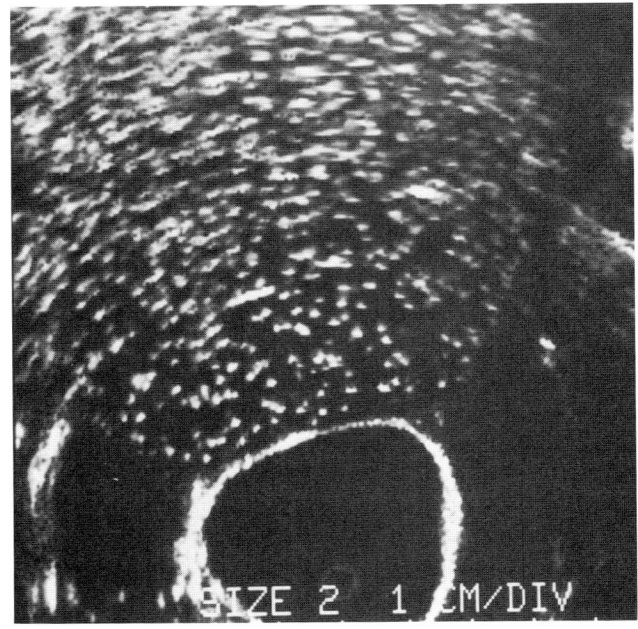

FIG. 3.8. Probe far from rectal wall. Image from a transducer focus phantom [PIRTO Phantom, Model 419, RMI, Inc., Middleton, WI] shows the transducer's 2–4-cm focal zone to be adjacent to the rectal wall for optimum visualization of the peripheral zone. The position of the probe in the dilated condom is shown by the small circle.

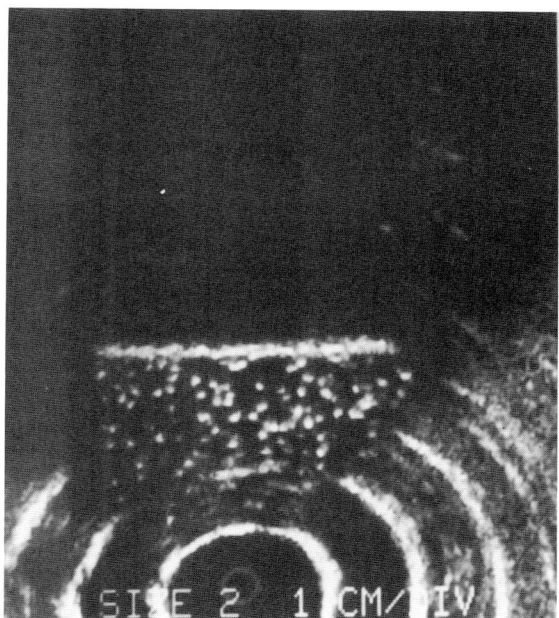

FIG. 3.9. Scan-plane thickness at prostate. A new transducer scan-plane-thickness phantom [Model 421, RMI, Inc., Middleton, WI] shows the thickness of the scan plane at the prostate's clinical image depths. The width of the horizontal line is the scan-plane thickness at the image depth of the horizontal line.

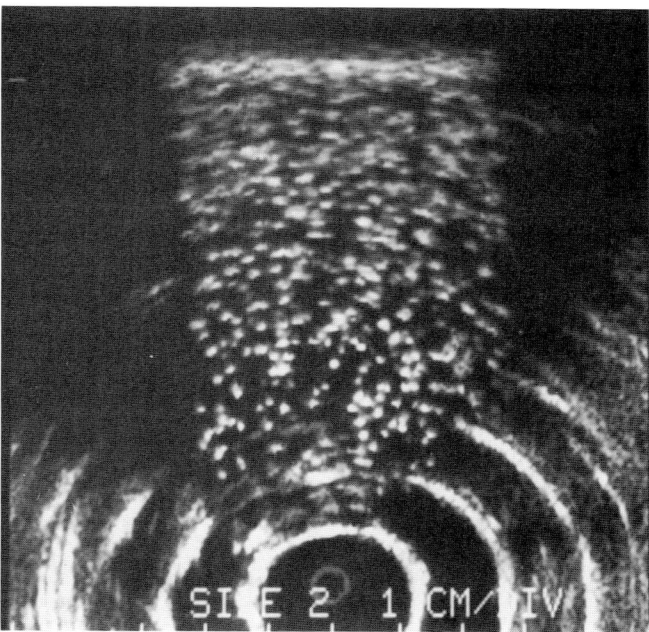

FIG. 3.10. Scan-plane thickness outside of prostate. A new transducer scan-plane-thickness phantom [Model 421, RMI, Inc., Middleton, WI] shows the thickness of the scan plane at the furthest images depths. The width of the horizontal line is the scan-plane thickness at the image depth of the horizontal line. A wide scan plane at this image depth is of no consequence in clinical imaging.

Fig. 3.8 is preferable because (a) the transducer's near zone is entirely in the water standoff and (b) the peripheral zone (adjacent to the rectal wall) is located in the transducer's focal zone.

The scan-plane thickness focal zone should also be located at the prostate's image depths for maximum certainty of observing small focal lesions. Figures 3.9 and 3.10 show the scan-plane thickness at two different image depths. They were acquired using a new ultrasound phantom (Scan-Plane Thickness Phantom, Model 421, RMI, Inc., Middleton, WI 53562) which demonstrates the thickness of the scan plane at selected image depths. The width of the horizontal line in these figures is the scan-plane thickness at the line's depth in the image. The scan plane is seen to be thinnest at the image depth that would be occupied by the prostate in a clinical scan. Single-element mechanical sector transducers have cylindrical beam patterns, so the scan-plane-thickness focal zone would be identical in depth to the in-plane focal zone. Multielement arrays, however, use cylindrical lenses to focus in the scan-plane-thickness direction. The image location of the scan-plane-thickness focal zone must be independently verified for these transducers.

4 // Scanning Techniques, Equipment, and Patient Preparation

Abdominal Approach	31
Transperineal Approach	33
Endourethral Approach	33
Endorectal Approach	34
Types of Equipment	
Transducer Preparation	
Patient Preparation	
Probe Insertion	
Technique of Examination—Axial Scanning	45
Technique of Examination—Sagittal Scanning	45
Image Preservation	46
Conclusion	49

There are various sonographic approaches that can be used to evaluate the prostate. The simplest approach, using conventional equipment, is the transabdominal route followed secondarily by the transperineal approach. Endourethral and endorectal scanning both require specialized equipment and techniques and obviously require different scanning approaches.

ABDOMINAL APPROACH

The suprapubic or abdominal examination is the easiest approach and may be performed using standard gray-scale ultrasound equipment. Both contact and real-time machines can be used successfully. The real-time examination can be performed with either a mechanical or a phased array sector unit or a linear array transducer. When performing this study, the urinary bladder must be distended with fluid (urine) prior to the examination. Either a 3.5- or 5.0-MHz transducer should be used. The transducer is placed on the lower abdomen, just superior to the symphysis pubis, and is angled so that the sound beam will traverse through the inferior portion of the bladder, identifying the prostate and seminal vesicles (Fig. 4.1). Images should be obtained in the transverse (axial) and longitudinal (sagittal and parasagittal) orientation. It is frequently necessary to also obtain various obliquely oriented images.

The normal prostate in this approach is slightly rounded. On the transverse image, the two lateral, the anterior and the posterior margins of the prostate are identified (see Chapter 5). By angling the transducer slightly less caudad, the seminal vesicles will be seen. Their sizes and shapes are variable and may appear as paired structures that are short or elongated,

32   *SCANNING TECHNIQUES, EQUIPMENT, AND PATIENT PREPARATION*

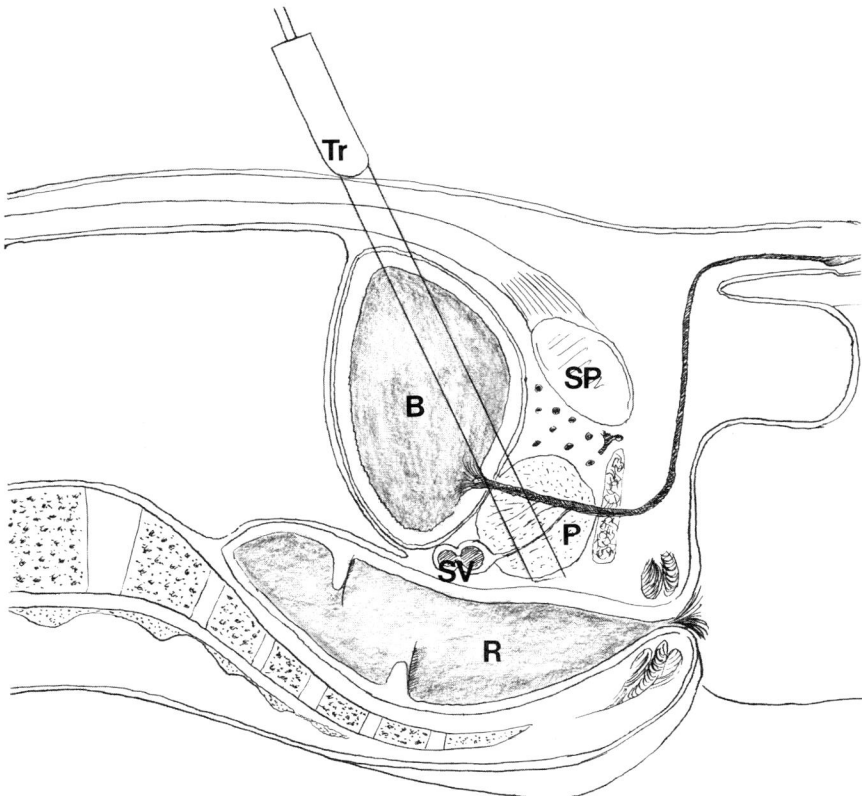

FIG. 4.1. Schematic diagram of transabdominal ultrasound scanning. The transducer (Tr) is placed superior to the symphysis pubis (SP) and is angled steeply caudad to visualize the prostate through a fluid-filled urinary bladder (B); a slightly less caudad view will visualize the seminal vesicle (SV). The rectum (R) will usually not be directly identified by this approach because of intraluminal air.

bow-tie- or dumbbell-shaped, thin or thick. While their absolute size and shape varies from one individual to another, they should, when normal, be symmetrical (in a single subject) to one another in size and shape. In the axial orientation, they are seen parallel to their long axis.

When obtaining sagittal or longitudinal images, the cephalad and caudad margins of the prostate are identified. The anterior and posterior margins should be clearly seen. The seminal vesicles will be delineated in cross section as slightly rounded structures situated just superior to the posterior aspect of the prostate between the rectum and the fluid-filled urinary bladder. To evaluate the entirety of both seminal vesicles, scans must be obtained from an area more lateral to the right side of the prostate to an area more lateral to the left side of the prostate. In many instances, the seminal vesicles in the oblique longitudinal image extend lateral to the most lateral portion of the prostate.

In general, the prostate is sonographically of homogeneous echogenicity. The various zones of the prostate cannot be distinguished from one another. The prostatic urethra is usually not clearly identified, although the bladder neck may be seen as a small fluid-filled area indenting the base of the prostate. This is true particularly if the bladder is overdistended. The seminal vesicles are homogeneous in size, shape, and echogenicity and are usually slightly less echogenic than the prostate.

TRANSPERINEAL APPROACH

Theoretically, the transperineal approach should be slightly more diagnostic than the abdominal approach, since the prostate is situated closer to the perineum (the area between the scrotum and the anus) than it is to the anterior abdominal wall. This has not proven to be true.

When using the transperineal approach, standard ultrasound equipment (contact or real-time units) is utilized. The transducer, optimally a 3.5- or 5.0-MHz unit, is placed on the perineum with acoustic gel used for coupling. The transducer is angled cephalad, and the prostate is identified. Better delineation of the prostate is obtained by having the urinary bladder at least partially filled with fluid (urine) prior to the examination.

A major limitation of this study is poor definition of the posterior margins of the prostate, since the rectum (particularly when empty) and prostate may not be clearly differentiable from one another. Prostatic enlargement or distinctly abnormal echogenic foci (particularly when highly echogenic) may be identified, but subtle lesions will often not be seen.

Transverse and longitudinal scans should be obtained for complete evaluation.

ENDOURETHRAL APPROACH

The endo- or transurethral approach, where a transducer is placed through the urethra into the urinary bladder, can also be used to identify the prostate (Fig. 4.2). This technique, which is a more recently introduced approach as compared to the conventional transabdominal

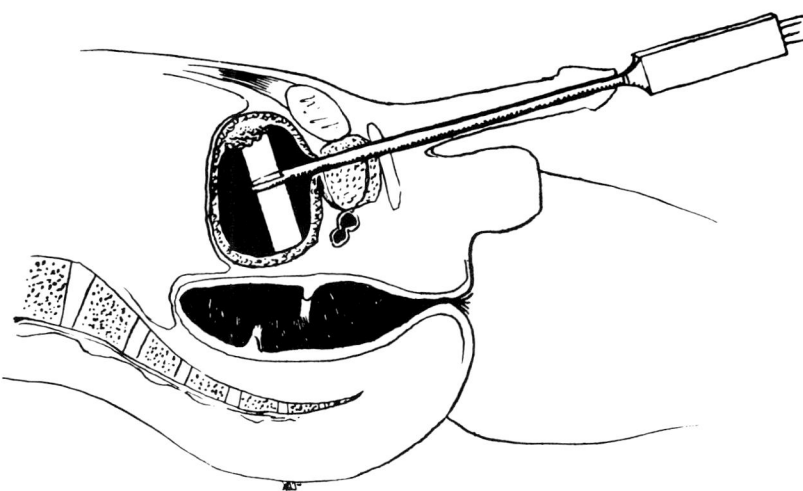

FIG. 4.2. Diagram of endourethral scanning. The transducer is placed through the penile urethra into the urinary bladder. Axially oriented images are visualized, and then the transducer is withdrawn slowly to visualize the prostate from the prostatic urethra. This technique was initially developed to identify and stage bladder cancers.

scan, requires special endosonographic probes that are smaller (thinner) than conventional transducers. The endourethral approach utilizes small (commercially available) probes and transducers that will be placed either directly into the urethra or through a cystoscope. The size of these instruments varies, but it usually ranges between 18 and 24 French.

The transurethral examination is used infrequently for primary evaluation of the prostate because of a number of theoretical complications involved. These include: (a) risks associated with the need for heavy sedation or general anesthesia; (b) possible post-examination infection or nonspecific urethritis; (c) evaluation of equal accuracy and efficacy with equipment that is technically easier to use and less uncomfortable to the patient; and (d) the fact that portions of the prostate are not always within the sharpest zone of focus of the transducer.

The endourethral probes presently available have transducers that will rotate in a 360° fashion (Fig. 4.3). These have appropriately been termed *radial scanners*. Various frequencies are available, but those between 5.5 and 8.0 MHz are most useful. The probe is usually placed either directly into the urethra or through a cystoscope into the urethra during a cystoscopic examination. The urinary bladder should be partially distended prior to insertion to avoid possible rupture or tear of the vesical wall. The transducer tip is placed within the urinary bladder. Scanning is commenced, and the transducer is removed slowly until the prostatic portion of the urethra is reached. At that time, sequential scans of the prostate are obtained as the probe is withdrawn in subcentimeter increments. Since the sharpest focal zone of these transducers is usually between 1 and 4 cm from the crystal, a small portion of the periurethral area of the prostate may not be imaged.

Because the endourethral approach is performed during routine cystoscopic examination of the urinary bladder, conventional sterile technique is required. These instruments can usually be either gas sterilized or placed in a liquid sterilizing solution (e.g., Cidex).

ENDORECTAL APPROACH

Endosonographic studies from the rectum have become a popular and clinically important technique. Although it was developed initially in the 1960s, the equipment has become more highly sophisticated during the past few years, and many of the diagnostic sonographic characteristics have been identified with the increased resolution capabilities of the equipment.

In conventional sonography, a transducer can be manually moved, and thus rotated, to obtain the longitudinal and axial orientation. However, the rectum is small, and conventional-sized transducers cannot be rotated manually. Thus, until recently, the transducers were too large to rotate. Imaging with a single probe was obtained with a single orientation. The transducers were usually oriented either in an axial orientation or in a longitudinal fashion. Recently (see below), several types of biplane tranducers (i.e., those able to image in two orientations) have been developed.

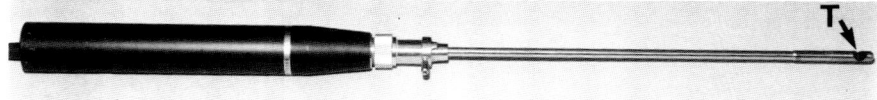

FIG. 4.3. Endourethral transducer. A commercially available endourethral probe is thin to enable placement through a resectoscope. The transducer at the tip of the probe (T) rotates in a 360° arc.

Types of Equipment

The earliest of the commercially available endorectal probes were radial scanners that utilized a specifically designed chair in which the patient would sit (Fig. 4.4). The probe was placed through a central hole in the chair and into the patient's rectum, with the patient seated throughout the study. These units used transducers yielding an axially oriented imager.

A larger variety of equipment is available with the hand-held units. The axially oriented scanner utilizes several types of transducers. A rotating transducer is similar to that used for endourethral sonography (Fig. 4.5). The transducer rotates in a 360° radius and is termed *radial scanner*. Rotation is usually relatively slow, so that 1 to 10 images/sec are obtained. Sector scanners have the transducer placed at the tip of these axially oriented imagers. The sector scanners have been developed in a variety of probes including mechanical-sector and phased-array technology. Additionally, curved linear technology has been applied to some of these devices that also yield a "pie-shaped" sector-type image.

The longitudinally oriented scanners images were initially developed utilizing a linear array real-time system. In these transducers, the crystals are arranged in a longitudinal fashion at the tip of the transducer, which is placed into the rectum (Fig. 4.6). Sagittal, oblique, parasagittal, and coronal images can be obtained. More recently, sector scanners have been developed (Fig. 4.7).

In the midline, a sagitally oriented scan is outlined. As the transducer is rotated clockwise and/or counterclockwise, oblique parasagittal images are obtained with a 90° rotation, and a coronal image is obtained. Sector scans have also been utilized to image in the longitudinal plane.

Recently, biplane probes have been introduced. These probes may have two distinctly different transducers in the tip, one to image in the transverse orientation and the other to image in the longitudinal orientation. These have been produced with a variety of techniques. One type of production model has two 90% pie-shaped sector-type scanners adjacent to each other (Fig. 4.8). Others have a pie-shaped sector for the axially oriented image and have a

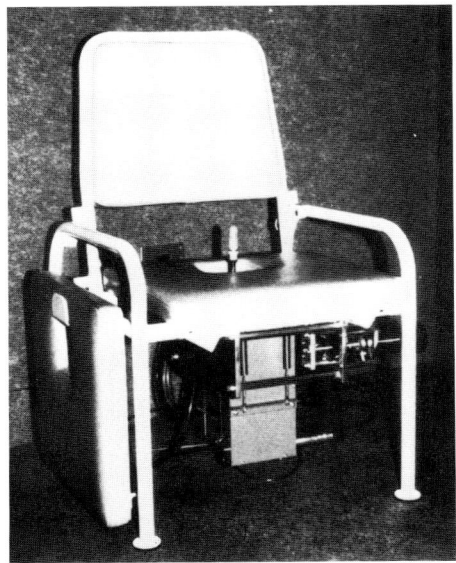

FIG. 4.4. Endorectal scan—chair. Initial endorectal scanning was developed with the use of a chair. A hole was situated in the seat of the chair for positioning of the transducer into the rectum.

36   SCANNING TECHNIQUES, EQUIPMENT, AND PATIENT PREPARATION

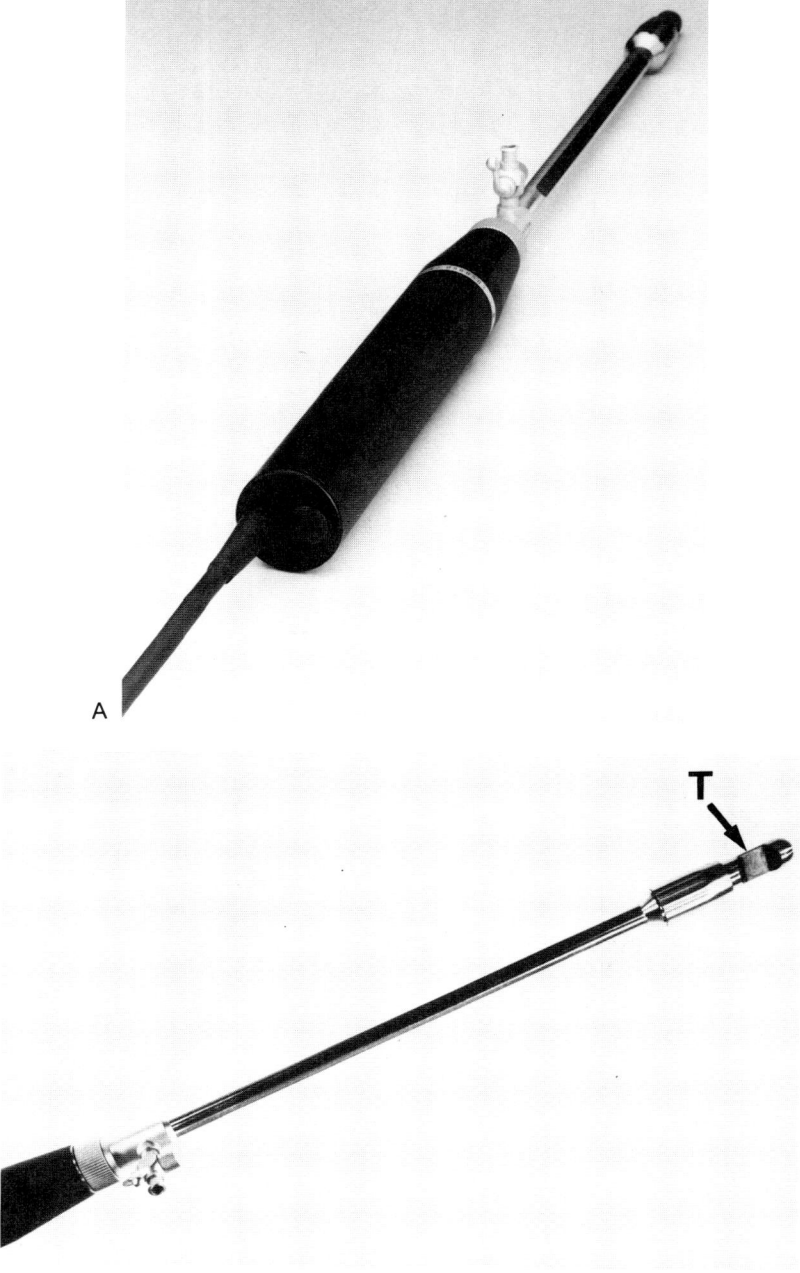

FIG. 4.5. Axially oriented endorectal radial scans. The radial scanner (**A**) is usually long and thin. The transducer (T) is placed at the tip (**B**) and rotates in a 360° radius, which is why the term *radial scanning* is used.

SCANNING TECHNIQUES, EQUIPMENT, AND PATIENT PREPARATION 37

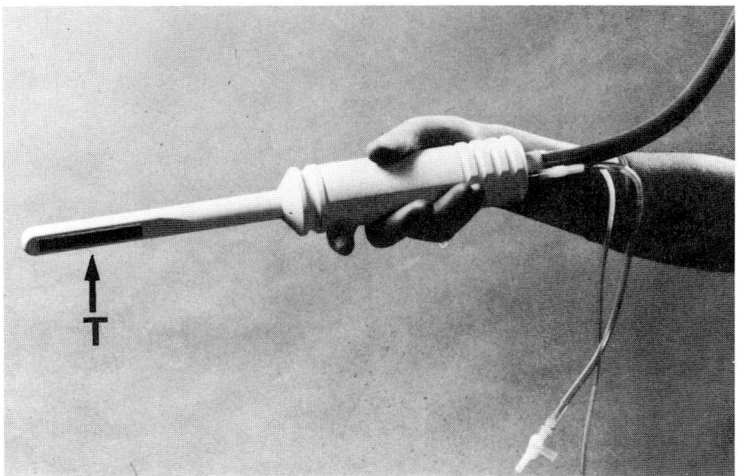

FIG. 4.6. Longitudinally oriented linear array endorectal transducer. This type of transducer has the crystals situated in a longitudinal fashion at the tip (T) of the probe. This is one type of configuration.

linear array for the longitudinal image (Fig. 4.9). A third variety uses both a curved linear-array transducer and an adjacent flat-faced one (Fig. 4.10). Some use a single mechanical sector transducer that can also be mechanically rotated to give an image in any direction. As more work in this field is undertaken, additional attempts at multioriented images will probably result in even more arrangements and types of transducers for these endorectal probes.

The early transducers utilized 3.5-MHz crystals. However, resolution was limited, and the sharpest zone of focus was not optimally situated in the posterior portion of the prostate. The development of more highly sophisticated 5-, 6-, 7-, and 8-MHz transducers has since ensued. More superficially focused with better axial and lateral resolution, they can more clearly and more accurately define smaller areas within the prostate.

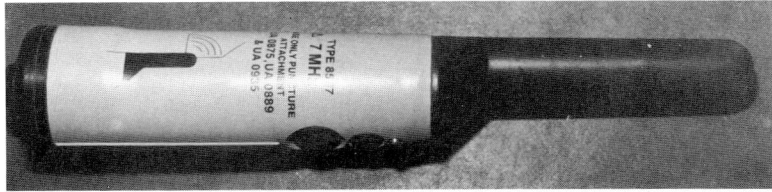

FIG. 4.7. Longitudinally oriented endorectal sector scan. A variety of sector scanners have been developed. This is an illustration of one type where the transducer is placed at the tip of the instrument. The images have an angulated pie-shaped configuration as demonstrated on the handle of the probe.

38 SCANNING TECHNIQUES, EQUIPMENT, AND PATIENT PREPARATION

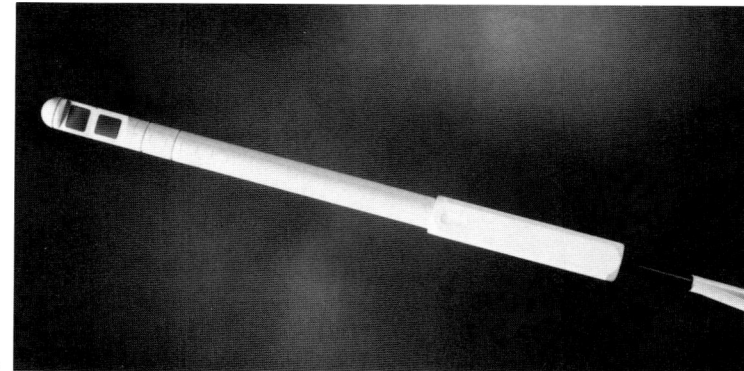

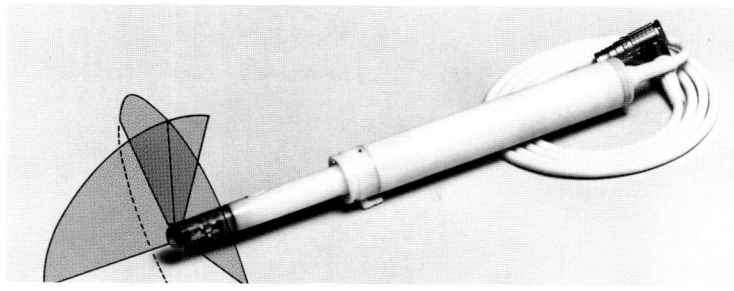

FIG. 4.8. Biplane endorectal probe with two sector scanners. Two different varieties of commercially available sector scanners are illustrated. One (**A**) has two separate crystals positioned at the tip of the probe. A second (**B**) has the crystals covered at the tip, but a schematic diagram overlay demonstrates the orientation of the visualized images. (Part A, courtesy of General Electric Medical Systems, Milwaukee, Wisconsin; part B, courtesy of Teknar, Inc., Fenton, Missouri.)

Transducer Preparation

Almost all of the transducers produced to date are prepared for the patient examination in a similar fashion.

The Single-Sheath (Cover) Technique (Fig. 4.11)

Although each unit is fashioned slightly differently, probe preparation for each one is similar. A disposable latex or rubber cover (also known as a *condom* or *sheath*) is placed over the entire portion of the transducer that will be placed within the rectum. This generally eliminates possible contamination of the transducer and therefore eliminates spread of disease. These covers are usually secured with a rubber band placed over a portion of the transducer or within specially produced grooves within the transducer. All of these tranducers have either one or two specially designed openings (orifices) so that water can be instilled from the external aspect of the probe into the area between the transducer crystals and the cover. This is done for better acoustic contact and for placement of the prostate in the sharpest zone of focus. Nonaerated water is inserted through the specially designed orifice. The water mixes with the residual air between the cover and the probe. Then the water and

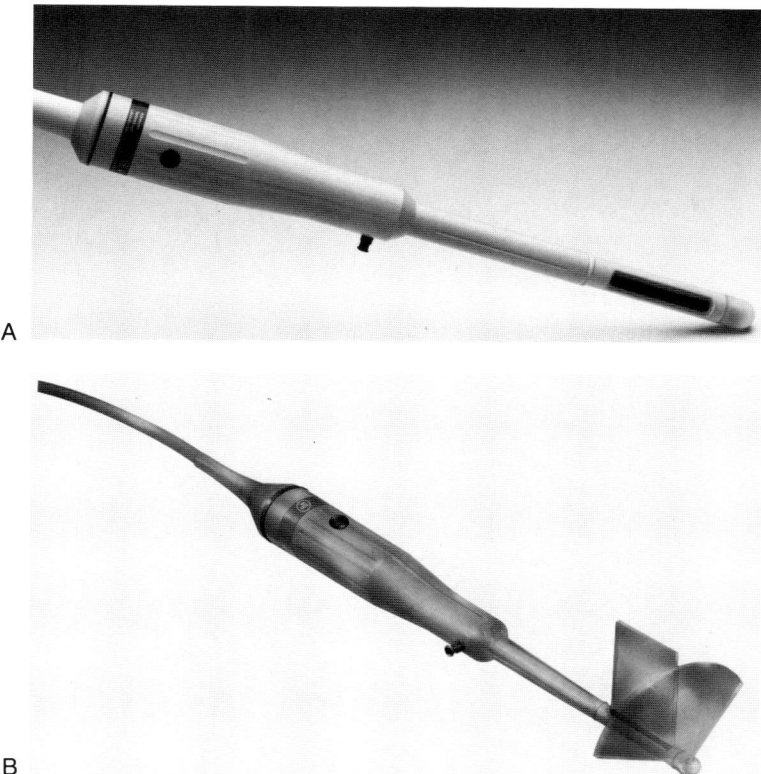

FIG. 4.9. Biplane endorectal probe with a sector and a linear transducer. Another variety of a biplane probe demonstrates a longitudinally oriented linear-array configuration and a pie-shaped sector axially oriented image placed at the tip of the transducer (**A**). Schematic overlay (**B**) demonstrates the orientation of the images. (Courtesy of Advanced Technology Laboratories, Bothell, Washington.)

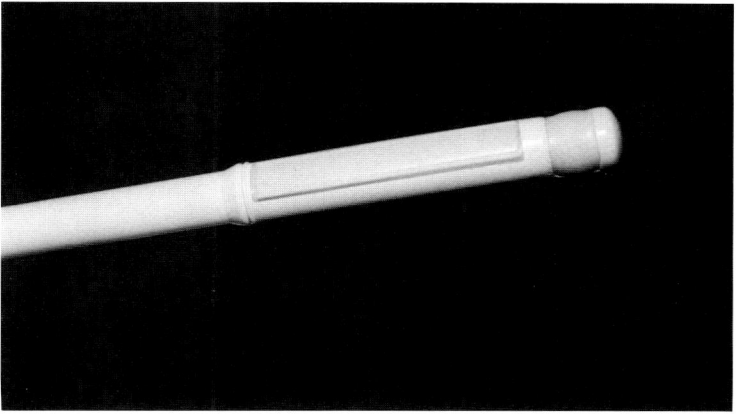

FIG. 4.10. Biplane endorectal probe with one curved and one flat-faced linear-array transducer. This biplane configuration incorporates a longitudinally oriented linear-array transducer for the sagittal orientation and a curved linear-array transducer for the axial scans.

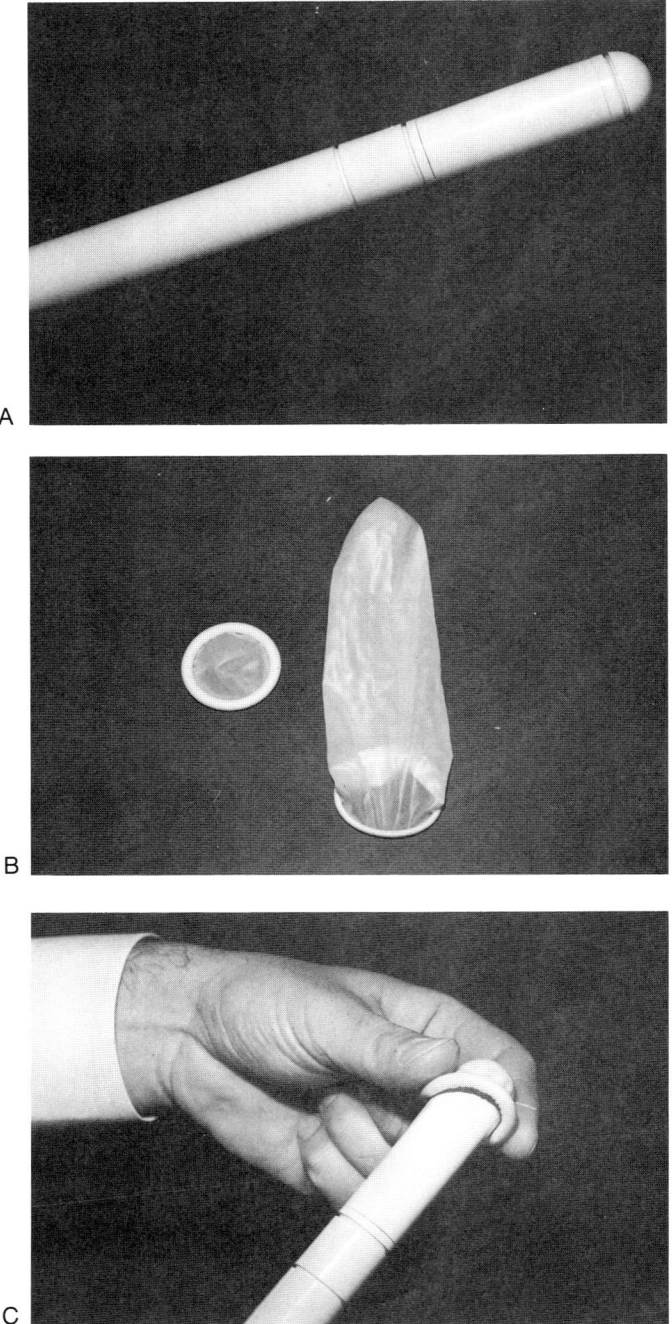

FIG. 4.11. Endorectal probe preparation. Almost all endorectal transducers are prepared in a similar fashion. One technique is as follows. The probe (**A**) must be covered by a condom (**B**). This can be a commercially available condom (part B, left), which is usually unrolled (part B, right) either during or prior to placement over the transducer. The condom (without the use of gel) is placed over the transducer (**C**).

SCANNING TECHNIQUES, EQUIPMENT, AND PATIENT PREPARATION

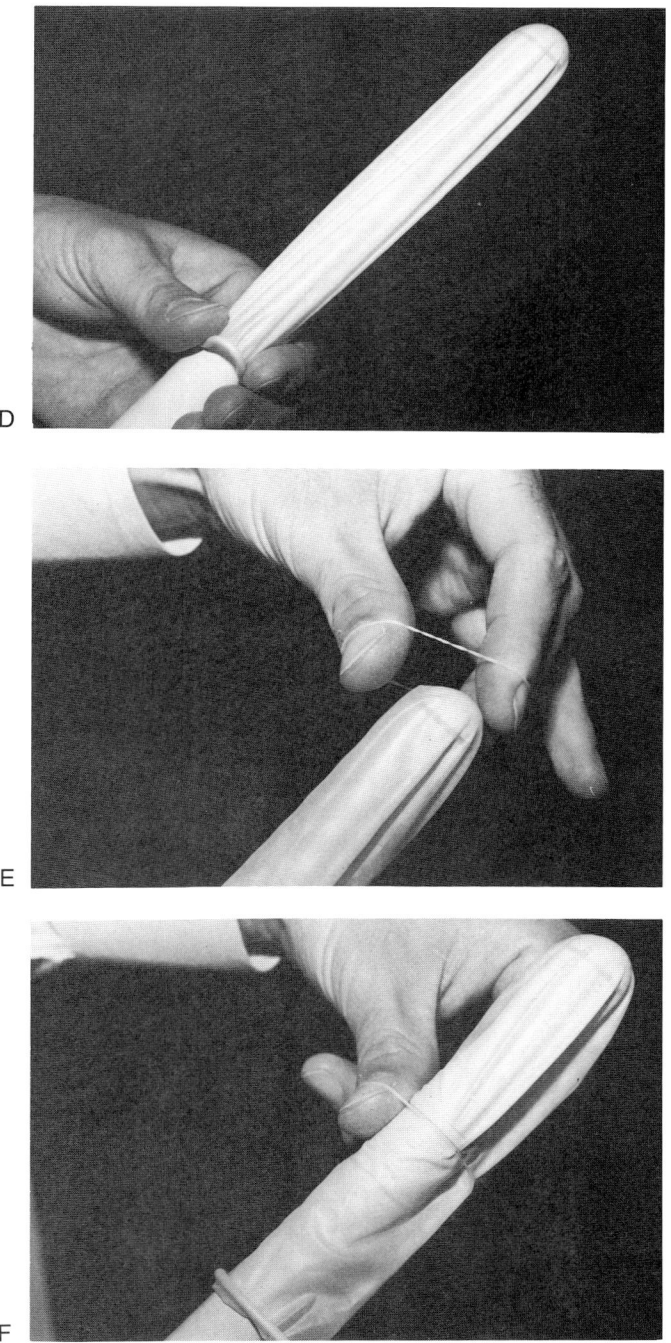

FIG. 4.11. *Continued*. The entire condom (**D**) is then uncurled. One or more rubber bands (**E**) are placed over the condom-probe complex and are secured in place (**F**).

all residual air are removed (Fig. 4.12). In this manner, acoustic contact between the transducer's crystals and the cover is optimized. Once the probe is properly prepared and inserted in the rectum, nonaerated water can be placed back through the orifice. This distends the cover and increases the distance between the prostate and the transducer, thereby allowing variability in placement of the sharpest zone of focus. The major limitation of the single-cover technique is that the cover must be discarded after each use. Then the probe must be cleansed, and a new cover must be replaced after each patient. Although gel, instead of water, can be used, it is not appropriate interfacing for the cover and the probe in the single-cover technique. The distance between the transducer and its cover cannot be varied once the probe is placed in position in the rectum.

Double-Cover Technique

This technique utilizes two covers. The distance between the transducer and cover cannot be varied. The first (inner cover) is placed on the transducer, secured, and prepared in a fashion that is similar to the single-cover technique (Fig. 4.12). Gel is then placed over the first cover and probe, and a second cover is positioned over the probe (Fig. 4.13). All air is squeezed from between the two cover interface before the outer (second) cover is secured to the probe. This technique theoretically allows reuse of the inner-cover–transducer complex following removal of the outer cover. From a practical standpoint, it is necessary to ensure that no contamination occurs. Additionally, because the sound beam must traverse two covers, some slight image degradation may result.

Patient Preparation

Patient preparation is usually not required prior to an endorectal sonogram, although occasionally a cleansing enema can remove fecal material that may obscure some sonographic

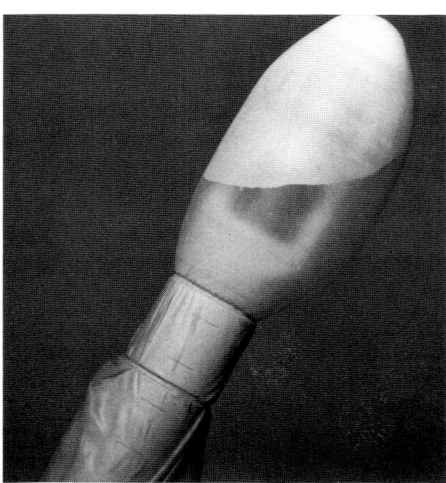
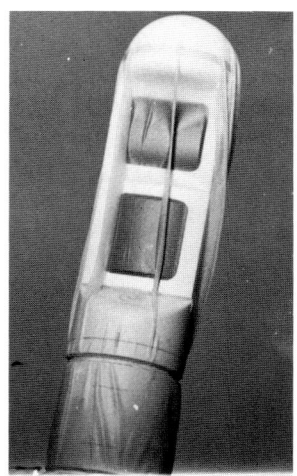

FIG. 4.12. Water placement into the probe-condom complex. Following placement of one disposable condom, water is placed via extension tubing into the probe-condom complex. It is important to ensure that no air is placed within the water (**A**). If this occurs, then the air must be removed (**B**).

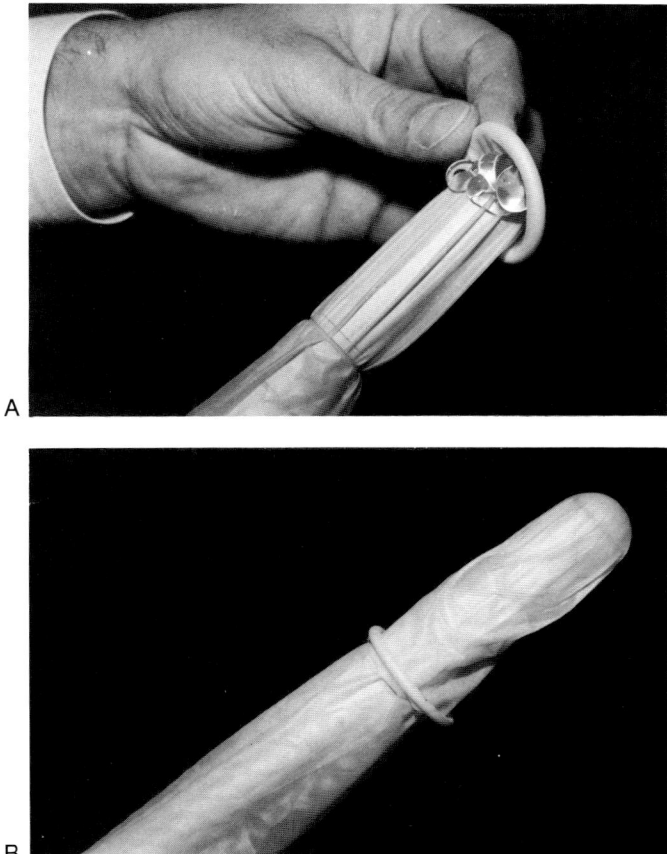

FIG. 4.13. Double-cover technique. This technique can be utilized for more rapid reusability of the probe. The first condom is installed in a fashion similar to that described in Fig. 4.12. Then, following placement of a small amount of gel (**A**), a second disposable condom can be placed over the first condom (**B**).

detail. The patient can be examined in the lateral decubitus, lithotomy, or knee-chest positions (Fig. 4.14). For optimal visualization of the base of the prostate and base of the urinary bladder, the urinary bladder should be partially distended with fluid (urine) prior to the examination. In general, a digital rectal examination should be performed prior to probe insertion to exclude any contraindications for this study (i.e., an obstructing lesion, rectal fissures, or other pathology). The anus and the tip of the probe are then adequately lubricated with gel, and the sonoendoscope is placed into the rectum. Nonaerated water is then placed between the condom and the transducer crystals so that proper imaging of the rectum is possible.

Since many of these endorectal transducers have the sharpest zone of focus from approximately 2 to 6 cm from the transducer crystal, a small area of separation (with water) between the transducer surface and the rectal wall is beneficial in order to evaluate the posterior portions of the prostate.

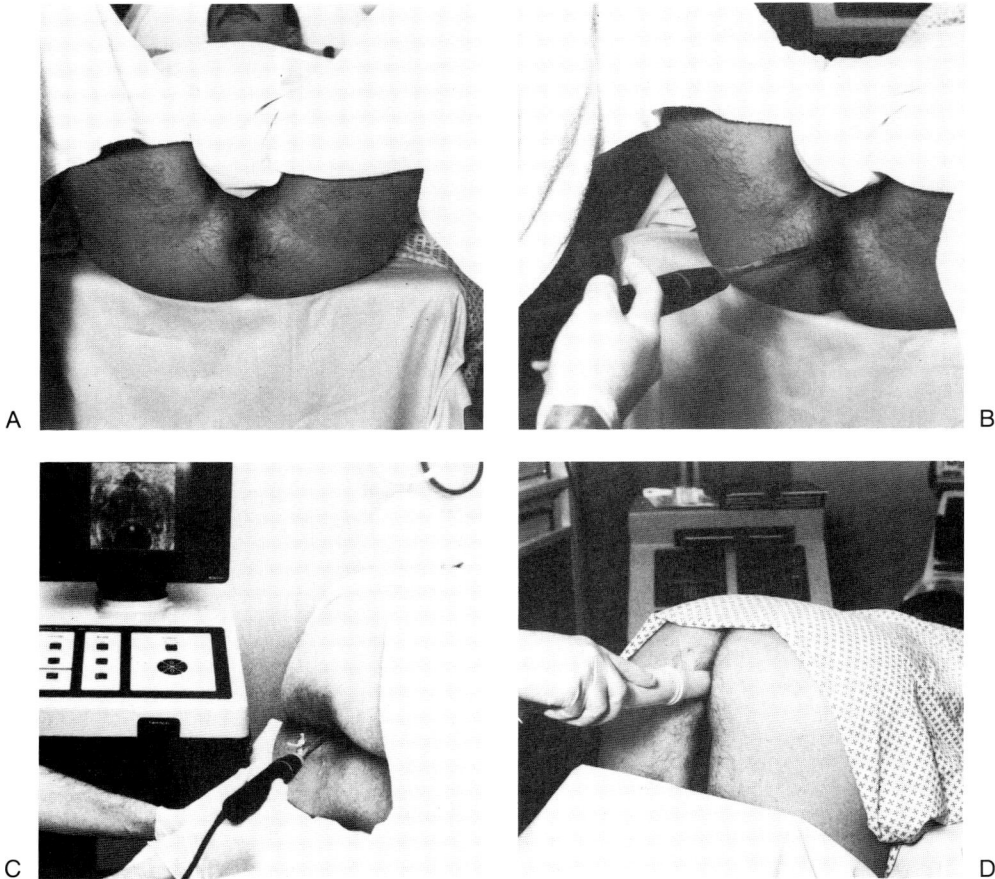

FIG. 4.14. Technique of endorectal ultrasound examination. The patient can be positioned in a variety of positions. The lithotomy position is seen prior to probe insertion (**A**) and during the examination (**B**). The left lateral decubitus (**C**) or the knee-chest (**D**) positions can also be used. Any of these positions are adequate, and personal preference by the physician and patient is suggested. (From reference 393.)

In general, the endorectal examination of the prostate may be slightly uncomfortable for the patient but should not be painful. The examination length will vary, depending upon the complexity of the study and the experience of the examiner, but is usually completed within 5 to 15 min.

Probe Insertion

The endorectal units vary in size. The longest can theoretically be inserted as deep as 25 cm from the anal verge. However, because of the blind fashion of insertion, it is preferable that these transducers be placed no more than 15 to 20 cm deep to the anus so that the risk of perforation is minimized. The diameters of the probes also vary, usually between 1.2 and 2.0 cm.

TECHNIQUE OF EXAMINATION—AXIAL SCANNING

When an axially oriented transducer is used, the transducer is usually placed up to the superior aspects of insertion (i.e., to the seminal vesicles or just above). At this level, the urinary bladder will be defined. The probe is then withdrawn in subcentimeter increments; the vas deferens, seminal vesicles, base of the prostate, body of the prostate, and finally the apex of the gland are imaged sequentially (Fig. 4.15). When a radial- or rotating-type transducer is used, the entire prostate is identified in a single sweep. When a sector scan device with a small angle of information (i.e., 90° or less) is utilized, the transducer may have to be rotated slightly to the right and then to the left side at each depth in order to image the entire gland. A reverse sequence (i.e., imaging of the apex of the prostate first and the seminal vesicles last) is equally acceptable and diagnostic.

TECHNIQUE OF EXAMINATION—SAGITTAL SCANNING

When a sagittally oriented transducer is employed, the prostate is imaged in long axis. Once the transducer is placed into the rectum, the entire prostate, including portions of the seminal vesicles, is usually seen from apex to base (Fig. 4.16). The midline of the prostate is usually identified first, and the probe is then rotated slightly clockwise or counterclockwise. All portions of the right side of the prostate and the right seminal vesicle are seen in counterclockwise rotation with the left side of the prostate and the left seminal vesicle in the clockwise rotation (Fig. 4.17). In certain circumstances, when the prostate is larger (in a cephalocaudad dimension) than the image size, the probe may have to be withdrawn slightly to identify the apex of the gland (with the probe placed more deeply into the rectal

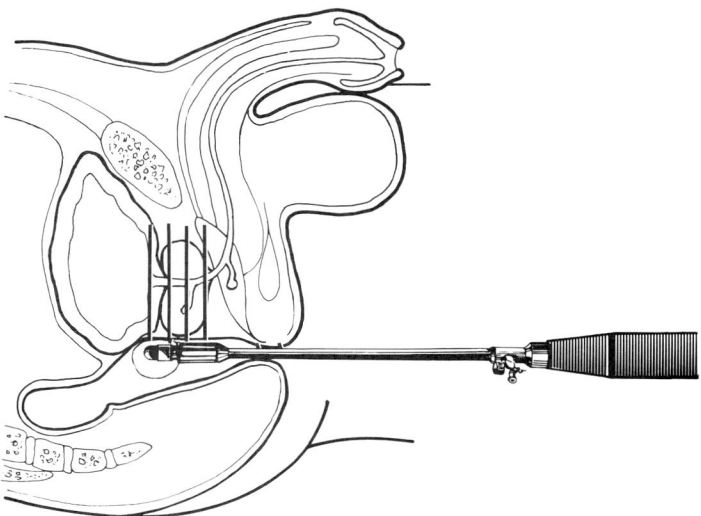

FIG. 4.15. Axially oriented scans—endorectal approach. With the transducer placed into the rectum, the seminal vesicles may be examined initially; the probe is withdrawn slightly at sequential increments to examine the remainder of the gland to the apex. The reverse order is equally adequate.

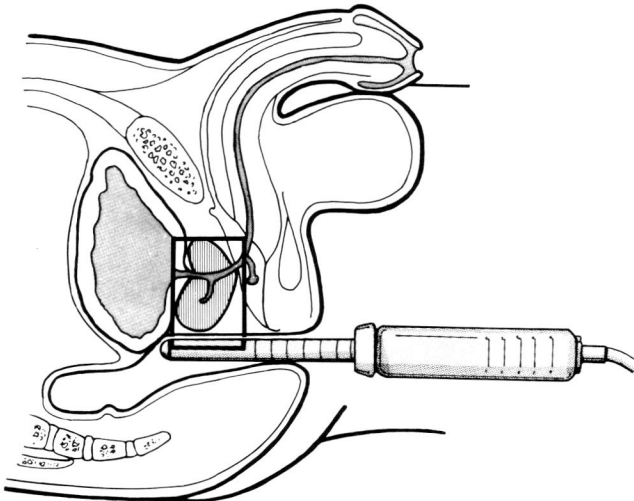

FIG. 4.16. Longitudinal orientation scans—endorectal approach. The longitudinal orientation requires the transducer be placed in the rectum. In general, the entire prostate will be identified from the apex to the base.

lumen) following initial imaging of the base and superior portions. In these cases, a repeat examination of the lower portion of the gland is undertaken.

Regardless of the orientation, when using a sector scanner, because the pie-shaped image in the near field is less than the rectangular linear-array design or the radial scanner, more water may have to be placed between the probe and anterior rectal wall to visualize the posterior portion of the prostate than when using other transducer designs (Fig. 4.18).

IMAGE PRESERVATION

A permanent record of each study should be made. This can be done by a number of methods, including the following:

1. *Hard-copy imaging.*
   a. Film—X-ray film is utilized. This requires an imager and developer capabilities. This has the highest initial cost but probably has the highest-quality images.
   b. Polaroid film—An imager is attached directly to the ultrasound machine. The imager is inexpensive to purchase, but the costs mount because of the substantially higher price of the polaroid film as compared to X-ray film. Resolution is also limited as is gray-scale delineation.
   c. Paper images—This new technique is inexpensive in terms of both the initial costs and the expense of the paper. Images have minimal resolution degradation.
2. *Videotape.* This requires a moderate cost of equipment. It produces high-quality images, but retrieval of a specific image can be time-consuming. It may be the preferable technique if the physician does not specifically perform the examination.

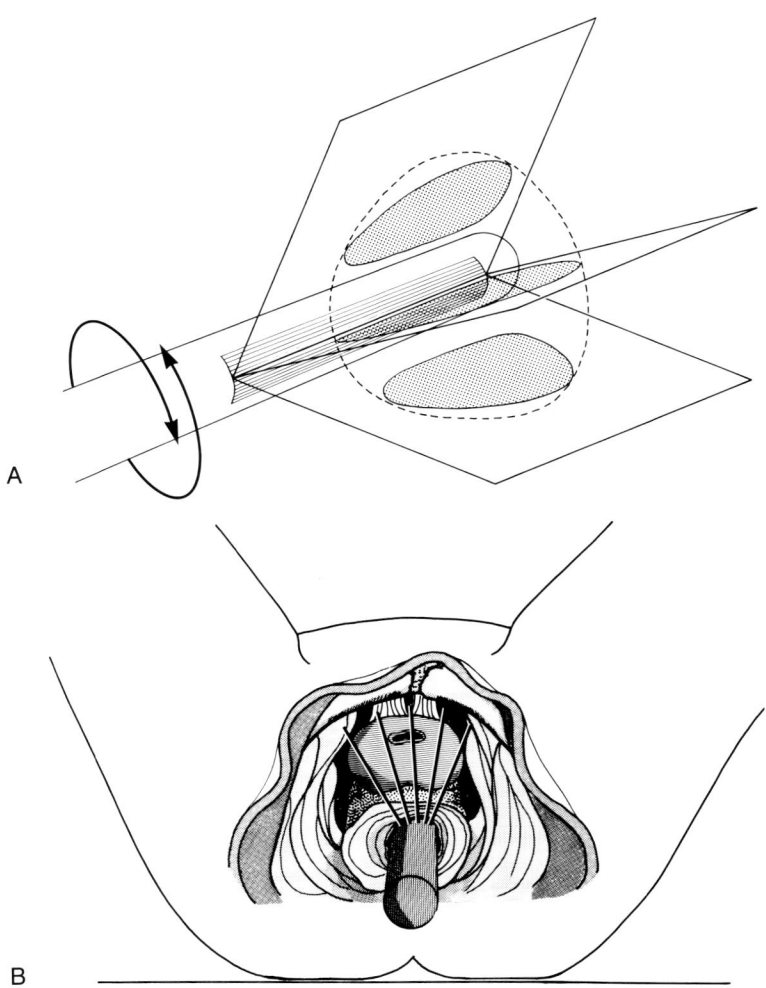

FIG. 4.17. Longitudinal orientation technique for endorectal examination. The longitudinal orientation requires movement of the transducer and probe in clockwise and/or counterclockwise rotation (**A**). By performing this, the lateral portions of the prostate (**B**) will be seen.

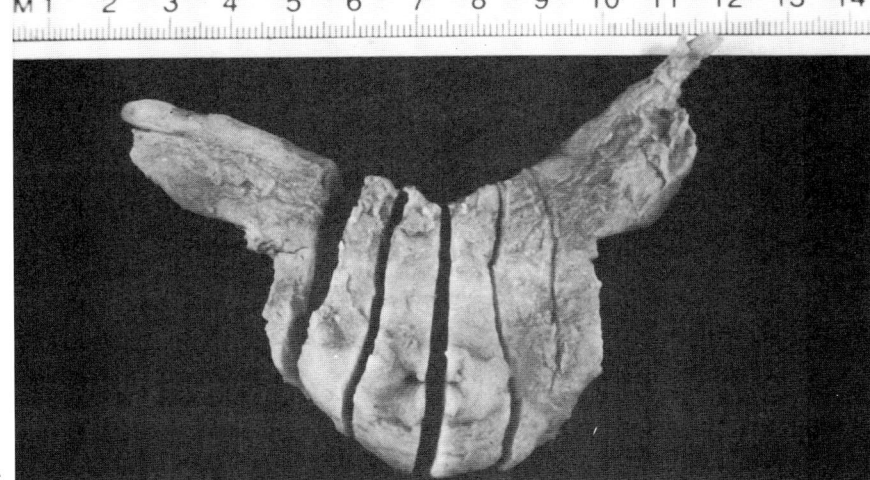

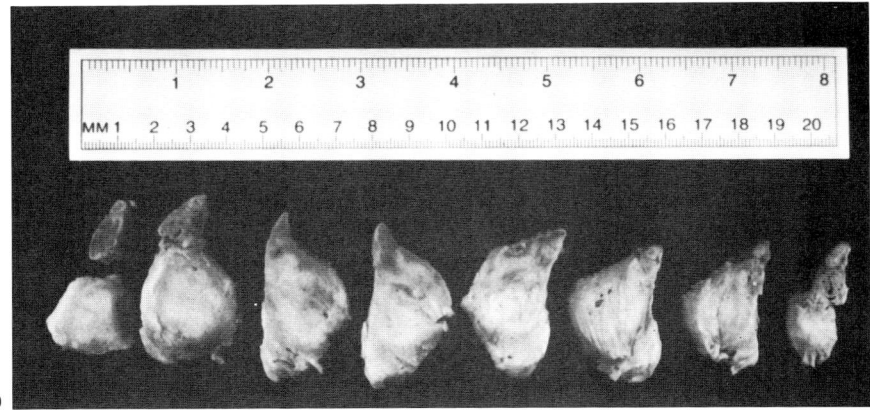

FIG. 4.17. *Continued.* The prostate will then be identified in obliquely oriented longitudinal sections, and is seen in a cut specimen of the prostate (**C**). The prostate (as seen in the gross specimen sections) will be seen in longitudinal orientation, and the seminal vesicles will be identified in cross section (**D**).

SCANNING TECHNIQUES, EQUIPMENT, AND PATIENT PREPARATION

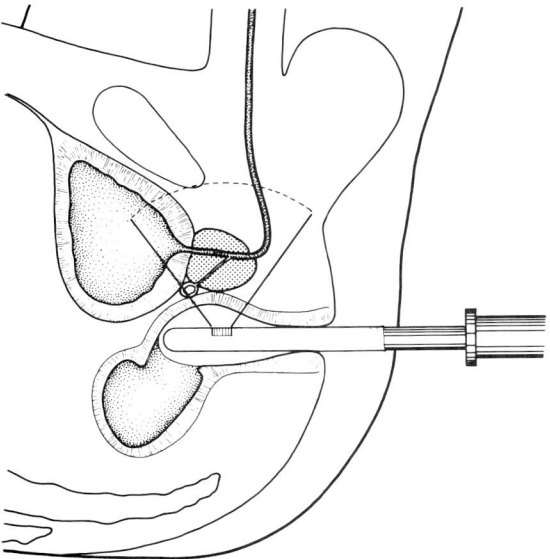

FIG. 4.18. Longitudinal orientation sector scanner. Because the pie-shaped sector image is smaller and closer to the transducer than the longitudinally oriented flat-faced linear scanner, more water needs to be placed into the condom to increase the depth of the posterior margin of the prostate from the transducer surface to enable a more adequate image.

CONCLUSION

Equipment is changing rapidly in the existing field of endosonographic imaging techniques. Almost daily, new units and updated machinery are being developed. Today, machines are already becoming obsolete (although not necessarily nondiagnostic) as newer concepts are introduced. As the field expands even further, we will see even more innovative models. Regardless of the future, today's equipment is certainly superb, and the images that are produced are of high diagnostic quality.

5 // *Normal Sonographic Anatomy*

Abdominal Approach	51
Perineal Approach	56
Endourethral Approach	56
Endorectal Approach	57
Comparison of Axial and Sagittal Endorectal Ultrasound Images	89

An understanding of the normal sonographic appearance of the prostate, seminal vesicles, and surrounding structures is essential before developing the ability to delineate pathologic processes within the gland. The normal prostate may have a different sonographic appearance at various ages and in different sonographic approaches. For example, a normal-appearing prostate is unusual in the elderly population because of the occurrence of benign hyperplasia. Truly normal glandular tissue, which will be defined below, is seen mostly in younger and middle-aged men.

ABDOMINAL APPROACH

When the abdominal approach is used, the orientation of the image is as advocated by the American Institute of Ultrasound in Medicine (AIUM). On the longitudinal image, the patient's head is oriented toward the left side of the screen; the feet are oriented toward the right side of the screen (Fig. 5.1). When the subject is studied in the supine position, the abdomen is at the top of the image; the posterior aspect of the patient is at the bottom of the image.

The transverse (axial) scan also orients the abdomen at the top of the screen and orients the back at the bottom of the screen. The patient's right side will be imaged on the left side of the image, and the patient's left side will be imaged on the right side of the image (Fig. 5.2).

The prostate is generally spheroid in shape and can be seen by imaging in both the sagittal (Fig. 5.3) and axial (Fig. 5.4) orientations. In the abdominal approach, the prostate will be identified through a fluid-filled urinary bladder and will appear to be homogeneously echogenic. The absolute degree of echogenicity depends upon the overall gain settings of the machine (Fig. 5.5). The time-gain–compensation (TGC) curves should be set appropriately so that, in the normal gland, homogeneous echogenicity is present. The normal seminal vesicles are slightly less echogenic in texture than the adjacent prostate (Fig. 5.3).

On the axial (transverse) image, the prostate is seen on the more steeply angled caudad views. As in the longitudinal view, most of the different normal tissues in the normal-

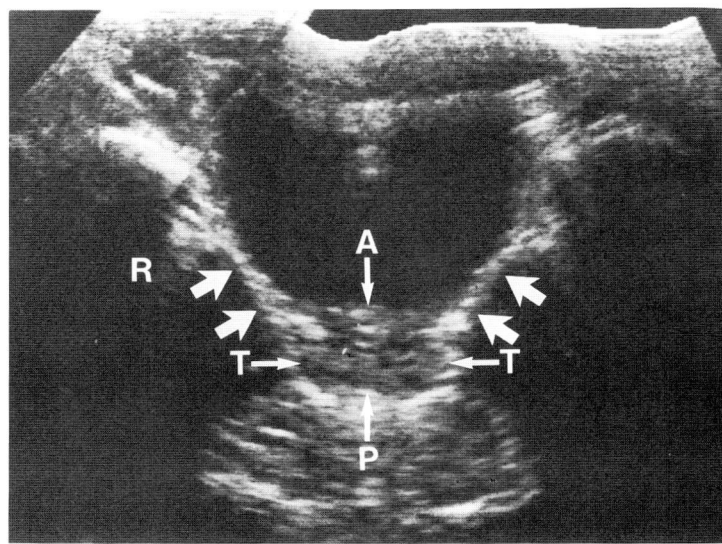

FIG. 5.1. Normal transverse transabdominal ultrasound of the prostate. The normal prostate will be seen in transverse orientation on the transabdominal scan as a rounded or ovoid structure. The anterior (A) to posterior (P) dimensions and the transverse (T–T) dimensions of the prostate will be identified. The prostate is best seen through a fluid-filled urinary bladder. The patient's right side (R) is on the left side of the image, and the patient's left side is on the right side of the image. Acoustic shadowing will be seen from the acetabulum and other pelvic bones (*arrows*).

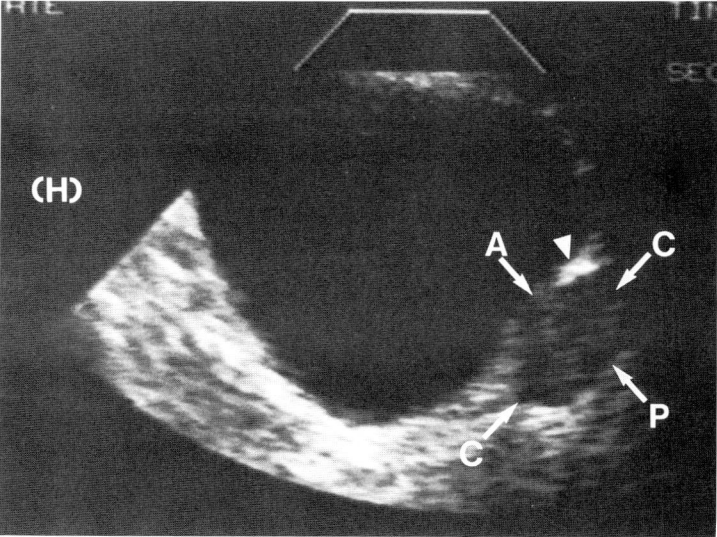

FIG. 5.2. Normal transabdominal longitudinally oriented sonogram. The prostate will be identified as a rounded or ovoid structure, and the anterior–posterior (A–P) dimension of the prostate will be identified. The cephalocaudad (C–C) dimensions will also be obtained. The urinary bladder should be identified as a fluid-filled structure anterior to the prostate. Occasionally, echogenic structures (*arrowhead*) within the prostate, calculi, may be delineated. (H) Toward patient's head.

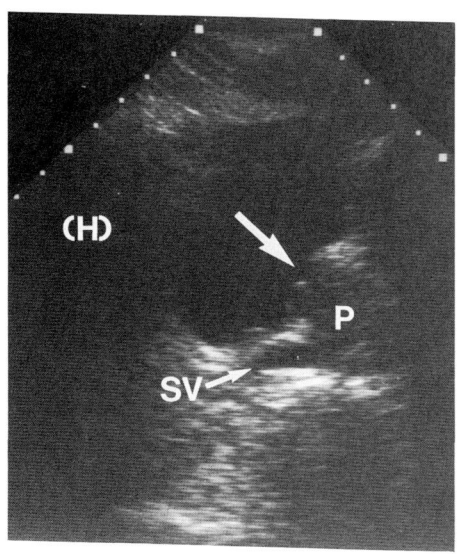

FIG. 5.3. Normal transabdominal ultrasound. The normal transabdominal ultrasound in longitudinal section will define the seminal vesicle (SV) superior to the cephalad margin of the prostate (P) on the longitudinal orientation. A slightly hypoechoic defect (larger *arrow*) may be identified, which is the periurethral tissues at the bladder neck. (H) Toward patient's head.

appearing rounded gland will not be delineated from one another. A slightly hypoechoic defect, a portion of the periurethral tissues, may occasionally be seen at the bladder neck (Fig. 5.3).

Differentiation of other internal structures of the prostate is not usually possible. By angling the transducer slightly more cephalad, the seminal vesicles will be seen. On the transverse orientation and using the abdominal approach, the seminal vesicles and prostate will not be identified on a single view. The seminal vesicles are paired structures which may be elongated or bow-tie-shaped (Fig. 5.6). Their echogenicity is slightly less than that

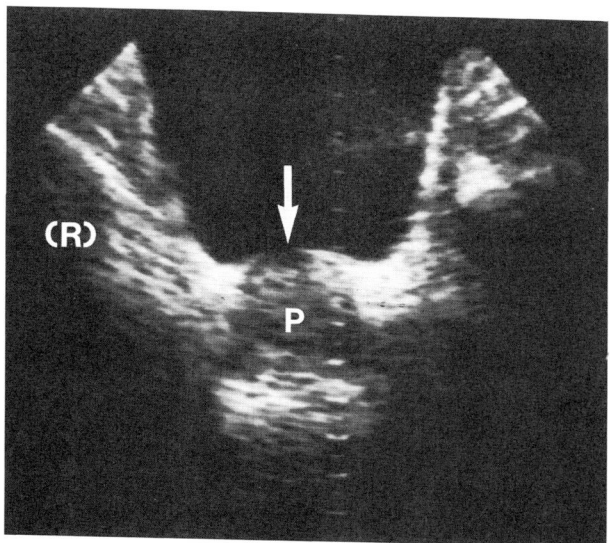

FIG. 5.4. Transabdominal prostate ultrasound. The prostate (P) is seen in longitudinal section with a hypoechoic defect (*arrow*) at the base of the bladder, the bladder neck. (R) Patient's right side.

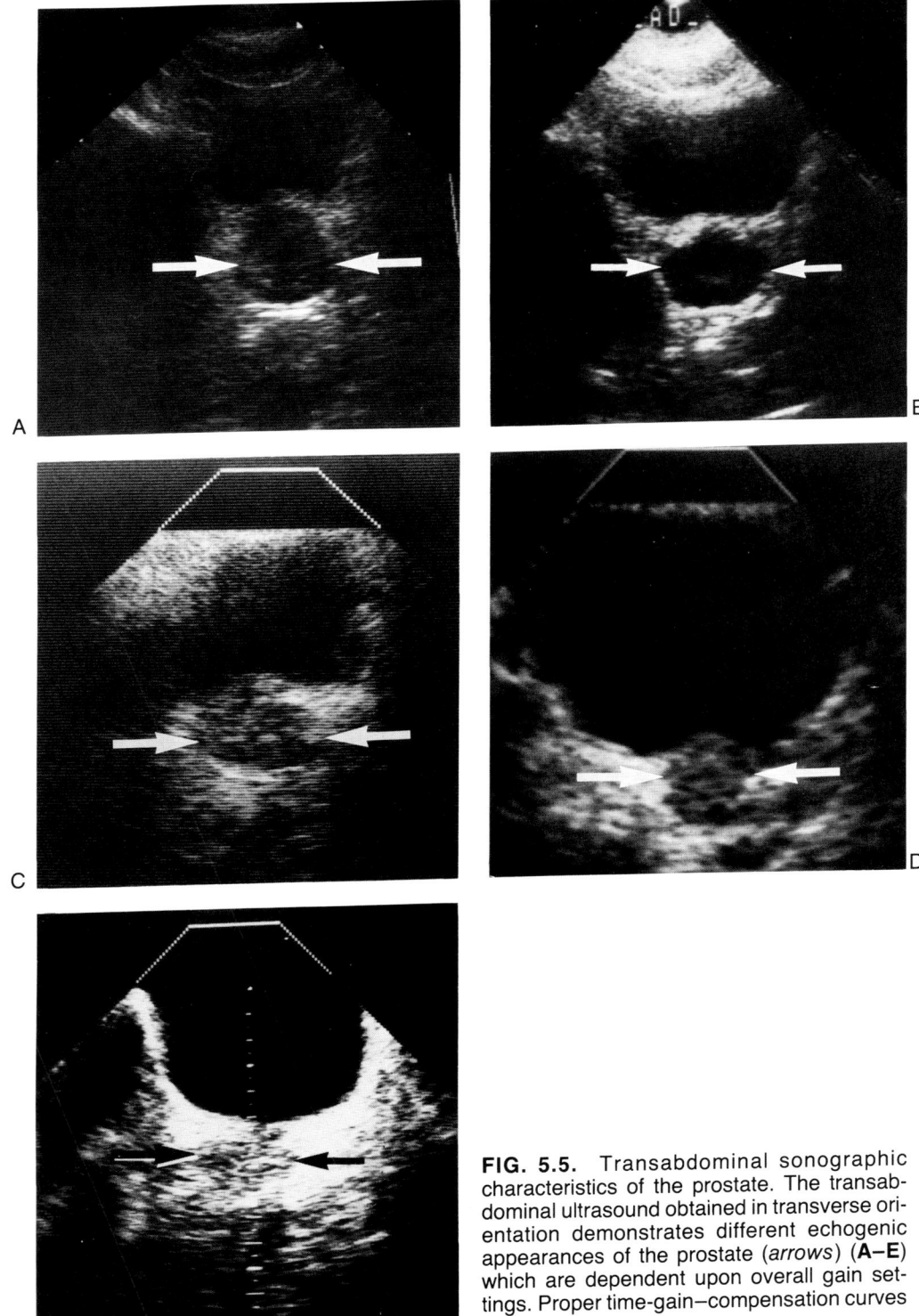

FIG. 5.5. Transabdominal sonographic characteristics of the prostate. The transabdominal ultrasound obtained in transverse orientation demonstrates different echogenic appearances of the prostate (arrows) (**A–E**) which are dependent upon overall gain settings. Proper time-gain–compensation curves are necessary.

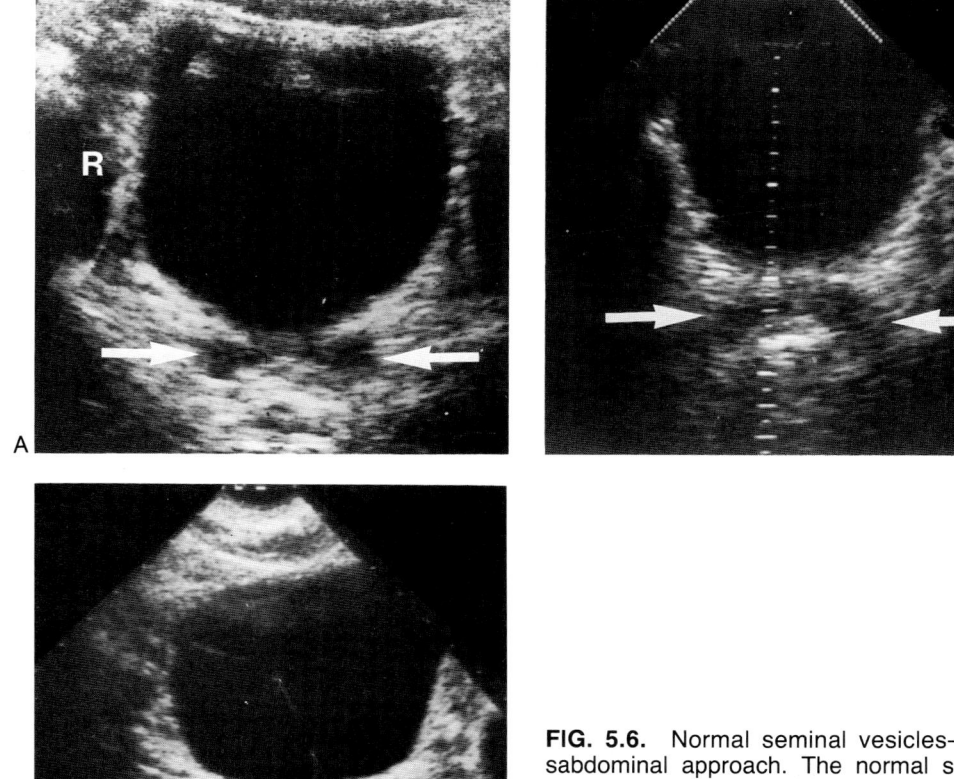

FIG. 5.6. Normal seminal vesicles—transabdominal approach. The normal seminal vesicles (*arrows*) can have a variety of appearances (**A–C**) and may appear bow-tie-shaped or elongated or may curve posteriorly. On the transverse image, the patient's right side (R) is on the left side of the image, and the patient's left side is on the right side of the image.

of the normal prostate; this is due, at least in part, to the higher fluid content of the seminal vesicles than the prostate.

On the longitudinal, sagittally oriented scan, the prostate will be seen in its cephalocaudad dimension as a homogeneously echogenic rounded structure. The seminal vesicles are identified in these images in cross section as rounded structures adjacent to the superior-posterior aspect of the prostate. The normal seminal vesicles are slightly less echogenic than the normal prostate. These structures and their differences in echogenicity will be identified in the sagittal and parasagittal images which show the more lateral portions of the prostate and seminal vesicles.

In general, the vas deferens and the majority of the prostatic urethra are not identified by the abdominal approach.

PERINEAL APPROACH

There is no convention for presenting images obtained by the transperineal approach. Other than on the axial scans, the patient's right side should be on the left side of the image, and the patient's left side should be on the right side of the image.

The transperineal sonogram of the prostate will define the gland only if the bladder is fluid-filled (Fig. 5.7). Echogenicity will be similar to the abdominal approach. There will be poor definition of the seminal vesicles; however, on the axial orientations, the seminal vesicles may be identified as bow-tie-shaped structures, and the prostate may be identified as being more caudad in position and rounded.

On longitudinal imaging, the prostate will appear rounded; a portion of the seminal vesicle, a smaller rounded structure sitting cephalad to the prostate, will also be seen in cross section.

A major deficiency in the perineal approach is delineating the posterior portion of the prostate from the adjacently placed rectum (which is often filled with air and/or fecal material).

ENDOURETHRAL APPROACH

All images in this approach are axially oriented. By convention, the patient's right side will be on the left side of the image, and the patient's left side will be on the right side of the image. The abdomen will be oriented toward the top of the image, and the back of the subject will be oriented toward the bottom of the image (Fig. 5.8).

The prostatic urethra may not be directly defined, but the transducer which is in the urethra will be seen, often as a bright echogenic reflector (which is the transducer) from which the ultrasound beam emanates. In the normal gland, there is poor differentiation between the periurethral and the acinar tissues, although the former are usually slightly less echogenic. In general, the central and the peripheral zones of the prostatic glandular tissues are not differentiable. Differences will be seen with enlargement (see Chapter 12). The prostate will appear to be rounded, with a depression in the posterior portion of the gland; this depression is called the *median furrow* or *median sulcus*. As the transducer is slightly removed, the

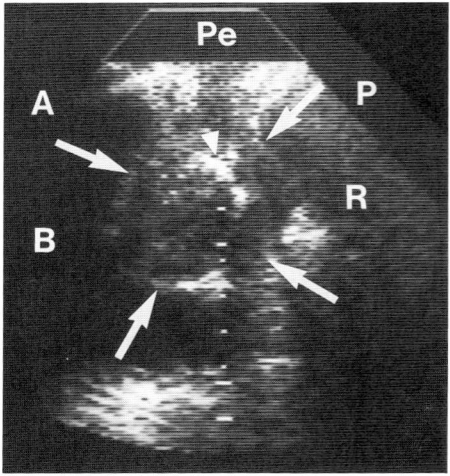

FIG. 5.7. Normal transperineal ultrasound of the prostate. With the transducer placed on the perineum (Pe), the prostate (*arrows*) may be identified as will a portion of the fluid-filled urinary bladder (B). The rectum (R) may not be clearly defined because of air and/or fecal material within the rectal lumen. An echogenic focus (*arrowhead*) with acoustic shadowing is seen which represents a calculus. The anterior aspect of the patient (A) is on the right side of the image, and the posterior aspect of the patient (P) is on the left side of the image.

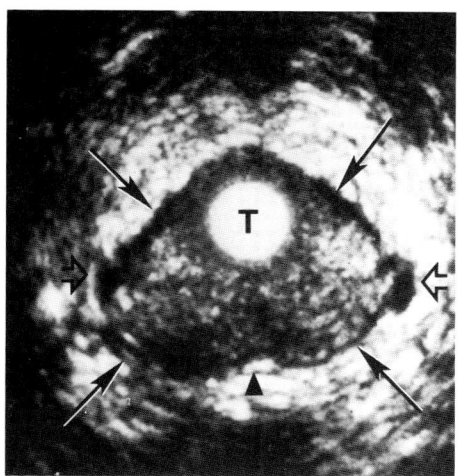

FIG. 5.8. Normal transurethral ultrasound of the prostate. With a transducer (T) placed within the prostatic urethra, the prostate (*arrows*) may be seen. The posterior aspect of the prostate may have an indentation (*arrowhead*), the median sulcus. Slight hypoechoic areas may be identified laterally (*open arrowheads*) which reflect the surrounding venous plexus. The anterior aspect of the patient is at the top of the image, and the posterior aspect of the patient is at the bottom of the image. The right side of the patient is on the left side of the image, and the left side of the patient is on the right side of the image. Courtesy of Dr. Hans Henrik Holm.

body (which is imaged as the largest portion) and the apex of the prostate (which is imaged as the smallest, more rounded portion) will be identified.

Homogeneous echogenicity of the prostate will usually be discerned, although some falloff of echogenicity may be noted in the more peripheral gland if the TGC curves are not set appropriately. Additionally, because these transducers are only sharply focused from 1 to 2 cm from the transducer tip, there may be a slight blurring of the most superficial periurethral tissues (i.e., those closest to the transducer).

ENDORECTAL APPROACH

The endorectal approach, which orients the prostate in either sagittal or transaxial orientation, demonstrates slightly different prostatic anatomy.

There has been no convention for imaging. In fact, the plethora of available equipment has made it difficult to obtain a similarly oriented image in all of the machines. For example, most (but not all machines) have a right-left image invert button that allows inverting the right and left side of the image. However, only a few companies to date have incorporated the possibility of a top-bottom image inversion.

Some machines orient the rectum at the top of the screen; others orient it at the bottom. This allows a theoretical possibility of having eight differently oriented images from the same scan (Figs. 5.9 and 5.10).

For purposes of consistency within this text, all images will be oriented in the following manner except where specifically noted:

1. *Axial scanners* (Fig. 5.9A).
   a. The rectum (and posterior structures of the patient) will be at the bottom of the image.
   b. The bladder (and anterior structures of the patient) will be at the top of the image.
   c. The patient's right side will be on the left side of the image.
   d. The patient's left side will be on the right side of the image.

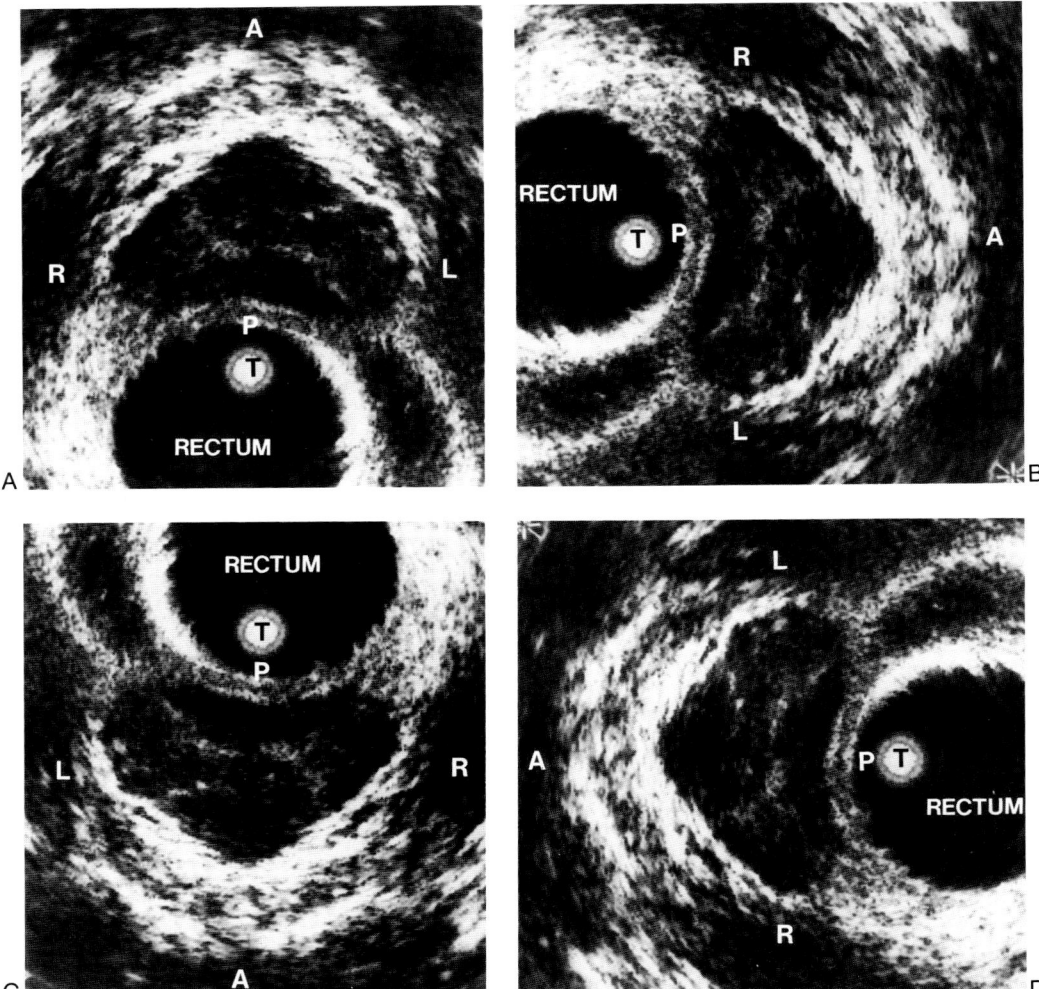

FIG. 5.9. Transverse orientation—endorectal ultrasound of the prostate, anatomic orientation. There are eight different ways in which the prostate can be oriented on an endorectal ultrasound of the prostate in the axial orientation (**A–H**). (R) Patient's right side; (L) patient's left side; (A) anterior aspect of patient; (P) posterior aspect of patient; (T) transducer. For purposes of this text, for all axially oriented images, the patient's right side will be on the left side of the image, the patient's left side will be on the right side of the image, the anterior aspect of the patient will be at the top of the image, and the posterior aspect of the patient will be at the bottom of the image (**A**).

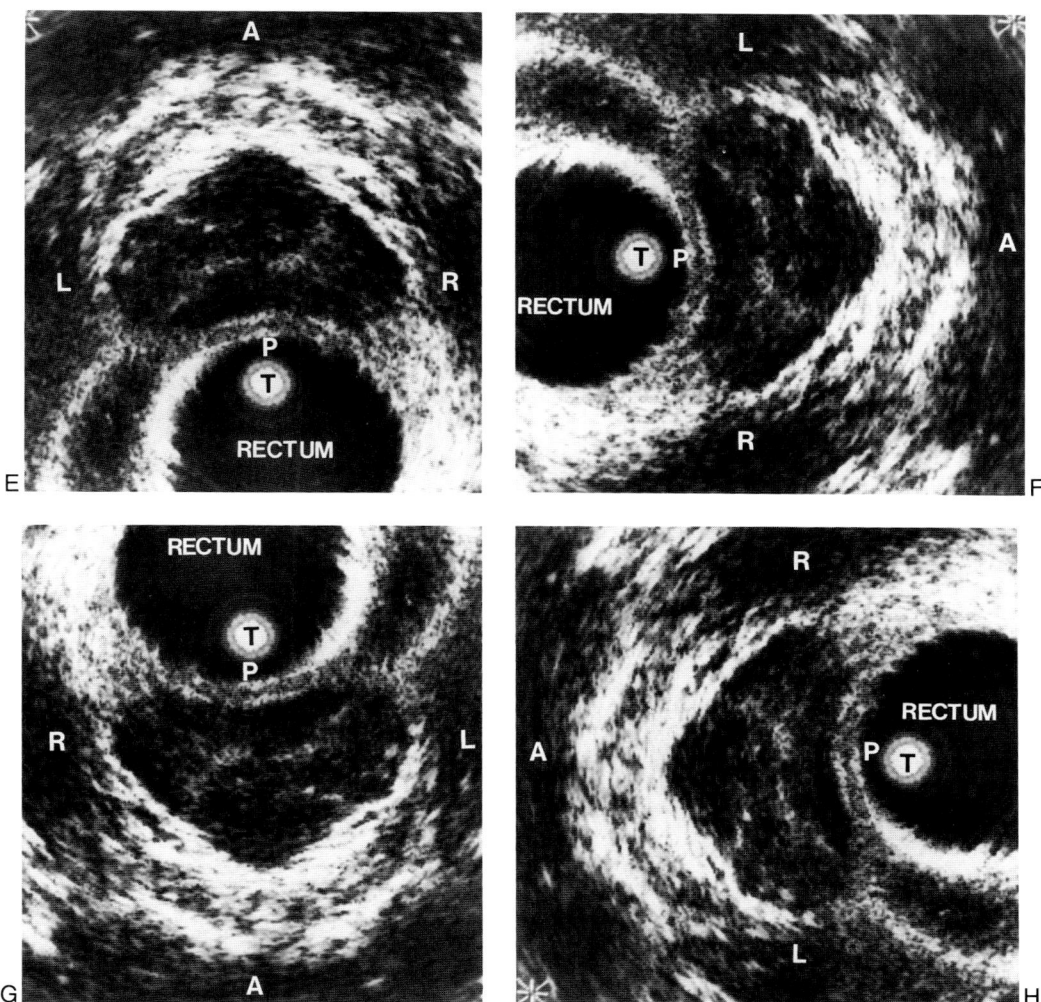

FIG. 5.9. *Continued.*

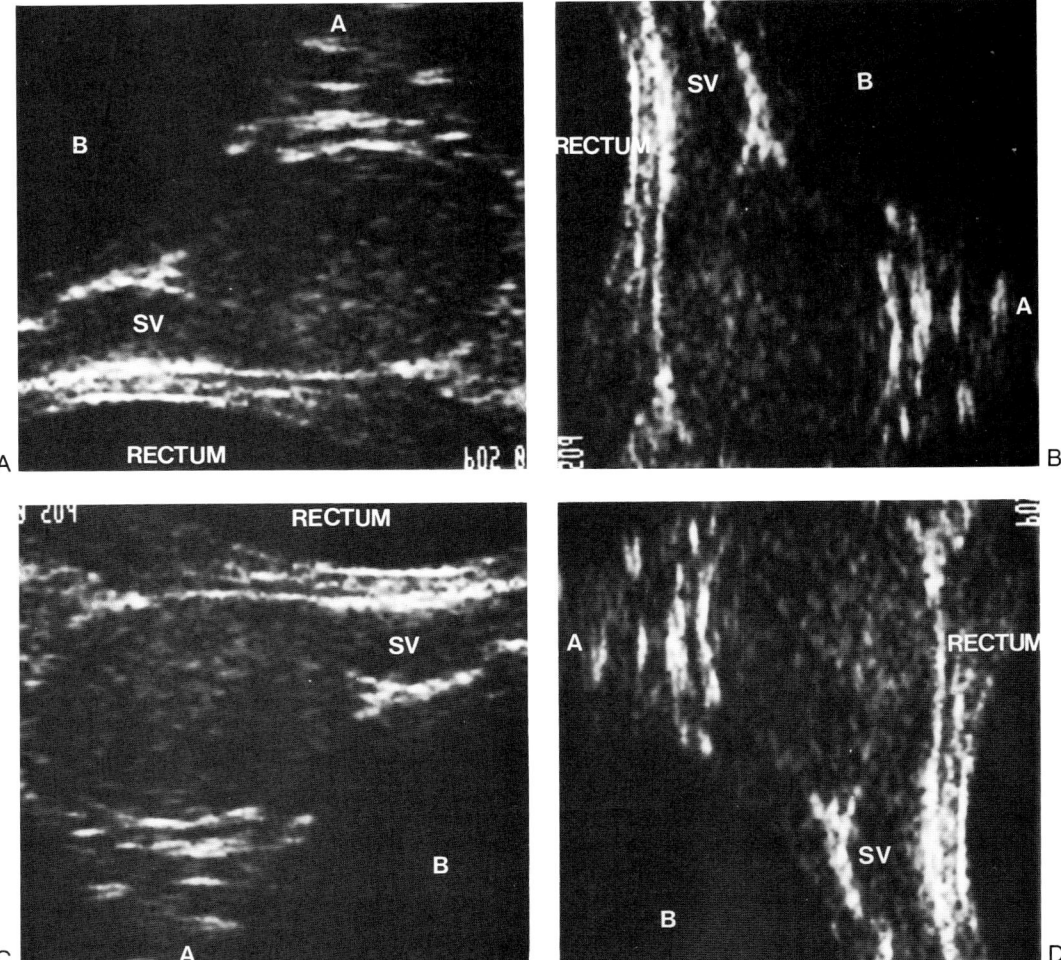

FIG. 5.10. Longitudinal orientation—endorectal ultrasound of the prostate, anatomic orientation. For the longitudinally oriented endorectal sonogram of the prostate, there are eight different orientations in which the image can be shown (**A–H**). For purposes of this text, although not all the machines orient the images in a similar fashion, all prostates will be shown on the endorectal sonogram with the rectum at the bottom of the screen and with the seminal vesicles (SV) and urinary bladder (B) to the left of the screen. The apex of the prostate will be oriented to the right of the screen, with the anterior (A) aspect of the patient at the top of the image (**A**).

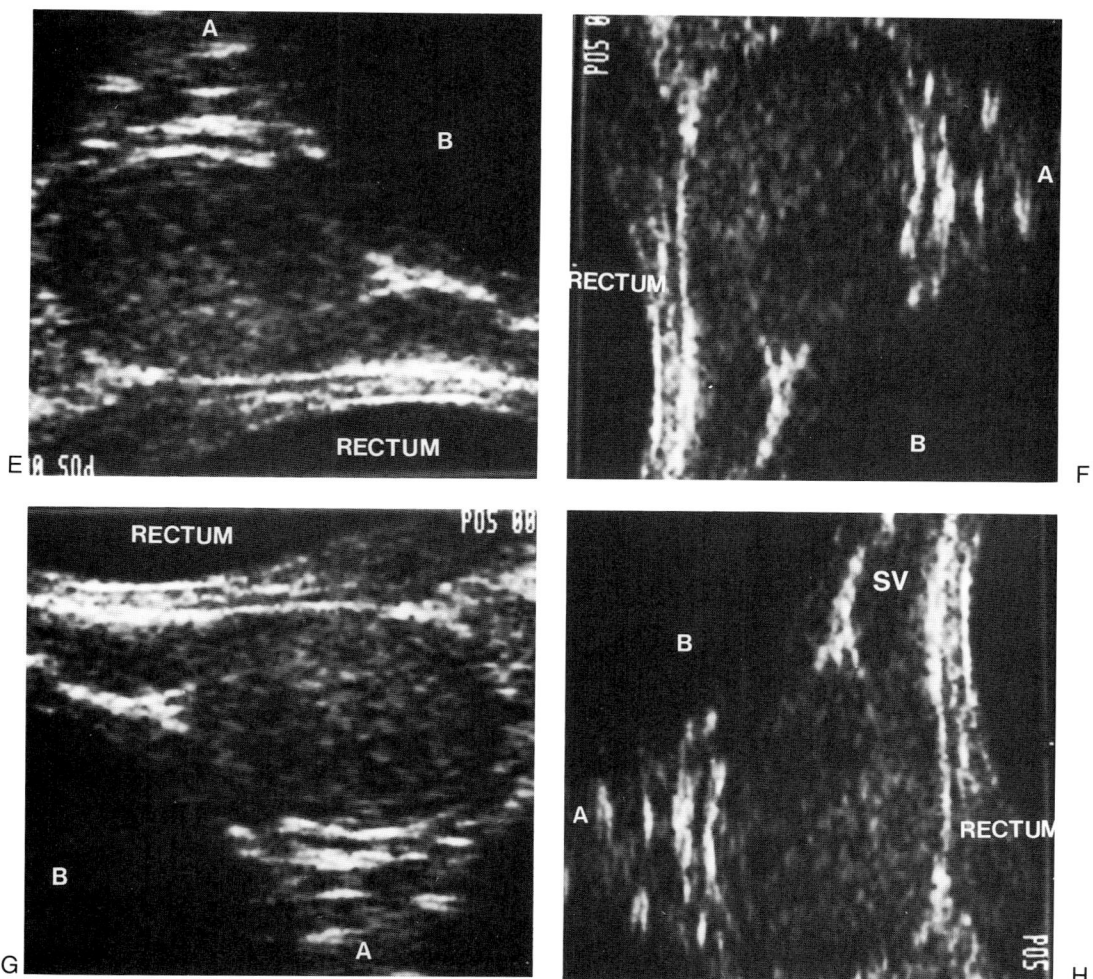

FIG. 5.10. Continued.

2. *Sagittal scanners* (Fig. 5.10A).
   a. The rectum (and posterior structures of the patient) will be at the bottom of the screen.
   b. The anterior structures of the patient will be at the top of the screen.
   c. The bladder (and cephalad structures of the patient) will be to the left side of the image.
   d. The apex (and caudad structures of the patient) will be to the right side of the image.

This orientation for the sagittal scanner is utilized for a number of reasons, including the following: (a) Simpler comparisons of the sagittal and axial orientations can be made; (b) AIUM nomenclature is preserved.

On the transaxial approach, the seminal vesicles and the prostate may be seen sequentially as the probe is withdrawn from the rectum (Fig. 5.11).

In the most cephalad views and in the most cephalad area of the examination, a portion of the seminal vesicles and the insertion of the vas deferens bilaterally, medially, and symmetrically may be discerned (Figs. 5.12 and 5.13). As the transducer is removed from the rectum slightly (i.e., more caudad), the seminal vesicles will be seen as paired structures (Fig. 5.14). They may be elongated, thin, thick, bow-tie-shaped, or dumbbell-shaped, or they may appear to frown (i.e., curve posteriorly). Of importance is the echogenicity, size, and shape, which should by symmetrical bilaterally. When a sector scanner with a pie-

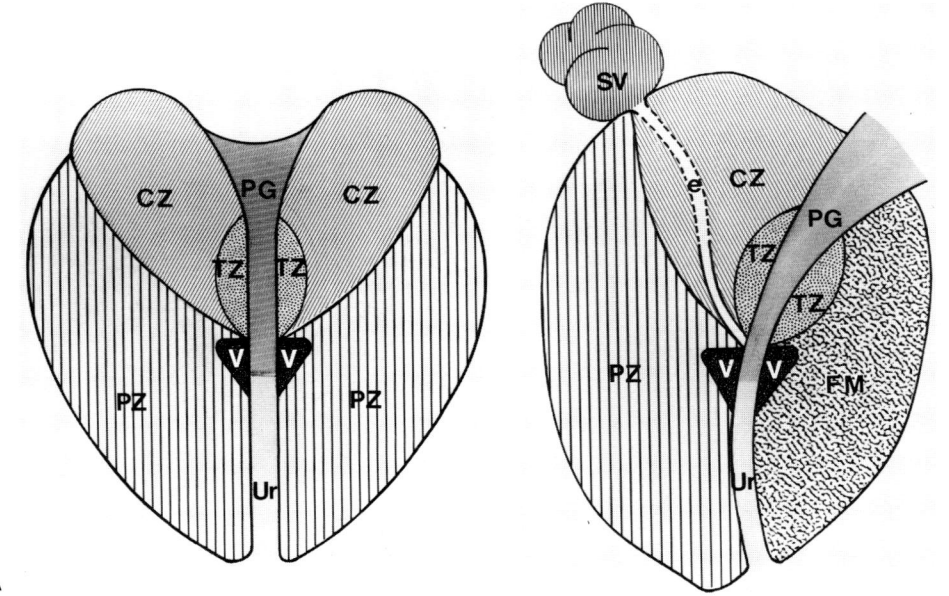

FIG. 5.11. Diagrams demonstrating histological orientation of anatomy. A curved coronal section, taken along the level of the prostatic urethra (**A**), along with a midline sagittally oriented line diagram (**B**), demonstrates the different histologic tissues. The periurethral glandular tissue (PG), the transition zone (TZ), the central zone (CZ), the peripheral zone (PZ), the verumontanum (V), the ejaculatory duct (e), the seminal vesicles (SV), the anterior fibromuscular stroma (FM), and the urethra (Ur) are seen.

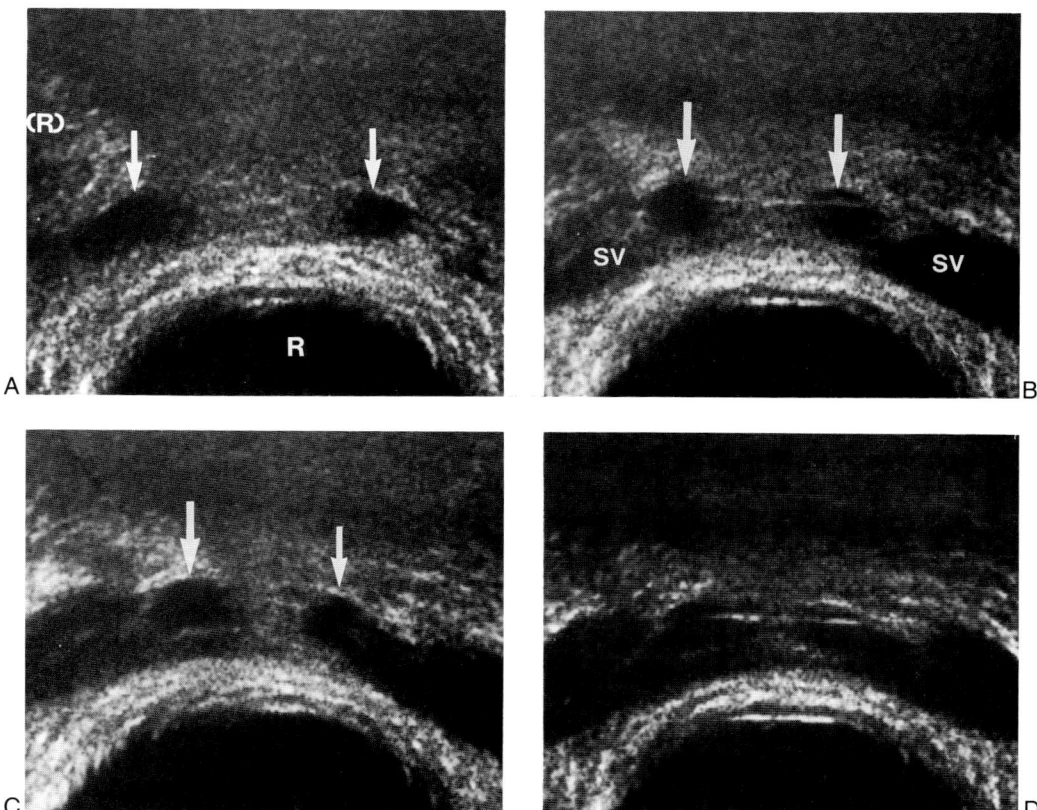

FIG. 5.12. Endorectal sonograms showing vas deferens and seminal vesicles. Axial orientation of the prostate using endorectal ultrasound approach demonstrates sequential scans from a level superior to the seminal vesicles (**A**) to the level of the seminal vesicles (**B**). The vas deferens (*arrows*) are identified as they join the seminal vesicles (SV). (R) Toward patient's right side; the R that is not inside parentheses represents the rectum.

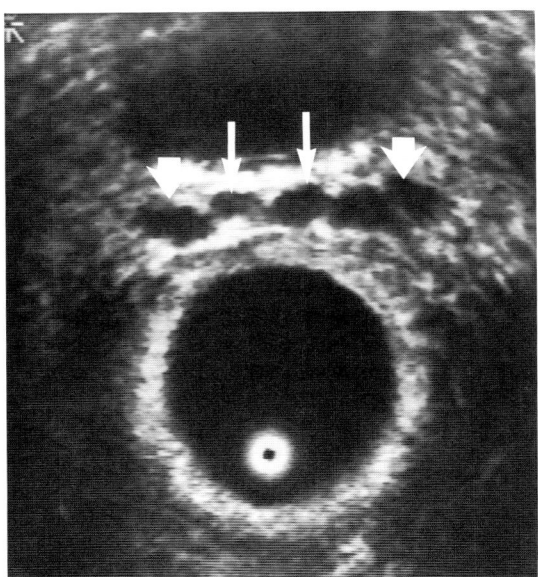

FIG. 5.13. Axial endorectal sonogram showing vas deferens and seminal vesicles. The vas deferens (*long arrows*) are seen as bilaterally paired structures joining the medial aspect of the seminal vesicles (*short arrows*).

shaped image is utilized to identify all of the seminal vesicles, images to the right and then (with probe rotation) to the left may be necessary (Fig. 5.15).

Occasionally, the vas deferens and the seminal vesicles will be seen with more tubular elements than solid components. This is normal, since the amount of fluid in the tubules of the seminal vesicles does vary over time.

If the transducer is angled slightly at this point, a section demonstrating the fluid-filled condom within the rectum, the seminal vesicles, a portion of the base of the prostate, and a portion of the fluid-filled urinary bladder may be identified (Fig. 5.16). On this section, it is difficult to differentiate echogenic characteristics of prostate and seminal vesicles because of the angulation of the transducer.

As the transducer is then moved slightly more cephalad, the prostate, at its base, may be defined as a semilunar-type structure. The normal indentation (i.e., the impression of the median sulcus of the prostate posteriorly) is not usually identified on the normal endorectal sonogram in the axial orientation. This is due to compression by the fluid-filled condom in the rectum upon the normal prostatic tissue. Thus, the normal anatomic landmark of the median sulcus is often lost. The normal prostate will appear to be slightly semilunar in shape in its more cephalad extent. It becomes more rounded towards the apex. The shape can also vary, depending upon the amount of distension of the condom. The glandular tissue of the prostate will appear to be slightly more echogenic than the normal seminal vesicles but will have homogeneous echogenicity.

In the anterior portion of the prostate at the base, situated in the midline, there will usually be a relatively well-defined, slightly hypoechoic structure (Fig. 5.17). This is not fluid-filled, but it has low-level echoes. This corresponds to the periurethral tissues (i.e., the transition zone and the periurethral glandular tissue) and the internal sphincter. The glandular tissues of the prostate (the peripheral and central zones) are more acoustically reflective (i.e., more echogenic) and, in the normal male, are not differentiable from one another. As

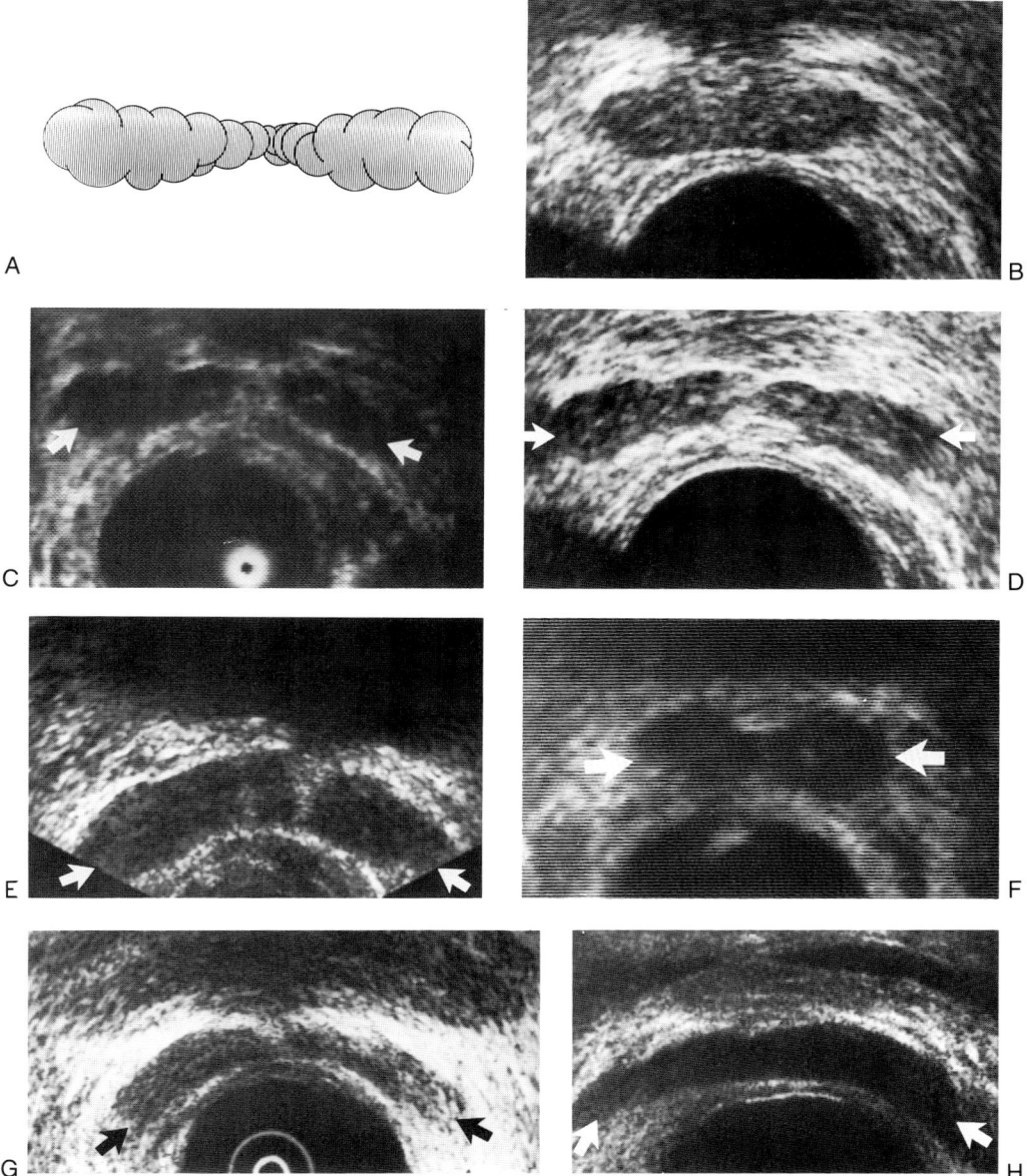

FIG. 5.14. Axial endorectal sonograms showing normal seminal vesicles. The seminal vesicles (arrows), identified in the axial orientation, may appear lobulated but bilaterally symmetrical as seen in the line diagram (**A**). The exact appearance of the seminal vesicles, however, is quite variable and can be bow-tie-shaped, thin, thick, rounded, more plump, or even dumbbell-shaped (**B–K**).

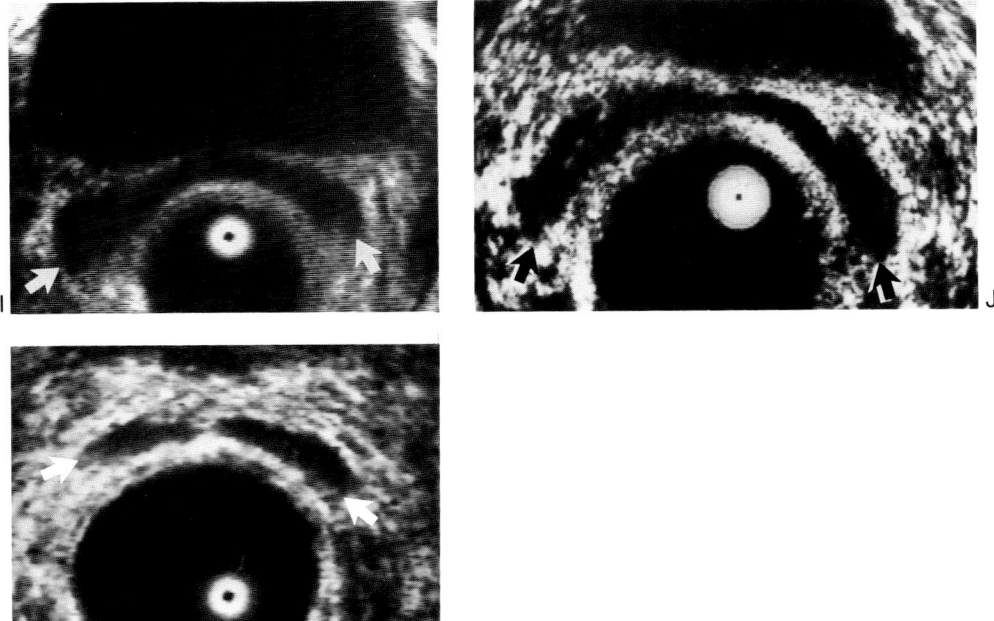

FIG. 5.14. *Continued.*

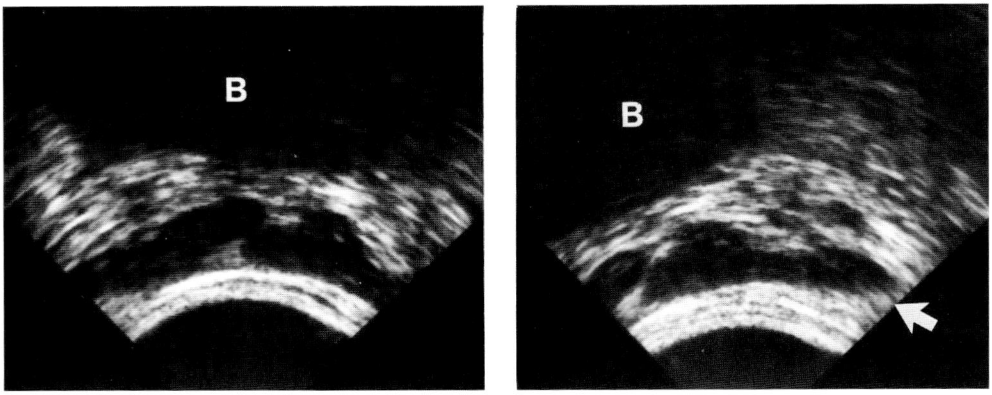

FIG. 5.15. Normal seminal vesicles seen on axial endorectal sonogram with sector scanner. A sector scanner may not identify the entire seminal vesicle in a single section (**A**). Thus, the probe may have to be rotated to the right and left (**B**) to identify the lateral margins (*arrow*). (B) Bladder.

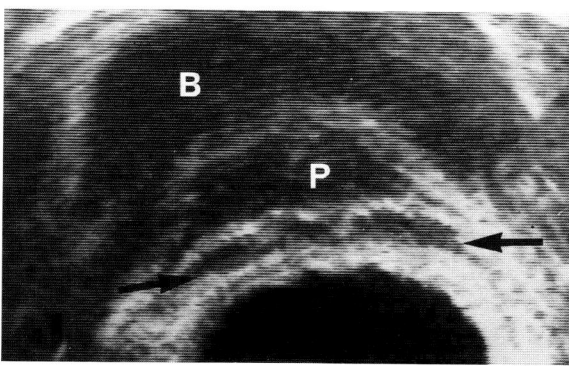

FIG. 5.16. Prostate, bladder, and seminal vesicles seen on axially oriented endorectal sonogram. The endorectal ultrasound approach is used with the transducer angled so that a portion of the fluid-filled urinary bladder (B), a small amount of the base of the prostate (P), and a small segment of both seminal vesicles (*arrows*) are identified. This image can only be obtained in the axial orientation with angulation of the tranducer.

the probe is withdrawn, sequential images (Fig. 5.18) to the level of the verumontanum will be identified (Fig. 5.19).

As the transducer is then removed slightly more caudad, the body of the prostate will be seen. The prostate will become echogenically more homogeneous. The overall echogenicity, however, is dependent upon overall gain settings. Here, special attention to quality technique is essential. At this level, the periurethral glandular tissue is much smaller. The anterior fibromuscular stroma may have sonographic characteristics similar to, or slightly more echogenic than, the periurethral tissues; that is, they may have a slight decrease in acoustic reflectivity as compared to the peripheral zone (Fig. 5.19).

As the probe is withdrawn further to beyond the level of the verumontanum, central tissues will not be present, but some anterior fibromuscular structures may be seen. In the normal individual, the central or peripheral zones of the glandular tissue are sonographically quite similar (Figs. 5.20 and 5.21).

As the prostate is then moved slightly more caudad, the apex of the gland, which will be smaller and more rounded in shape, will be discerned (Fig. 5.22).

The periprostatic tissues identified include the following:

1. The urinary bladder, which should be at least partially fluid-filled, is identified in the superior position. Subtle internal echoes may be defined if the overall gain settings are higher than necessary.

2. Laterally placed, the obturator internus muscles, which can be seen in all scans, will be identified. They are most pronounced in the lower section.

3. Additionally, towards the apex, the bilaterally paired levator ani muscles may be seen. Muscles, in general, are slightly hypoechoic in nature.

4. Anterior to the prostate, situated between the prostate and the symphysis pubis and pubic bones, is the anterior prostatic fat and fascia, which is usually defined as a mixed (but slightly less echogenic) area as compared to fat in general.

5. The prostatic capsule, which is not a true capsule, is usually seen surrounding the prostate as an echogenic band. This band is variable in thickness and is probably a com-

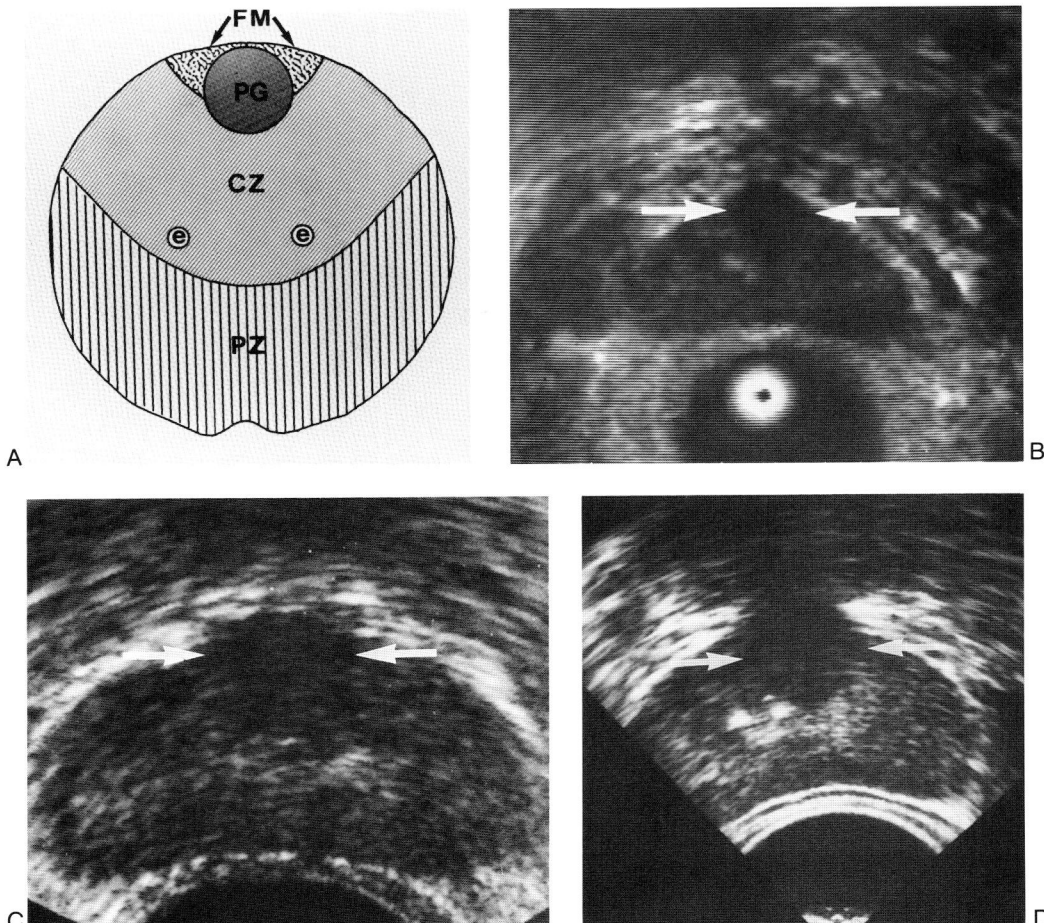

FIG. 5.17. Normal prostate at the level of the base of the gland—axial endorectal sonogram. The diagram of the base of the prostate (**A**) demonstrates the areas that would be identified. The anterior fibromuscular stroma (FM), the periurethral glandular tissue (PG), the central zone (CZ), the peripheral zone (PZ), and the two paired ejaculatory ducts (e) are identified. A radial image (**B**) demonstrates the relatively hypoechoic periurethral glandular tissue (*arrows*) and the internal sphincter in the anterior-superior aspect of the gland. The similar hypoechoic area is identified on a 110° axially oriented sector scan (**C**) and a 90° sector scan (**D**) image of the base of the prostate.

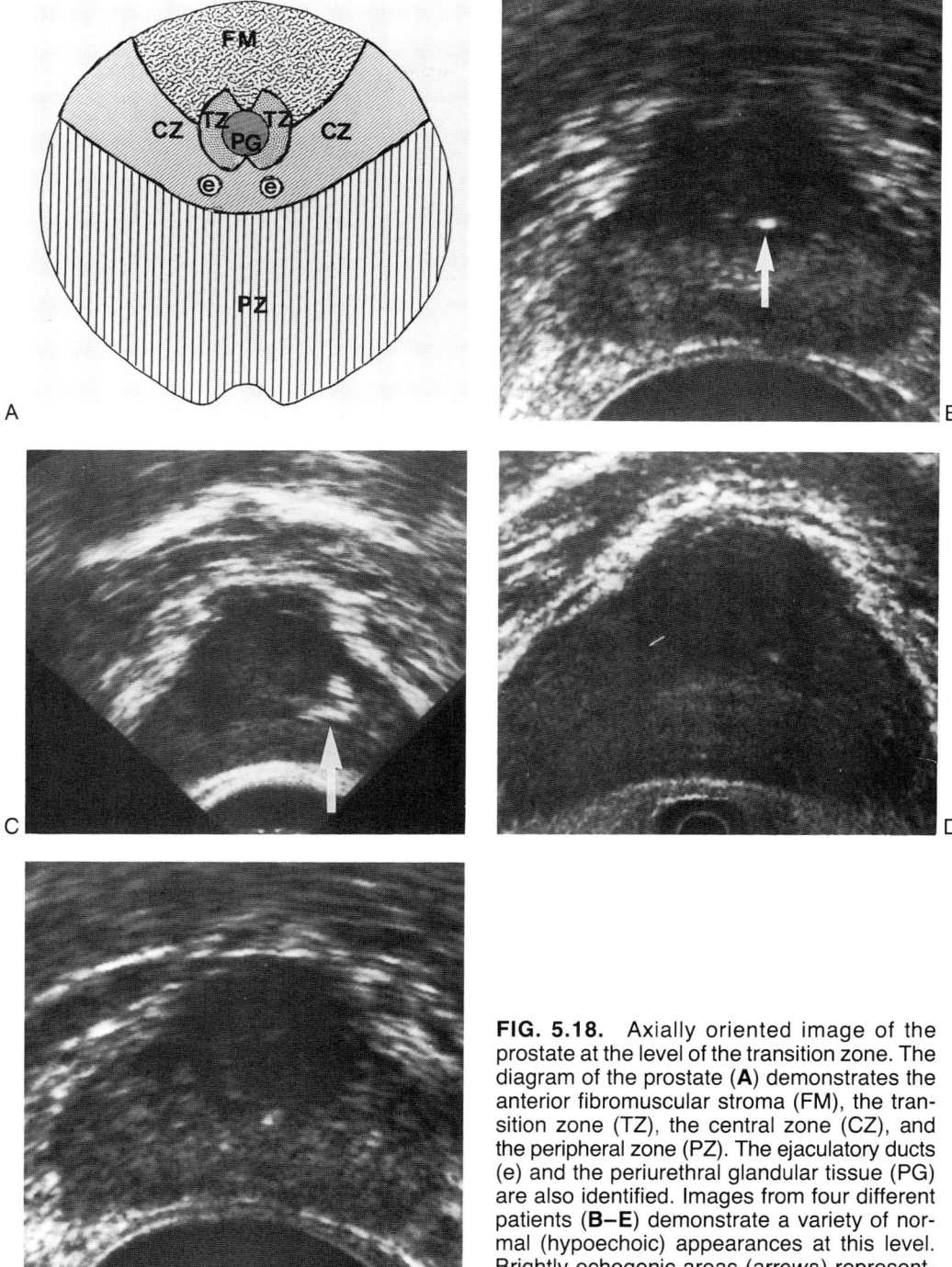

FIG. 5.18. Axially oriented image of the prostate at the level of the transition zone. The diagram of the prostate (**A**) demonstrates the anterior fibromuscular stroma (FM), the transition zone (TZ), the central zone (CZ), and the peripheral zone (PZ). The ejaculatory ducts (e) and the periurethral glandular tissue (PG) are also identified. Images from four different patients (**B–E**) demonstrate a variety of normal (hypoechoic) appearances at this level. Brightly echogenic areas (*arrows*) representing a calculi are also seen.

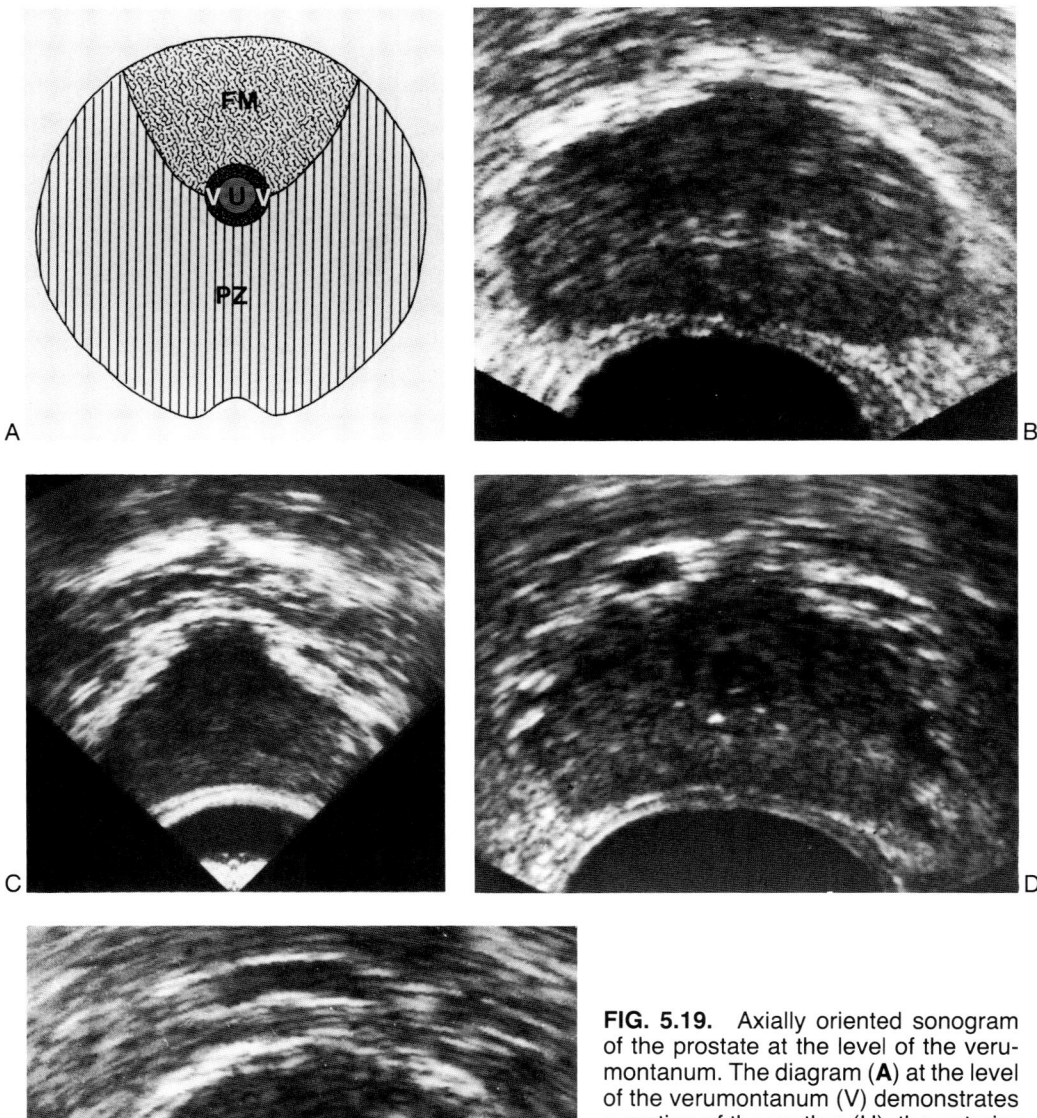

FIG. 5.19. Axially oriented sonogram of the prostate at the level of the verumontanum. The diagram (**A**) at the level of the verumontanum (V) demonstrates a portion of the urethra (U), the anterior fibromuscular stroma (FM), and the peripheral zone (PZ). Four different images (**B–E**) demonstrate a varied appearance in different normal individuals at this level. Note that the fibromuscular stroma, in general, is slightly less echogenic than the periurethral glandular tissue and the normal transition zone.

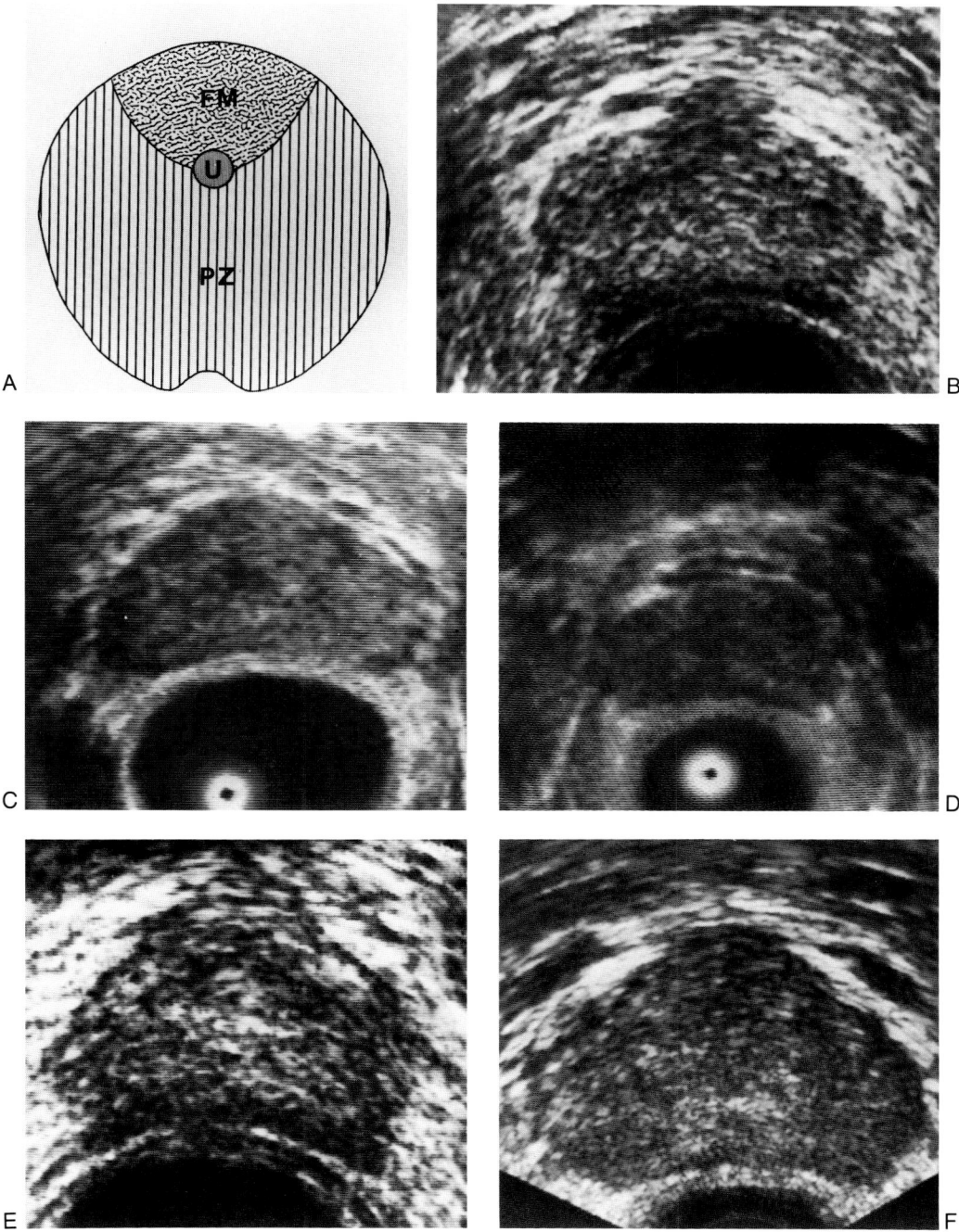

FIG. 5.20. Axially oriented image of the prostate just caudad to the verumontanum. A line diagram (**A**) at the level just inferior (caudad) to the verumontanum demonstrates the anterior fibromuscular stroma (FM), the prostatic urethra (U), and the peripheral zone (PZ). Images of five different normal males (**B–F**) demonstrate the varied appearance in these normal individuals ranging from a completely isoechoic (i.e., equally echogenic) fibromuscular area to a slightly hypoechoic zone.

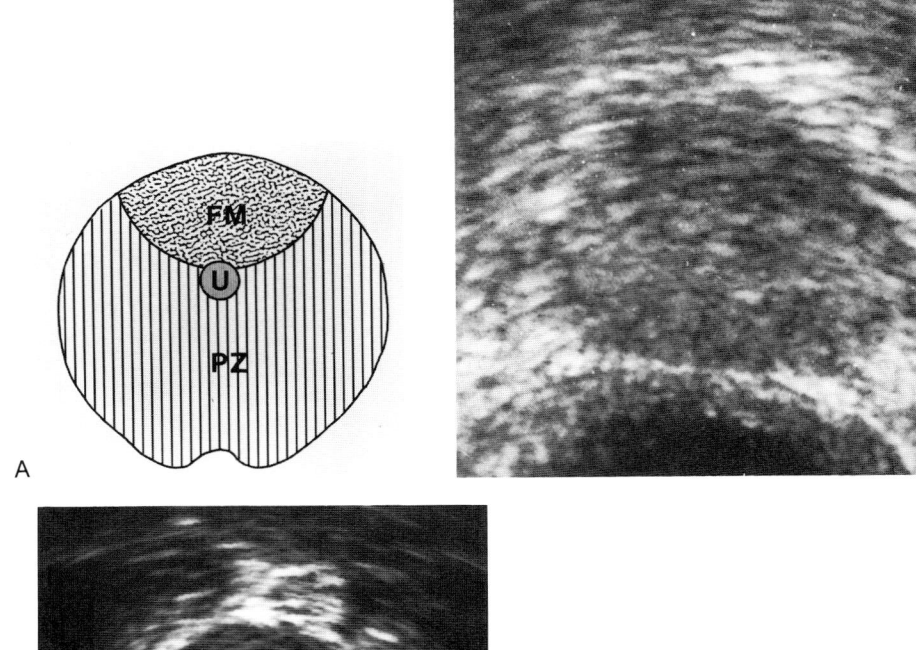

FIG. 5.21. Axially oriented image of the prostate superior to the apex. A line diagram (**A**) of the area just inferior to the level obtained in Fig. 5.20 shows the anterior fibromuscular zone (FM), the prostatic urethra (U), and the peripheral zone (PZ). The prostate in two normal patients (**B** and **C**) demonstrates relatively homogeneous echogenicity of the normal structures at this level.

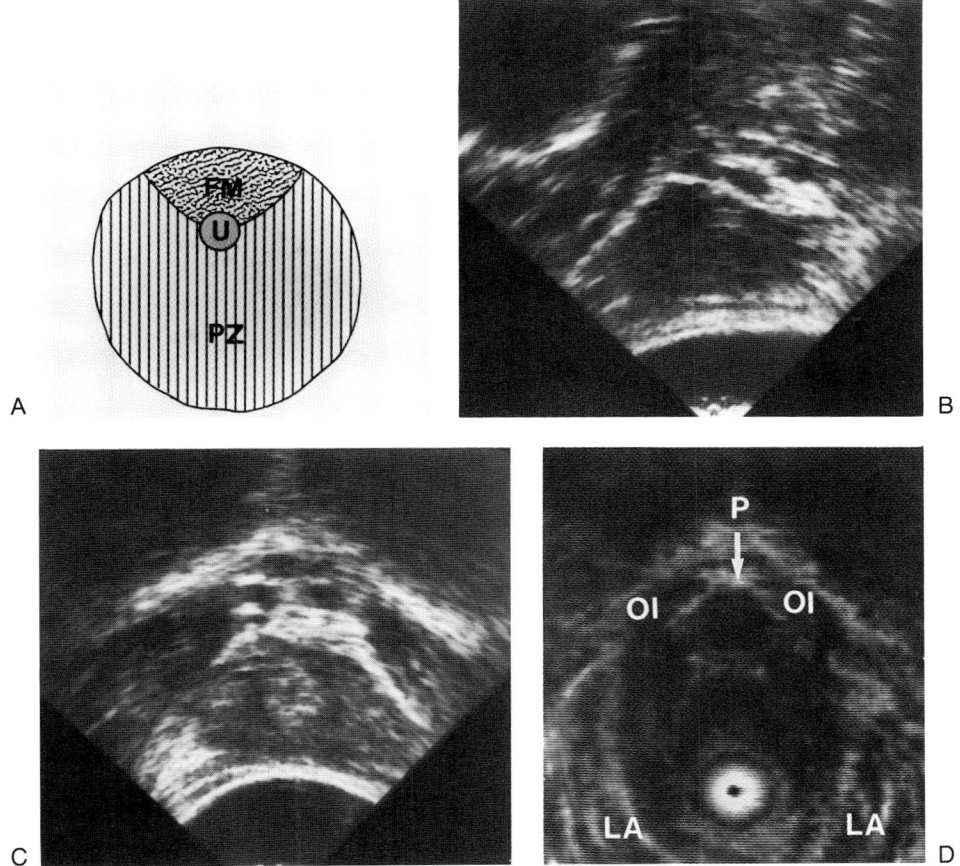

FIG. 5.22. Axially oriented image at the level of the apex. A line diagram (**A**) of the apex demonstrates the anterior fibromuscular stroma (FM) and the prostatic urethra (U); it also demonstrates the peripheral zone (PZ), which encompasses most of the prostate at this level. The prostate (P) at this level appears to be relatively homogeneous (**B** and **C**). The surrounding levator ani (LA) and obturator internus (OI) muscles may also be well-delineated at this level (**D**).

bination of periprostatic fat and the fascia of the capsule. As the gain settings are increased, it may appear thicker.

In the normal male, the sagitally oriented image is very different in appearance and is slightly more confusing (for the neophyte) than the axial orientation.

The prostate in the midline will be identified from cephalad to caudad extent. At the base, or cephalad extent of the prostate, the slightly hypoechoic periurethral tissues and internal sphincter may be identified (Fig. 5.23). Additionally, the proximal urethra may be seen as a small nipple or indentation upon the periurethral tissue (Fig. 5.24). The anterior fibromuscular stroma will be seen adjacent to the periurethral tissues, frequently with no difference in echogenicity. The central and the peripheral zones of the prostatic glandular tissue will be defined on this midline image as inseparable from each other. Homogeneous echogenicity will be noted, and no differentiation of these acinar tissues will be possible. Portions of the prostatic urethra, when empty, may be defined as relatively parallel lines extending from the base of the prostate, with either the bladder neck or the periurethral tissues extending toward the apex of the gland in the midline. These are acoustic reflections of the empty apposed wall of the urethra.

The seminal vesicles in the midline images will be seen as small, semirounded structures that are slightly less echogenic than the prostate. In the midline, they are usually smaller than in the lateral aspects and more closely situated to the superior-posterior aspect of the prostate. There is variable appearance to the seminal vesicles. They may be large or small, but bilateral symmetry should be present. They may be situated immediately adjacent to the prostate, or occasionally they may appear (particularly in the lateral aspects) to be slightly separated.

Toward the midline (but slightly lateral), bilaterally, each of the vas deferens may be identified where they join into the medial aspect of the seminal vesicle as two parallel, relatively hypoechoic structures (Fig. 5.25).

The ejaculatory ducts, when empty, may be seen as slightly hyperechoic lines coursing from the seminal vesicles into the urethra, joining at the area of the verumontanum (Fig. 5.26). This acoustic reflectivity is a reflection off the empty walls of the tubular structures. Since these structures do not course in a true sagittal orientation, they are usually seen segmentally.

As the transducer is rotated slightly clockwise or counterclockwise, the hypoechoic periurethral glandular tissues and the relatively hypoechoic anterior fibromuscular tissue are lost. The acinar tissue of the peripheral and central zones are inseparable and have indifferentiable homogeneous echogenicity. The seminal vesicles, situated superior and posterior to the prostate, are often larger laterally than their medial portions (Figs. 5.27 and 5.28).

The relationship between the prostate and the seminal vesicles is best ascertained on the longitudinal scan. The seminal vesicles may be rounded or elongated within the male population and may also be adjacent to, or separated from, the prostate. Great difference in these parameters exist (Figs. 5.29–5.33). Right and left symmetry should be present to determine subtle changes. An evaluation of the space between the prostate and the seminal vesicles is essential. The fat anteriorly located between these structures has been termed the *prostatic–seminal-vesicle angle*. The angle is variable and can normally be acute, obtuse, or at right angles (Fig. 5.34). Regardless of the angle in a single individual, it should be the same bilaterally. A slightly echogenic space posteriorly between the seminal vesicle and

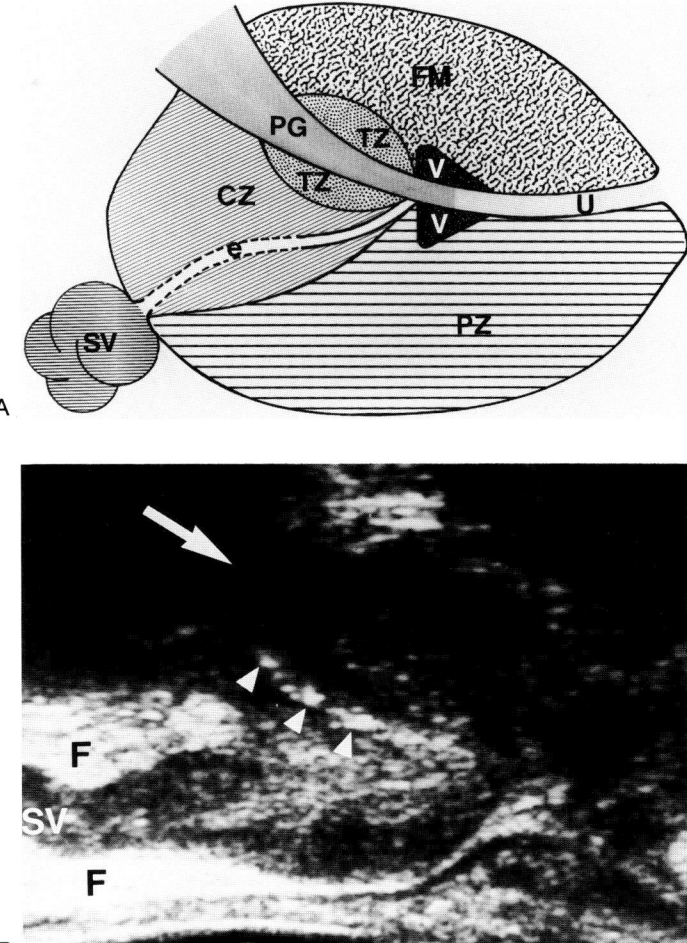

FIG. 5.23. Sagittally oriented endorectal sonogram in the midline. The line diagram of the prostate (**A**) demonstrates a cross section of the seminal vesicles (SV), a segment of the ejaculatory duct (e), the central zone (CZ), the transition zone (TZ), and the peripheral zone (PZ). The verumontanum (V), the periurethral glandular tissue (PG), the inferior aspect of the prostatic urethra (U), and the anterior fibromuscular stroma (FM) are identified. A longitudinally oriented endorectal sonogram utilizing a linear-array machine (**B**) identifies the prostate in a similar area. The brightly echogenic fat (F) surrounding the seminal vesicles (SV) is identified. Additionally, the hypoechoic area of the periurethral tissues (*arrow*) and internal sphincter is seen; subtle echogenic areas (*arrowheads*) lining the prostatic urethra (corpora amylacea) are also seen. There is no sonographic difference between the peripheral and central zones.

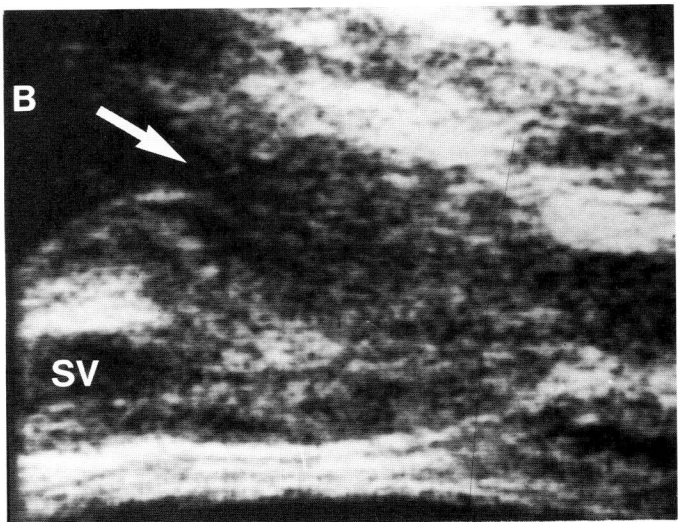

FIG. 5.24. Proximal urethra seen in the longitudinally oriented endorectal sonogram. This sonogram demonstrates indentation of fluid from the urinary bladder (B) into the proximal, nondilated urethra (*arrow*). The peripheral and central zones are not differentiable. The seminal vesicles (SV) are clearly seen.

the prostate has been referred to as the *nipple* (162). It should also be symmetrical bilaterally; however, it is not always seen, even in the normal individual. When present, the echogenic characteristics are probably due to the presence of fat.

The prostatic capsule will also be defined as a relatively hyperechoic area with some thickness, which is usually attributed to a combination of capsule and periprostatic fat. The symphysis pubis may be seen as an echogenic area as a result of shadowing from the bone, which will obscure all other sonographic information. Occasionally, when TGC curves are set inappropriately, the bright echogenic reflectors from the symphysis may not be seen; shadowing, however, will still be discerned.

The anterior prostatic fat and fascia will be seen between the echogenic symphysis pubis; the echogenic anterior aspect of the prostatic capsule will be seen as a mixed echogenic structure, consisting of a combination of fat, fascia, lymphatics, nerves, and vessels.

A fluid or partially fluid-filled prostatic urethra may be seen and will be discussed in more detail in Chapter 15.

The urogenital diaphragm may be seen on the longitudinal probe, just inferior to the apex of the gland. The urogenital diaphragm will be seen as a slightly low-level, but mixed, echogenic structure—a combination of its muscular and fibrous components.

NORMAL SONOGRAPHIC ANATOMY

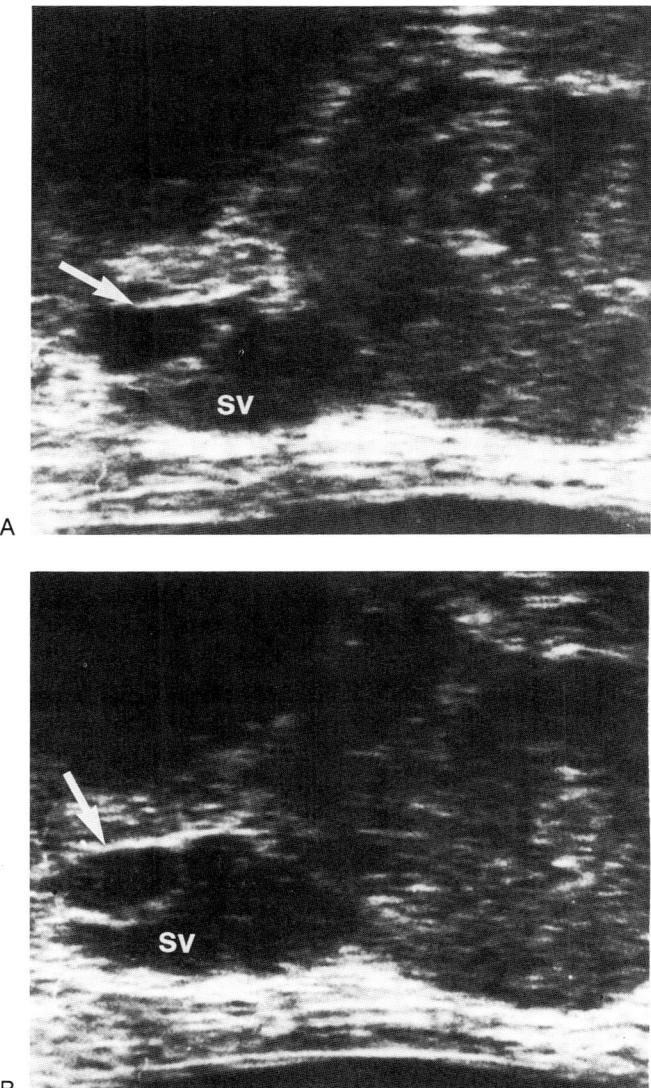

FIG. 5.25. Visualization of the seminal vesicle and vas deferens in the longitudinal orientation. Four images of the prostate in longitudinal orientation with varying degrees of angulation (**A–D**) demonstrate the orientation of the seminal vesicle (SV) and vas deferens (*arrows*) to the prostate (P).

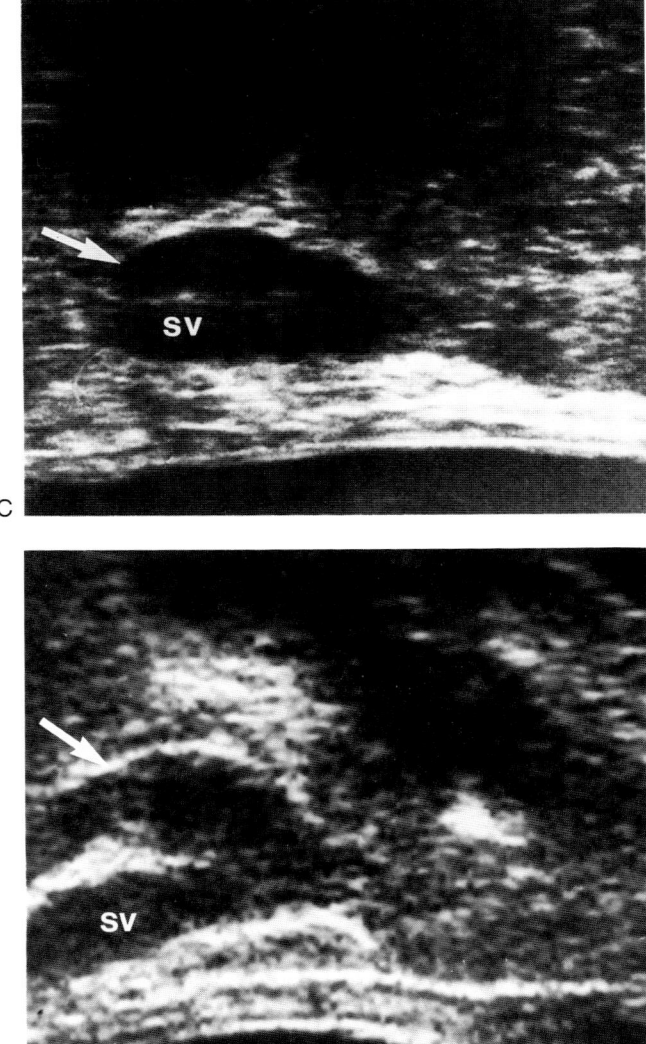

FIG. 5.25. Continued.

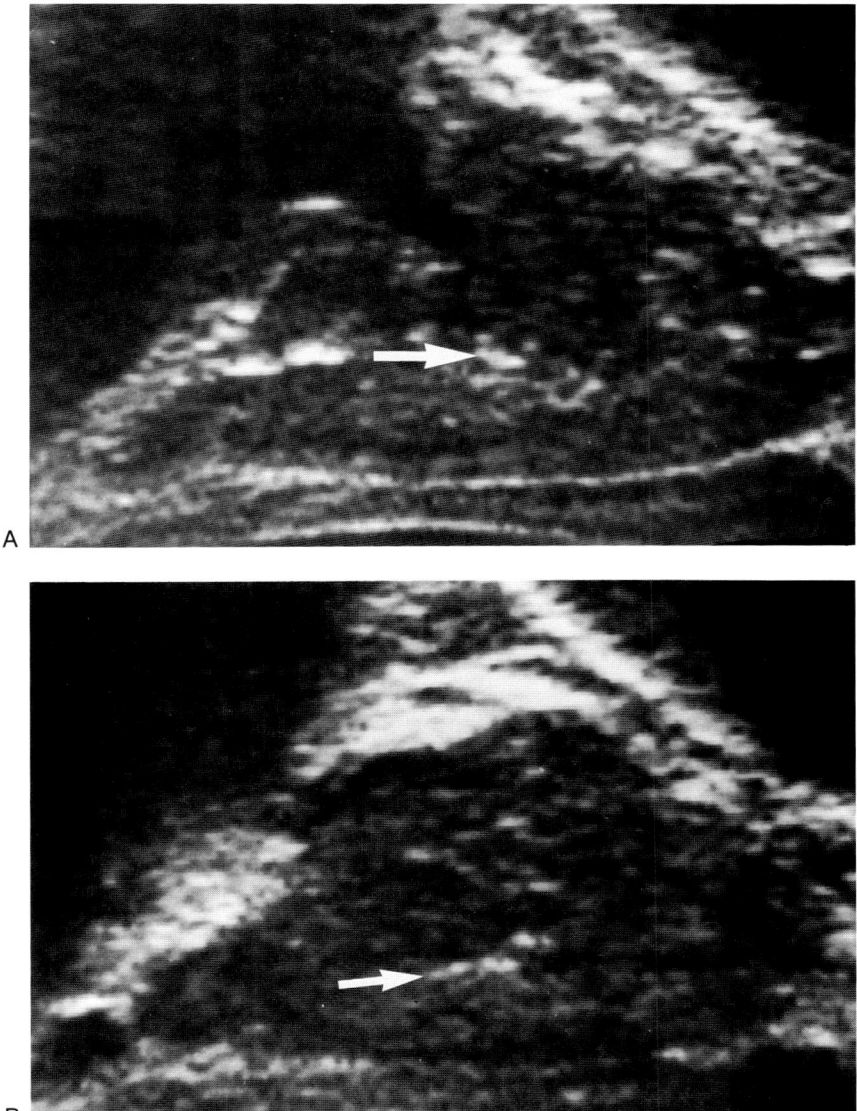

FIG. 5.26. Sagittal endorectal image of the ejaculatory ducts. The longitudinally oriented sonogram may demonstrate very subtle findings with regard to the ejaculatory duct (*arrows*). These may appear as subtle echogenic lines (**A**) or a more linear acoustic reflector (**B**) as the ejaculatory duct courses from the seminal vesicle to the verumontanum.

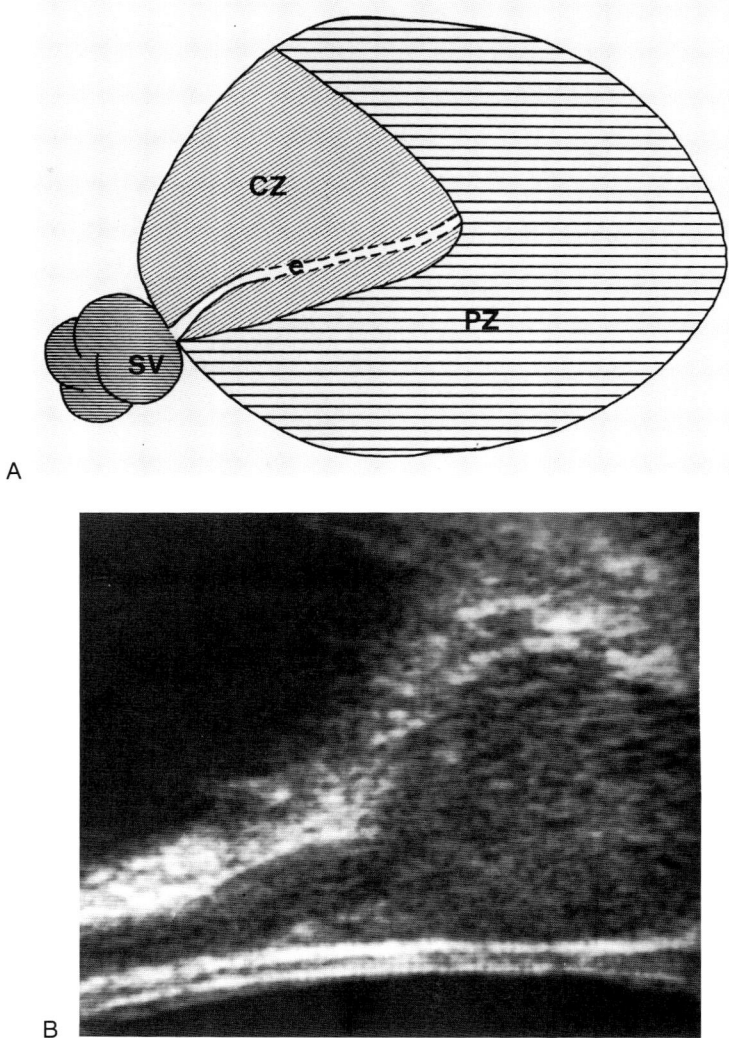

FIG. 5.27. Laterally placed longitudinally oriented sonogram of the prostate. The longitudinally oriented diagram of the prostate (**A**) demonstrates the seminal vesicle (SV), the peripheral zone (PZ), the central zone (CZ), and a portion of the ejaculatory duct (e). The endorectal ultrasound (**B**) demonstrates no differentiation between the central and peripheral zones.

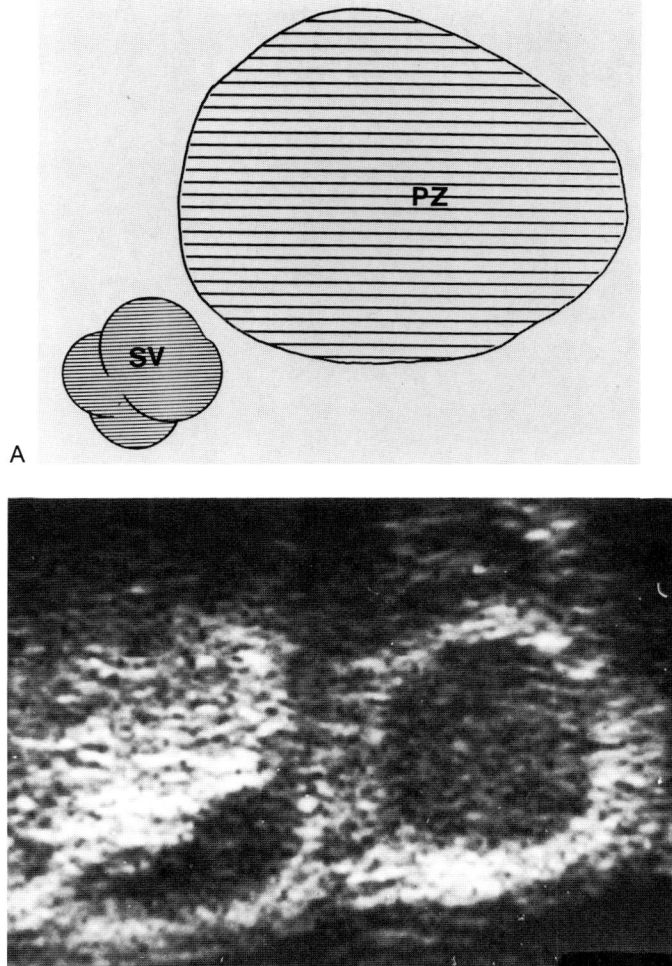

FIG. 5.28. Longitudinally oriented image of the prostate—far lateral aspect. The diagram of the obliquely oriented ultrasound image (**A**) demonstrates a cross section of the seminal vesicle (SV) and the peripheral zone (PZ) of the prostate. A corresponding endorectal sonogram with a linear array transducer (**B**) demonstrates a normal ultrasound image.

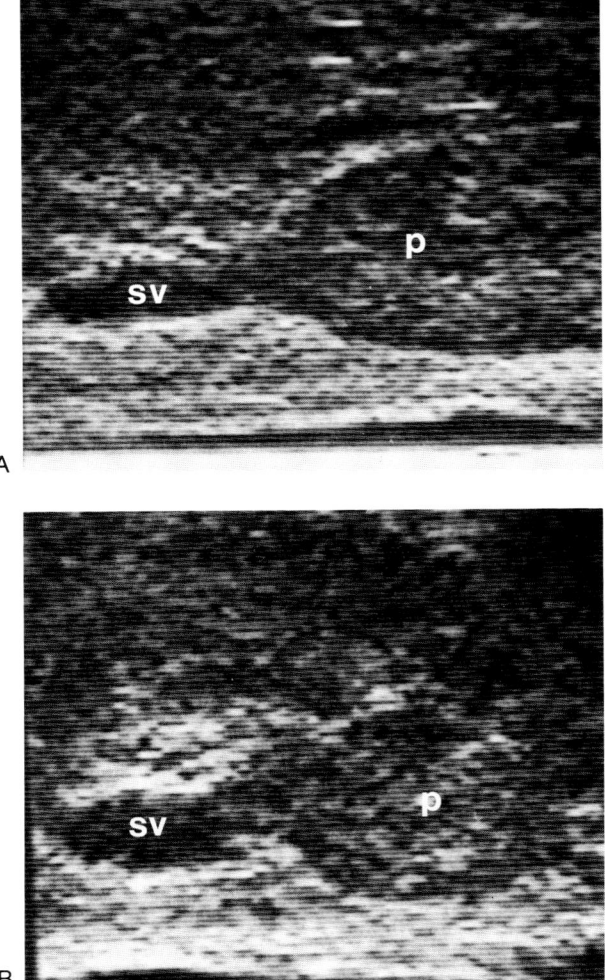

FIG. 5.29. Seminal vesicle prostatic relationship—longitudinal orientation. Sequential images of the prostate, close to midline (**A**), with slight (**B**) and with marked (**C**) rotation of the probe to the lateral portions of the prostate, demonstrate the seminal vesicle (SV) as it separates from the prostate (P). This may be a normal finding.

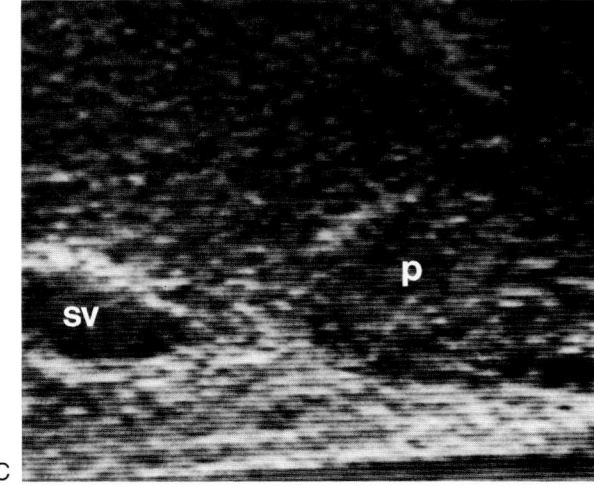

FIG. 5.29. Continued.

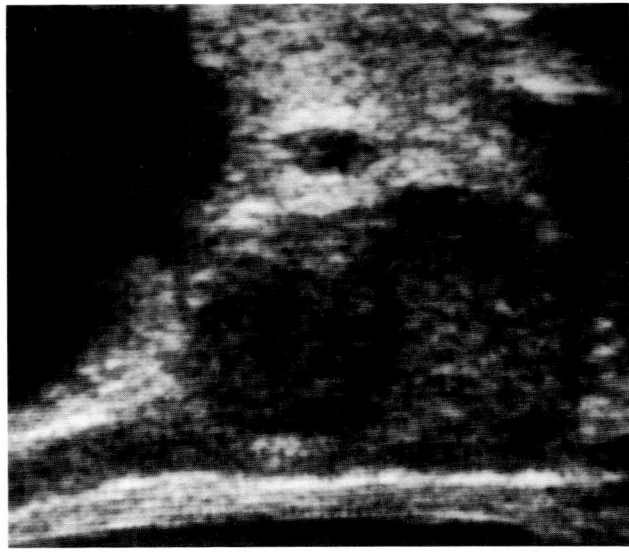

FIG. 5.30. Longitudinally oriented ultrasound—relationship between the prostate and the seminal vesicle. Sequential images of the prostate and seminal vesicle from near midline (**A**), along with progressive visualization of the lateral aspects of the prostate (**B** and **C**), demonstrate a different type of normal relationship between the prostate and the seminal vesicle; in this man, the seminal vesicle appears to elongate.

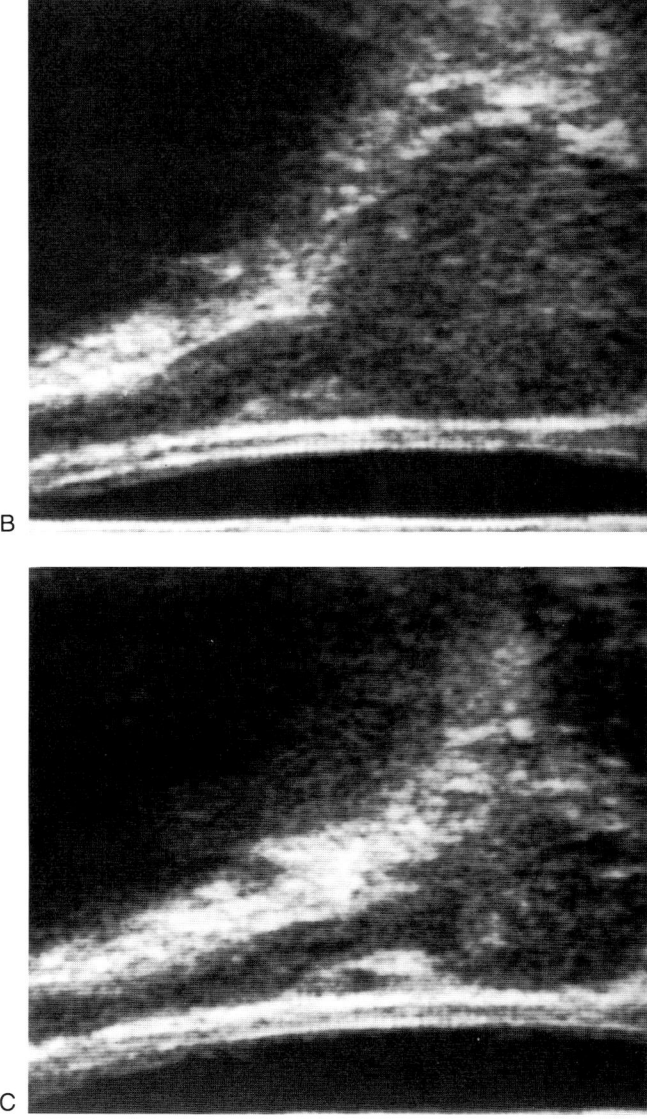

FIG. 5.30. Continued.

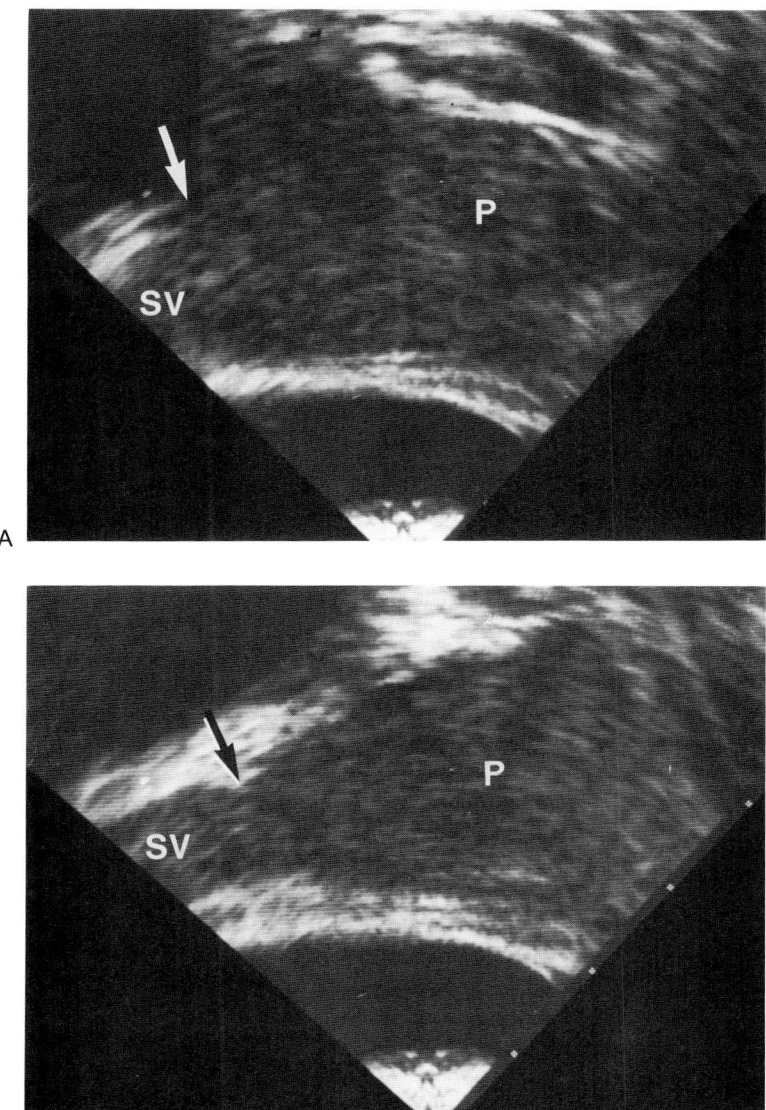

FIG. 5.31. Normal prostate–seminal-vesicle "angle". A longitudinal image in the midline (**A**) demonstrates a relatively acute angle (*arrow*) between the seminal vesicle (SV) and the medial aspect of the base of prostate (P). In the lateral aspect of the prostate (**B**), the angle has become more obtuse.

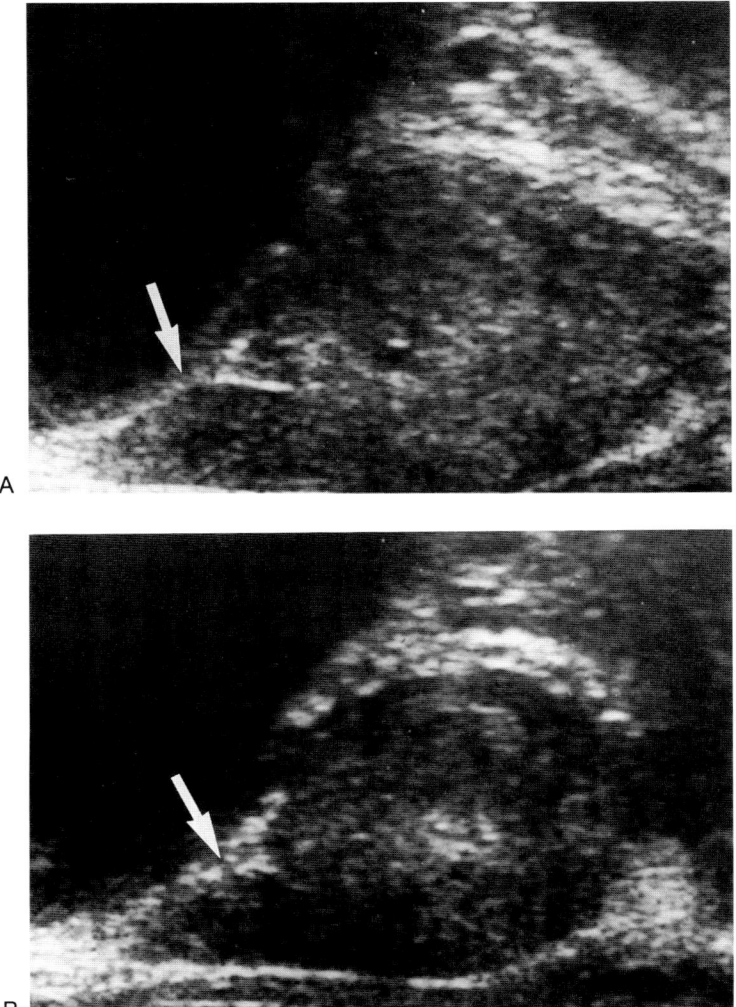

FIG. 5.32. Normal seminal-vesicle–prostate "angle" (*arrow*). Longitudinally oriented images of the prostate from the midline (**A**) and progressively lateral (**B–D**) demonstrate the relationship between the normal seminal vesicle and the prostate.

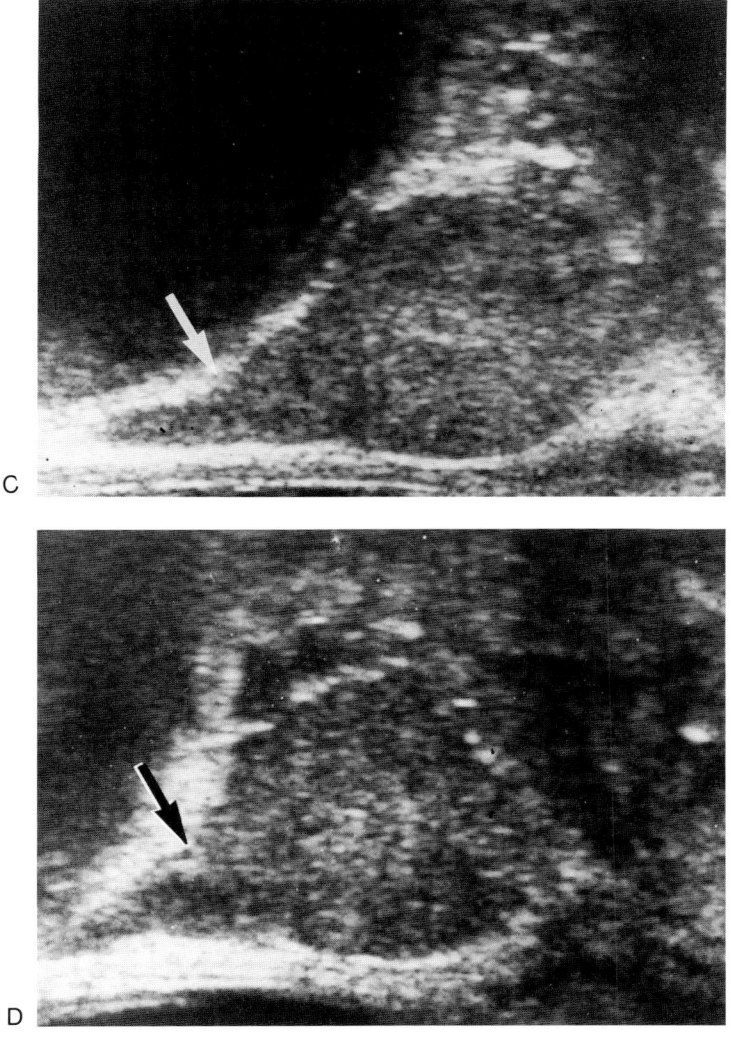

FIG. 5.32. Continued.

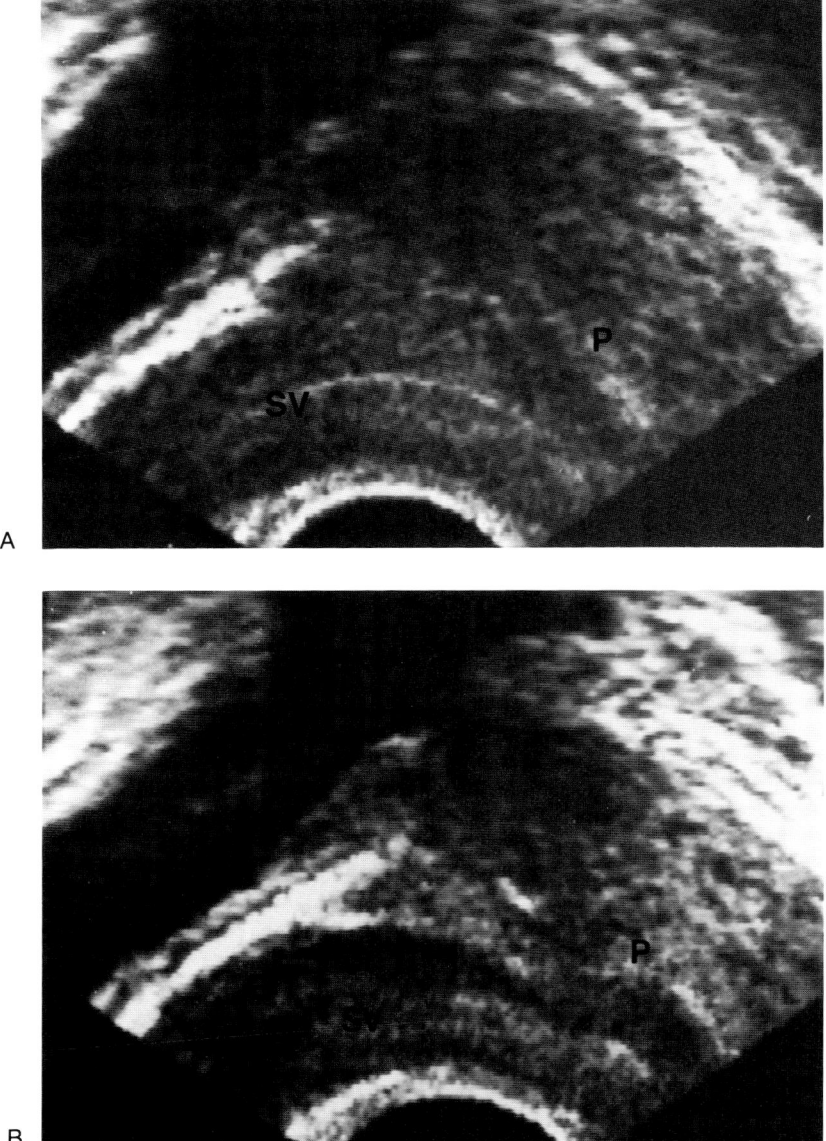

FIG. 5.33. A normal seminal-vesicle–prostate relationship. A longitudinally oriented sector scan of the prostate from the midline (**A**) with progressive lateralization (**B–D**) of the prostate demonstrates one of many normal seminal-vesicle (SV)–prostate (P) relationships.

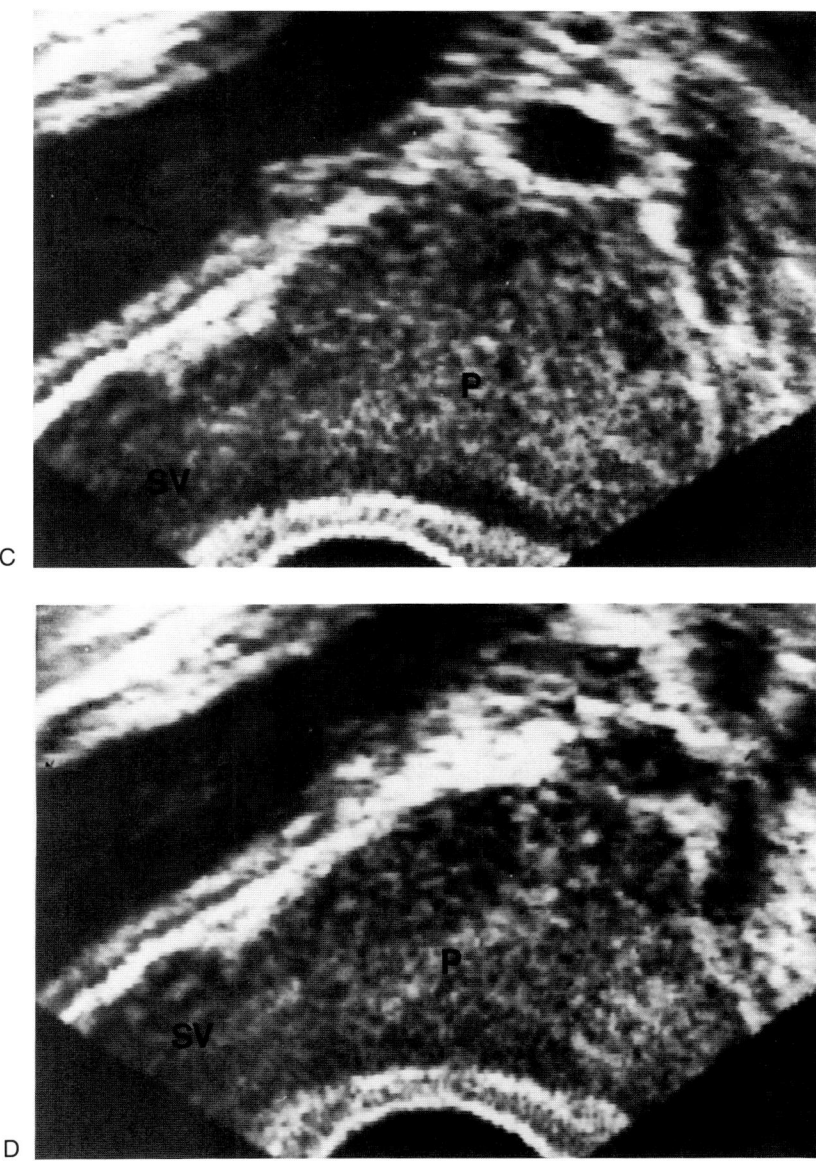

FIG. 5.33. *Continued.*

COMPARISON OF AXIAL AND SAGITTAL ENDORECTAL ULTRASOUND IMAGES

As shown previously, the prostate and its surrounding structures appear very different on the longitudinally and axially oriented endorectal sonograms. Although many prostatic abnormalities will have similar sonographic chracteristics on both orientations, their appearance

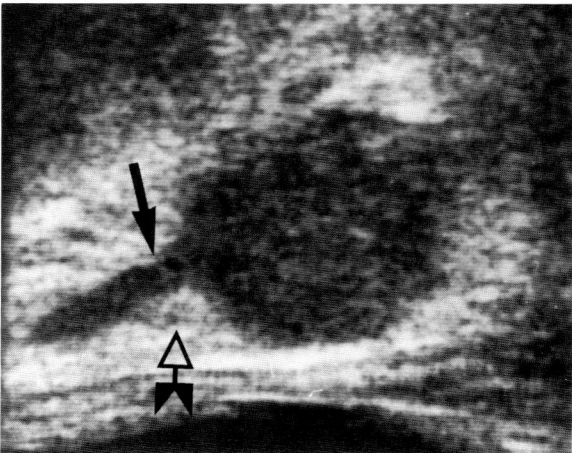

FIG. 5.34. Prostate–seminal-vesicle "angle" (*closed arrow*) and "nipple" (*open arrow*).

may be quite different. Thus, an evaluation of the differences in the axial and the sagittal images is necessary to understand the importance of both orientations.

The axial orientation obtained with either a radial or pie-shaped or linear array sector scanner yields a true transversely oriented image. This characterizes the anatomic shape and configuration of the gland quite clearly and is similar in appearance to that seen on computed tomography and magnetic resonance imaging. The presence of either a symmetrical architectural pattern or asymmetrical findings in the prostate is clearly defined. Right versus left comparisons are easy to ascertain.

The longitudinally oriented scan appears to be slightly more difficult for an initial evaluation. Although asymmetrical involvement of the prostate can be ascertained, it requires close comparison of an image of the right and left sides. Technical expertise during the scanning process is essential.

In general, the following are comparative characteristics of the two orientations (also see Table 5.1) (401):

1. Symmetrical versus asymmetrical internal architecture of the prostate is usually better and more easily defined with the axial orientation.

2. The lateral margins of the prostate are more clearly delineated on the axial orientation.

3. The apex and the base of the prostate are usually better defined on the longitudinal orientation.

4. Impingement upon the bladder base by prostatic disease (i.e., hyperplastic nodules) is better seen on the longitudinal orientation.

5. The prostatic urethra (and its course) and ejaculatory ducts are more clearly defined on the sagittal orientation because of the ability to image these tubular structures parallel to their long axis.

6. Lateral bulges of the capsule are better defined by the axial orientation.

7. Ultrasound guided biopsies, either transperineal or transrectally performed, are more accurately performed with the sagittally oriented scanner for guidance. With this technique, the entire needle and area of tissue extraction is defined. In the axial approach, only the needle tip during initial insertion into the area of abnormality is delineated. The exact tissue biopsied is incompletely identified (see Chapter 8).

TABLE 5.1. Comparison of the axial and sagittal image

Feature	Which identifies feature best
Asymmetry	Axial orientation
Base	Sagittal orientation
Apex	Sagittal orientation
Anterior margin	Equal
Posterior margin	Equal
Right side	Axial orientation
Left side	Axial orientation
Tumor	Equal
Capsule bulge	
Apex, base	Sagittal orientation
Lateral margin	Axial orientation
Anterior, posterior margin	Equal
Calculi	Equal except for radial scanner
Cyst	Equal except for radial scanner
Biopsies	Sagittal orientation
Urethra	Sagittal orientation
Ejaculatory duct	Sagittal orientation
Seminal vesicle involvement by tumor	Sagittal orientation

8. The anterior and posterior margins of the prostate are equally well-defined on both orientations.

9. Gross symmetry of the seminal vesicles is better defined on the axial scanner, but subtle changes may be more clearly seen by the longitudinal scan.

There are other issues that should also be addressed with regard to the strengths and weaknesses of each scan plane. Not all of these relate to orientation per se, but instead they relate to the type of scanner. If either a linear array scanner or a sector scanner is used, prostatic cysts and prostatic calculi are generally equally well-defined on both orientations. The internal sonographic characteristics of cysts (i.e., sharp back walls, good through-transmission, and no internal echoes) will be seen. Calculi, despite their size, either large or small, will be brightly echogenic and will cause some acoustic shadowing. Some manipulation of the gain settings may be necessary to demonstrate shadowing (i.e., from smaller calculi).

With the radial (rotating) probe, cysts and calculi and their secondary characteristics may not be as clearly defined on the axial image. This is probably due to the technical deficiencies with the slow rotation of the transducer crystal. Perhaps reflection of the sound beam off the latex cover, the rectal wall, or other intervening structures, coupled with a slow scan speed, may result in poor definition of the secondary sonographic characteristics (i.e., acoustic enhancement or sonographic shadowing) that are seen with these types of lesions.

The ability to define internal differences, prostatic lesions, or homogeneous echogenicity is usually a property of the transducer, not the orientation. Transducers that have good resolution, small pixel size, and sharply focused near-fields are generally equivalent. Increased frequency is not always "better" or more diagnostic. However, the earlier 3.5-MHz transducers are usually less accurate and less diagnostic than the newly developed, highly sophisticated 5-, 6-, 7-, and 8-MHz units. This is not always due to frequency alone, but to other physical characteristics of the machinery as well.

In general, a complete prostatic examination should include both an axial and a sagittal orientation. Although an adequate study can usually result from the use of a single orientation, the more subtle areas may not be clearly discerned. Both images should be used in examining the prostate.

6 // Prostate and Seminal Vesicle Size Determination

Techniques of Size Determination	93
Ultrasonic Measurements	
Planimetric Calculation	
Evaluation of Seminal Vesicle Size	98

Accurate estimation of the size and weight of the prostate is necessary so that the clinician and surgeon can plan proper medical intervention for patients who require treatment and surgery for symptomatology secondary to prostatic enlargement. The surgical approach may vary, depending upon the prostatic size. Although surgeons approach their patients according to individual therapeutic requirements, smaller glands (usually less than 50–60 g in weight) can, in general, be adequately and effectively resected using the transurethral approach (310). The larger gland, however, is often incompletely or inadequately resected by this method. In these cases, an open prostatectomy, accomplished by a retropubic or suprapubic approach, may be optimal. These surgical approaches are distinctly different from a radical prostatectomy used for definitive treatment for some prostatic cancers. These open procedures, which are technically more difficult to perform with small glands, frequently result in inadequate resection. When used inappropriately, complications and morbidity may occur.

TECHNIQUES OF SIZE DETERMINATION

The determination of prostate size can be performed by using a number of techniques:

1. Clinically, the digital rectal examination with palpation of the gland is inaccurate when estimating only prostatic size in symmetrically enlarged glands. Even in these cases, and particularly with an asymmetrically enlarged prostate, there can be a large degree of error (467).
2. Radiographic technique using cystography or intravenous pyelography to evaluate prostatic size by determining the amount of compression upon the bladder base is also inaccurate (40). Further inaccuracies in size assessment are compounded in glands that enlarge in an asymmetric fashion.
3. Ultrasound of the prostate has proven to be quite beneficial in estimating the dimensions, and thus the weight, of the gland. The suprapubic approach is the simplest method, although equally accurate measurements are obtained by the other (particularly the endorectal) techniques.

Ultrasonic Measurements

To assess accurate size of the gland, accurate measurement must be identified in all three dimensions; that is, the anterior-posterior, transverse, and cephalocaudad measurements must be obtained (Fig. 6.1 and 6.2).

Various formulas have been used to assess prostatic size and weight; all of them are relatively accurate. The weight of the prostate (in grams) is essentially equivalent to the size of the prostate (in cubic centimeters) because the specific gravity of a prostate is between 1.0 and 1.05.

The simplest method for assessing the prostatic size is by assuming the gland to be spheroid in shape. By imaging the radii of all three dimensions, the formula for a sphere can be used; that is, the weight $= \frac{4}{3}\pi r^3$.

If the prostate is irregularly shaped, all three radii—namely, that of the transverse (r_1), the cephalo-caudad (r_2), and the anterior-posterior (r_3) dimensions—are calculated separately. Accurate weight assessment, if the gland is asymmetrically enlarged, will be calculated by the formula

$$\text{Weight} = \frac{4}{3}\pi r_1 \times r_2 \times r_3$$

If symmetric enlargement is present and all three radii are equivalent, then the simpler formula

$$\text{Weight} = \frac{4}{3}\pi r^3$$

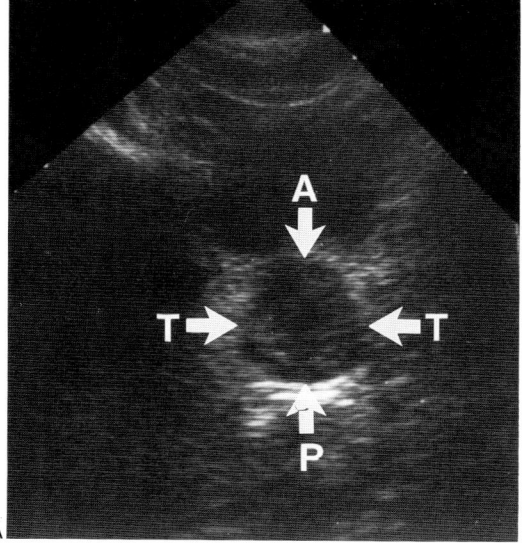
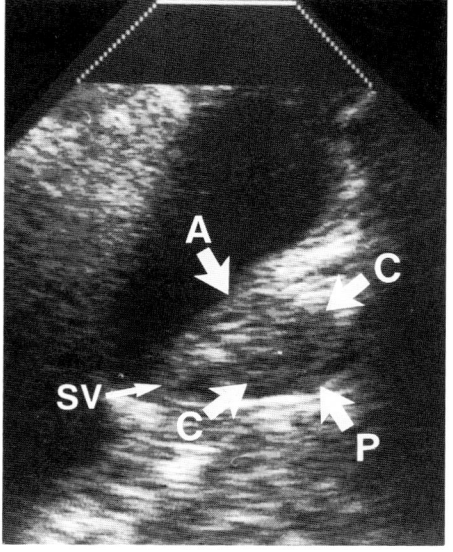

FIG. 6.1. Technique of measurements by use of ultrasound. Transabdominal ultrasound in the transverse (**A**) and longitudinal (**B**) orienations allows calculation of all three dimensions of the prostate. (A–P) Anterior–posterior measurement; (T–T) transverse measurement; (C–C) cephalo-caudad measurement; (SV) seminal vesicle.

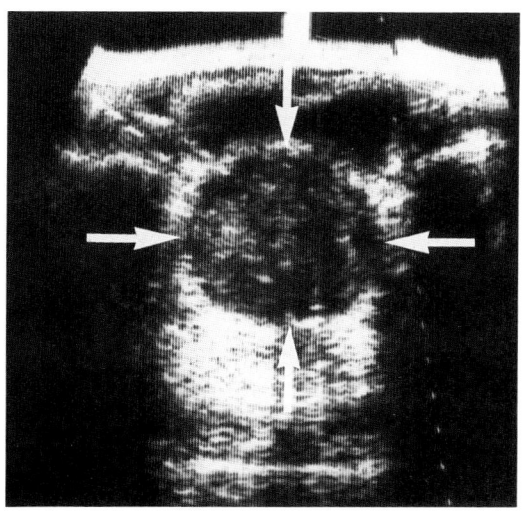 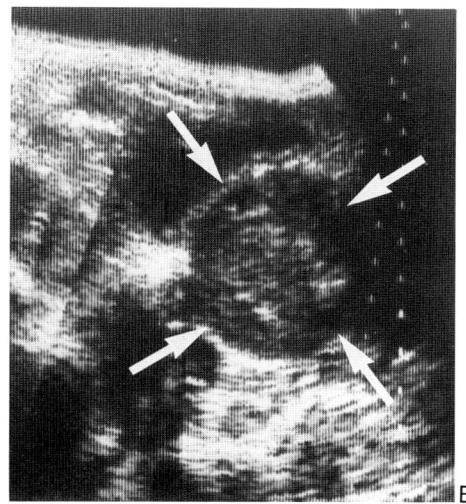

FIG. 6.2. Transverse (**A**) and longitudinal (**B**) transabdominal images show margin of an enlarged prostate. The *arrows* indicate where measurements are taken.

can be used (192). The weight of the prostate can also be assessed with a formula using the diameters (D). If the gland is asymmetrical in shape, then the above formulas can be simplified to

$$\text{Weight} = 0.5 \times D_1 \times D_2 \times D_3$$

with D_1 being the transverse, D_2 the cephalo-caudad, and D_3 the anterior-posterior dimension (5,518). If the gland is symmetrical in shape the following formula can be used

$$\text{Weight} = 0.5\, D^3$$

where D equals the average diameter.

If the prostate appears to be bilobed, accurate calculations can be made by assuming the gland to be two separate spheres and adding the two subsequent results (312).

Although these simple formulas can be used, many people prefer comparisons to tables. These tables have been calculated using a clinical grade of enlargement (Table 6.1) or estimate of weight (Table 6.2) (416). The transperineal approach can also be used with the same formula, which requires the measurements of the same three dimensions.

The endourethral and endorectal examinations can also be utilized for preoperative evaluation of gland size. A biplane approach must be used, and calculations of the anterior-posterior, the lateral, and the cephalo-caudad dimensions must be obtained (Fig. 6.3).

TABLE 6.1. Prostate size

Grade	Diameter (cm)	Weight (g)
I	3.0–3.8	<30
II	3.8–4.5	30–50
III	4.5–5.5	50–85
IV	>5.5	>85

Adapted from ref. 416.

TABLE 6.2. Prostate size

Diameter (cm)	Weight (g)
3.0–3.5	14–22
3.5–4.0	22–33
4.0–4.5	33–47
4.5–5.0	47–65
5.0–5.5	65–87
5.5–6.0	87–113
6.0–6.5	113–143
6.5–7.0	143–179
7.0–7.5	179–220
7.5–8.0	220–267

Adapted from ref. 416.

Planimetric Calculations

The axial orientation alone can also be used. However, in these cases, slightly more complicated arithmetic computation is required. The prostate is examined from apex to base at various subcentimeter intervals, the most common being 0.5-cm or 0.25-cm increments (Fig. 6.4). Using a computer, electronic planimetric calculations of the area of each section are then obtained, and all sections are summed to obtain a final result (29,190). If a "stepper"-type device (which automatically moves the transducer in or out of the prostate at set intervals) is used (Fig. 6.5), the accuracy of the technique is improved.

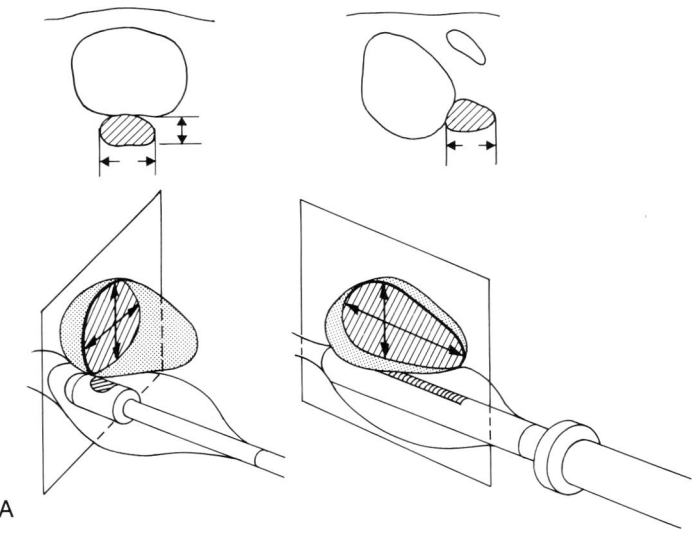

FIG. 6.3. Endorectal ultrasound approach for calculation of measurements. Two planes are required in order to calculate prostatic size using the endorectal approach (**A**). The axial image (*lower left*) will yield both the anterior–posterior and the transverse dimensions (*upper left*). The longitudinal scan (*lower left*) will confirm the anterior–posterior dimension and will also yield the cephalo-caudad dimension (*upper right*).

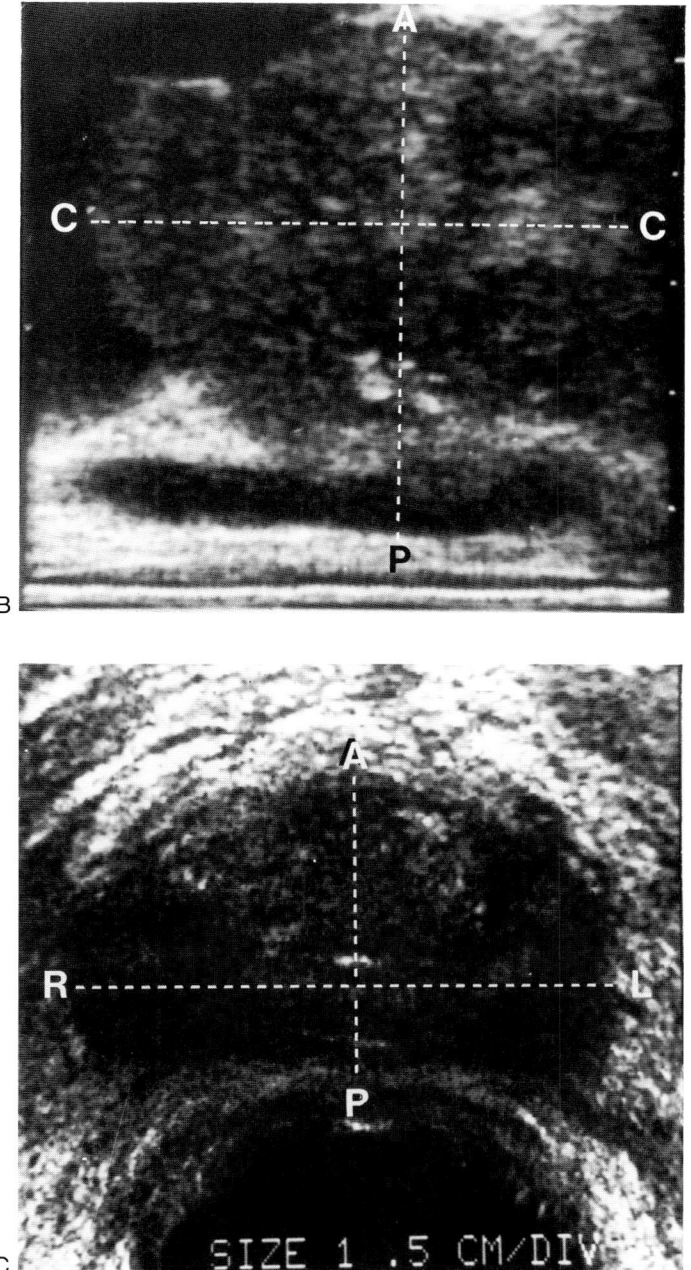

FIG. 6.3. *Continued.* A longitudinal view (**B**) and an axial view (**C**) shows the measurements. (R–L) Right–left measurements; (C–C) cephalo-caudad measurements; (A–P) anterior–posterior measurement.

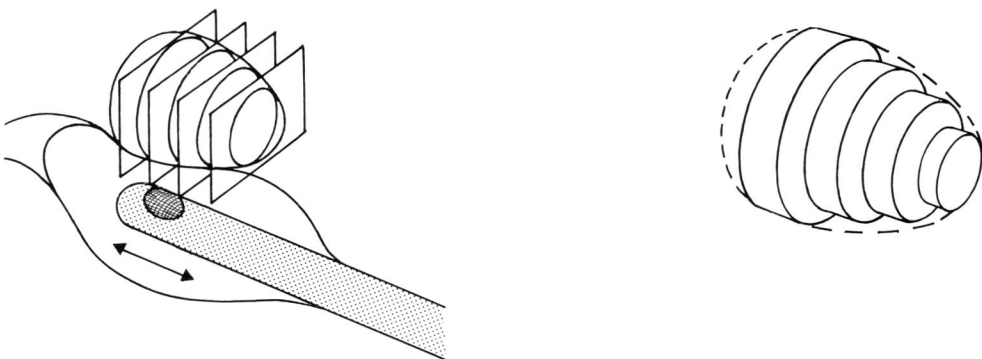

FIG. 6.4. Planimetric calculations using the endorectal approach. By using the longitudinally oriented endorectal ultrasound transducer, sequential images of the prostate can be obtained from base to apex (**left**). By summing the areas of each section, a cylindrical model, and thus a volume (**right**), can be obtained.

EVALUATION OF SEMINAL VESICLE SIZE

Calculation of seminal vesicle size can be ascertained by utilizing abdominal sonograms, axial and longitudinal transrectal ultrasound scans, or other techniques which will image three cross-sectional dimensions (Fig. 6.6). A normal range of measurements has been

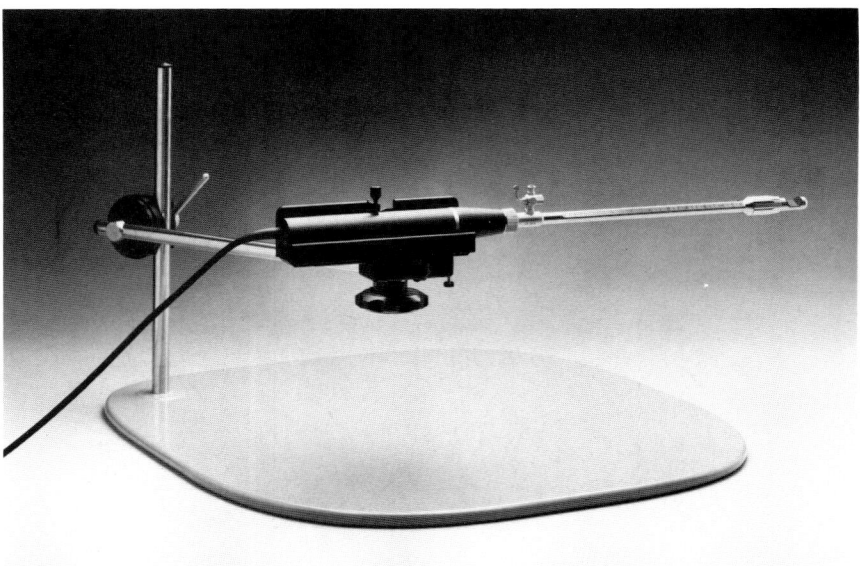

FIG. 6.5. Automated "stepper"-type device. The axially oriented endorectal probe is placed in a special device which is automatically programmed to move the transducer in or out of the prostate at subcentimeter increments. The calculated areas are then summed to obtain the volume. (Courtesy of Bruel & Kjaer Instruments, Marlborough, Massachusetts.)

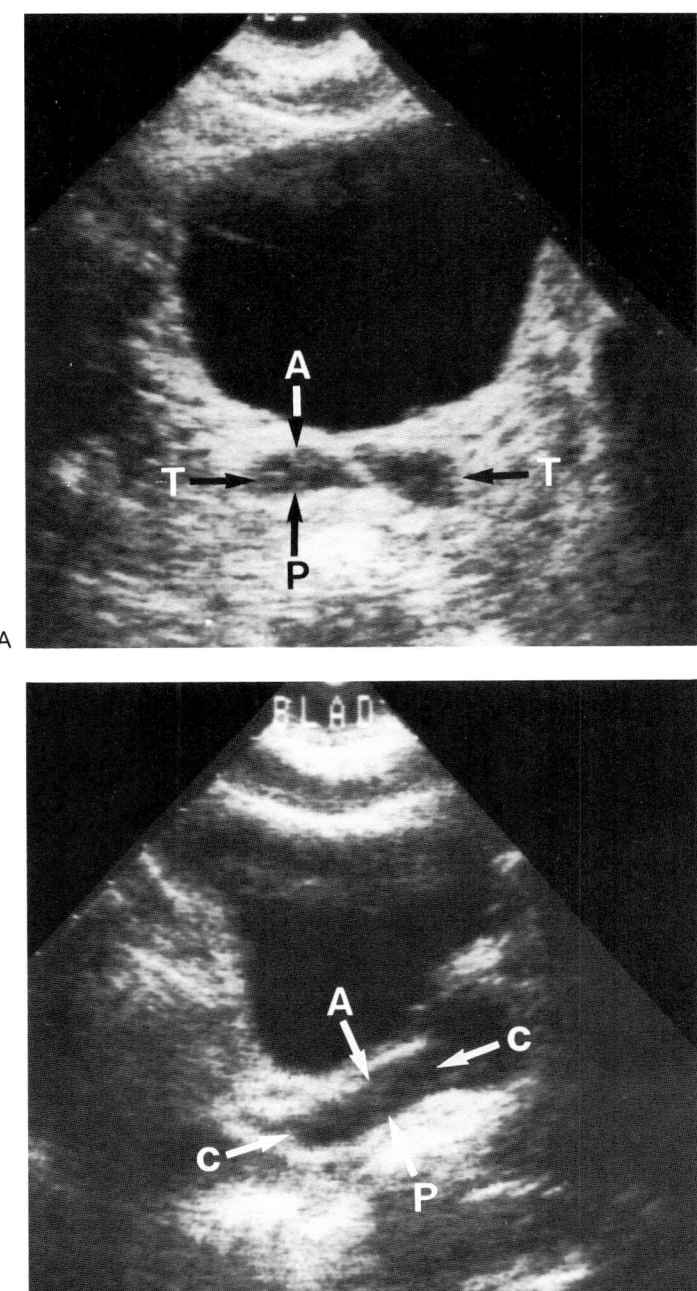

FIG. 6.6. Seminal vesicle measurements. A longitudinal image of the prostate obtained by using the transabdominal approach (**A**) yields the anterior–posterior (A–P) and the transverse (T–T) dimensions of the seminal vesicles. A longitudinal image obtained by using the abdominal approach (**B**) will confirm the anterior–posterior (A–P) and the cephalo-caudad (C–C) dimensions.

calculated (417). The average length of the seminal vesicles from the prostatic margin—i.e., the medial aspect to the fundus (the lateral aspect) of the seminal vesicle—is approximately 7.5 + 1.3 mm. The highest or thickest point of the fundus is 1.9 ± 0.16 mm. The broadest point (on transverse images) is 2.7 ± 0.45 mm, and the highest point (on longitudinal image) is 1.9 ± 0.19 cm. These calculations can be obtained using any of the various imaging devices. More complicated planimetric calculations can also be used for accurate assessment of seminal vesicle size with the examination by the transrectal radial approach. Summation of the size of each image requires the use of a microprocessor.

However, regardless of these various formulas, the most important evaluation of the seminal vesicle is symmetry. There is marked variation among the size of normal seminal vesicles of different normal male individuals. Absolute size is less important than symmetry between right and left side in terms of shape, position, and echogenicity. These findings are more imporant than the actual measurement.

7 // Sonographic Approach to the Diagnosis of Prostatic Disease

The Prostate	101
The Abnormal Area	101
The Periprostatic Space	103
Echogenicity	103
Anechoic Lesions	
Hypoechoic Lesions	
Isoechoic Lesions	
Hyperechoic Lesions	
Mixed Echogenic Lesions	
Summary	112

The diagnosis of disease by ultrasound requires a consistent technique for evaluating the prostate, seminal vesicles, and the surrounding structures. Although any approach that is methodical, systematic, and consistent is acceptable, the following is one suggested methodology.

Evaluation can be divided into that of (a) the prostate (Table 7.1), (b) the focus or area of abnormality (Table 7.2), and (c) the periprostatic tissues (Table 7.3).

THE PROSTATE

When evaluating the prostate, it is important to determine shape, size, and weight. Is there asymmetry in size and shape? The margins of the capsule should then be assessed for distortion, bulging, asymmetry, erosion, or destruction. Next, the internal architecture should be evaluated. Sonographic symmetry or asymmetry should be ascertained. Is architectural symmetry present or disrupted? Are there abnormalities within the gland?

THE ABNORMAL AREA

Once it has been determined that there is a demonstrable area of disease within the prostate, this (or these) should be further evaluated. Is there one or more than one area of abnormality? Where are the foci of disease located? Is the abnormal focus periurethral (which would suggest, but not necessarily be diagnostic of, benign disease) or peripherally placed? Is the focus of disease well-marginated or irregular? What is its echogenicity? Is it hypoechoic, hyperechoic, of mixed echogenicity, or isoechoic compared to the remaining prostatic tissue? Is the area of abnormality adjacent to the capsule that is causing distortion, or is there erosion through the capsule? Is the prostatic urethra identified? If so, does this focus of disease

Table 7.1. Evaluation of prostate

Margins of prostate
   Smooth
   Irregular

Capsule
   Intact
   Disrupted

Peripheral zone
   Identified   Yes
                        No
   Normal   Yes
                        No

Central gland
   Normal   Yes
                        No

Echogenicity
   Normal
   Abnormal   Diffuse
                        Focal

Architecture
   Symmetrical
   Asymmetrical

Focal abnormality
   Yes
   No

Urethra
   Normal position
   Abnormal position

Table 7.2. Evaluation of focal lesions of the prostate

Are focal abnormalities present?
   Yes
   No

How many?

Where are they found?
   Peripheral zone
   Central gland

Margins of focus
   Well-defined
   Poorly defined

Echogenicity of focus
   Anechoic
   Hypoechoic
   Isoechoic
   Hyperechoic
   Mixed echogenicity

Is there a halo sign present?

Are there any calculi present?
   Yes
   No
   Where?

Secondary sonographic characteristics
   Shadowing (attenuation)
   Enhancement

Table 7.3. Evaluation of periprostatic tissues

Capsule
  Normal
  Bulged but intact
  Eroded
  Invaded
Lymph nodes
  Absent
  Present
Seminal vesicles
  Symmetrical
  Asymmetrical
Seminal vesicle–prostate "nipple"
  Normal
  Abnormal
Seminal-vesicle–prostate "angle"
  Normal
  Abnormal

cause distortion upon the posterior urethra? Are there calculi present within the gland? Are there abnormal echogenic foci with or without acoustic shadowing within the gland? Are these echogenic areas periurethrally placed, or are they surrounding the lesion(s) in question? If an anechoic mass is present, is there is a sharp back wall without internal echoes and good sound through-transmission, thus suggesting the presence of a prostatic cyst? Are the ejaculatory ducts identified? If so, are they normal or dilated? Are other abnormalities of the ejaculatory ducts noted?

THE PERIPROSTATIC SPACE

The next step is identification of the periprostatic tissue.

Are the seminal vesicles normal? Are they symmetrical in size, shape, and position? Are the prostate–seminal-vesicle "angles" symmetrical? Is the prostate–seminal-vesicle "nipple" present? Is there mass effect? Is there erosion or enlargement into the seminal vesicles? Is the base of the bladder intact, or is there impingement upon the base of the bladder by a space-occupying lesion that may originate from the prostate? Is there adenopathy? That is, are there lymph nodes identified in the periprostatic areas?

ECHOGENICITY

Following these evaluations, the determination of the possible presence of disease can be made. Only then can differentiation into the possibility of benign versus malignant pathology be ascertained.

A comparison of echogenicity is essential but confusing. If one reviews all of the published literature, an apparent abundance of contradictory data will overwhelm the reader. A few concepts must be understood to help sort out this quagmire.

Careful reading of the literature will show that a basis of comparison may be difficult. For example, if one analyzes echogenicity, he or she will discover that different texts have used different bases of comparison (91,253,397,404,444,522). Some have used the symphysis pubis; others have used either the prostate capsule, the peripheral zone, or the central glandular areas.

Throughout this text, the sonographic characteristics of lesions of the prostate will be defined as follows:

Anechoic Lesions

These are lesions in which there are no echoes (Fig. 7.1). This is the classic finding in a fluid-filled collection; however, fluid will also have other secondary characteristics, including well-defined boundaries and sharp borders and good sound through-transmission. Anechoic solid masses will not have these secondary characteristics (Fig. 7.2).

Hypoechoic Lesions

These lesions are less echogenic than the remainder of the prostate of the same area (i.e., peripheral zone compared to peripheral zone) (Fig. 7.3). These may have subtle internal echoes (Fig. 7.4) or may have no internal echoes; that is, anechoic lesions are a subset of hypoechoic lesions. These foci will be less echogenic than the normal prostate; more importantly, however, they will be less echogenic than the surrounding tissue. There may be some inhomogeneous echogenicity within the lesion (Fig. 7.5). It is important to compare

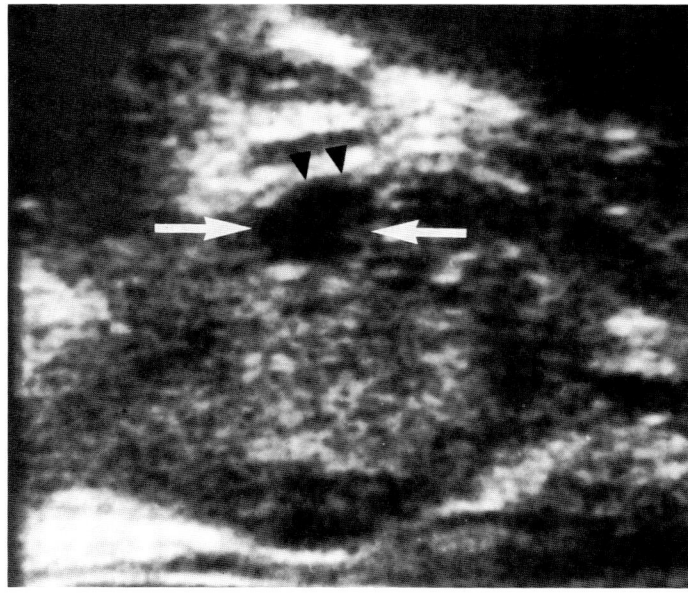

FIG. 7.1. Anechoic lesion. A longitudinally oriented linear array examination of the prostate demonstrates an anechoic lesion (*arrows*) without internal echoes. There are sharp back walls (*arrowheads*), suggesting that this is a fluid-filled lesion.

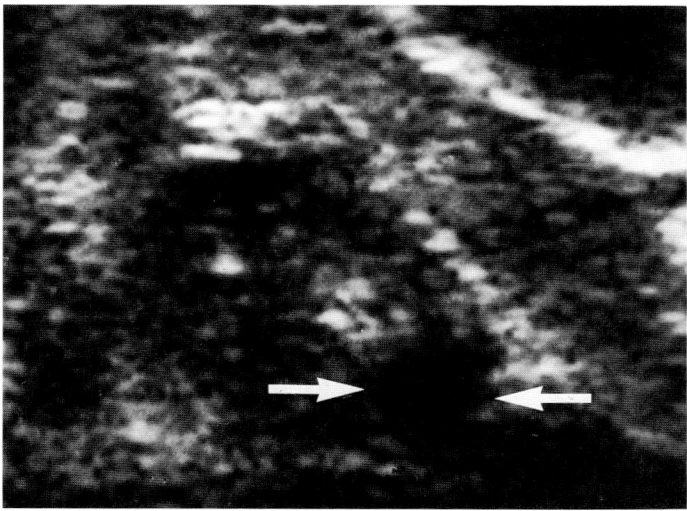

FIG. 7.2. Anechoic lesion. This solid mass in the apex (*arrows*) is seen on longitudinal ultrasound of the prostate. It is poorly marginated but without internal echoes. There are no sharp back walls seen.

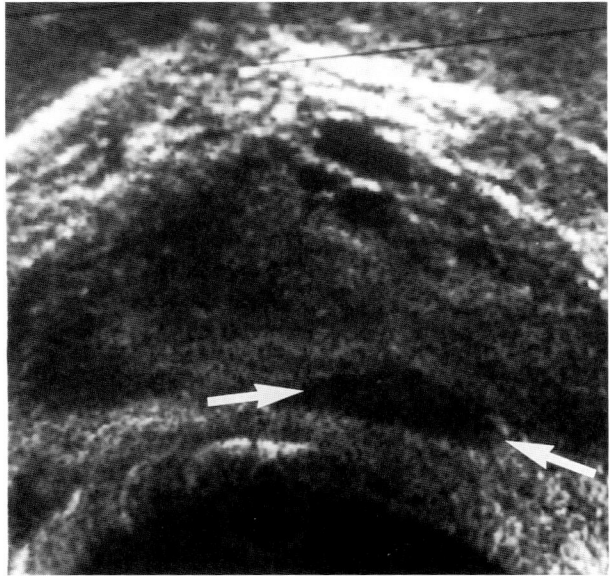

FIG. 7.3. Hypoechoic lesion. Transversely oriented ultrasound of the prostate demonstrates an anechoic lesion (*arrows*) that does have some subtle internal echogenicity. The back walls of the lesion are not clearly demarcated.

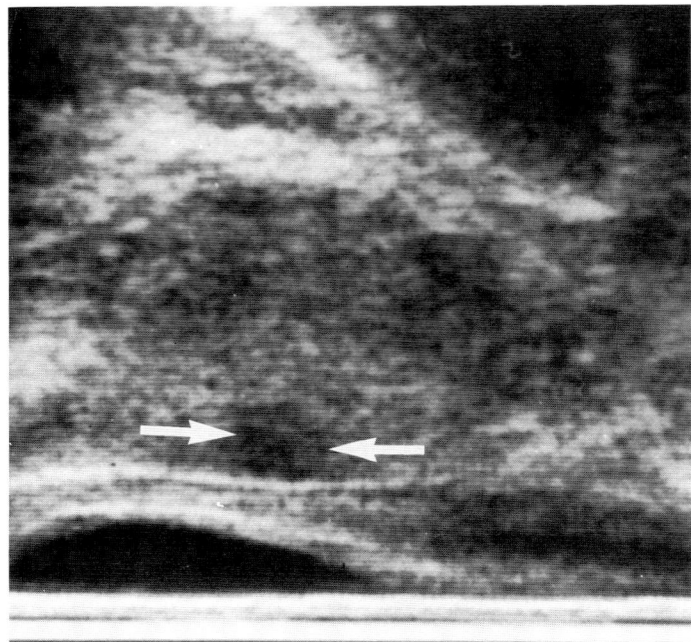

FIG. 7.4. Hypoechoic lesion. A longitudinally oriented linear array examination demonstrates a hypoechoic lesion (*arrows*) in the peripheral zone that is distinctly different sonographically from the remainder of the same area. The margins of the lesion are not clearly demarcated.

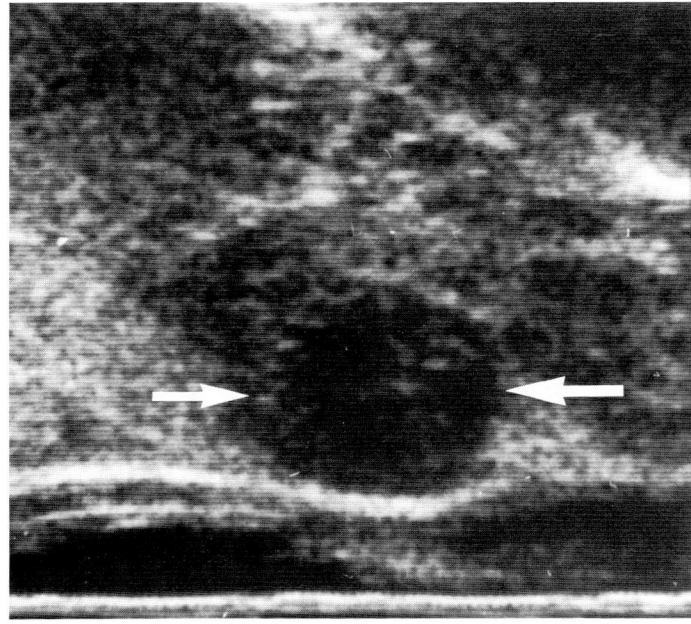

FIG. 7.5. Hypoechoic lesion. A longitudinally oriented linear array examination demonstrates a peripheral-zone hypoechoic lesion (*arrows*) with some subtle echogenicity. The overall sonographic findings are of low-level (*hypoechoic*) echogenicity.

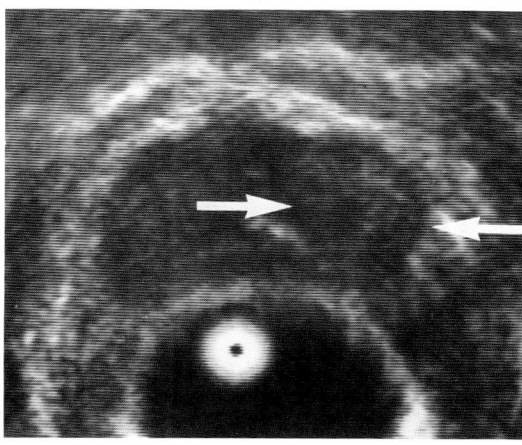

FIG. 7.6. Isoechoic lesion. A transversely oriented endorectal ultrasound of the prostate demonstrates a lesion in the left lateral margin of the gland (*arrows*) which sonographically has echogenicity identical to that of the right lateral margin of the prostate. The only identifiable abnormal area is the asymmetry in shape of the prostate with a large bulge off the left lateral margin.

similar tissue, (i.e., peripheral zone to peripheral zone, or central zone to central zone). If a peripheral zone lesion is compared to the central zone, confusion and misdiagnoses may result.

Isoechoic Lesions

These lesions have the same echogenicity as the remaining prostate (Fig. 7.6). Although they may not be clearly delineated by ultrasound, they will be identified by irregularities of their margin or a defined halo surrounding the lesion. An isoechoic lesion without a well-defined region of different echogenicity will, by definition, not be differentiated from normal tissue. Secondary characteristics may be the only delineating feature (Fig. 7.7). Although it is not pathognomonic, this area of diffuse echogenicity is suggestive of a benign lesion and may be termed a "halo" sign (Fig. 7.8).

Hyperechoic Lesions

These are lesions that are more echogenic than normal or residual prostate tissue. They can vary from subtle areas of increased echogenicity (Fig. 7.9) (i.e., a barely perceptible change in comparison to the normal or residual prostatic tissue) to areas that are brightly (Figs. 7.10 and 7.11) and thickly echogenic, which are usually calculi or occasionally corpora amylacea.

Mixed Echogenic Lesions

The acoustically mixed lesion will have areas of decreased, as well as increased, echogenicity (Fig. 7.12). They are usually less well defined than the purely hypoechoic lesion.

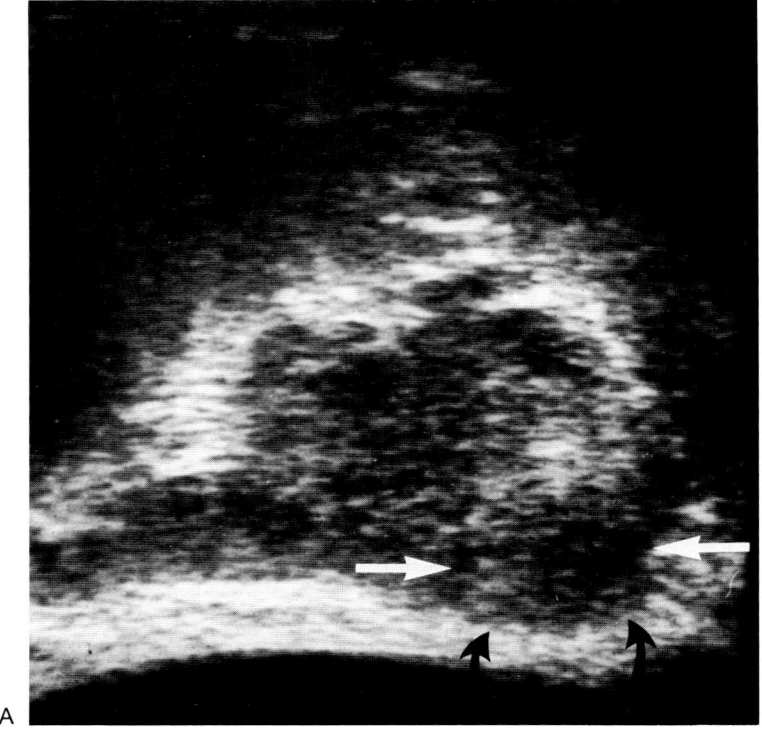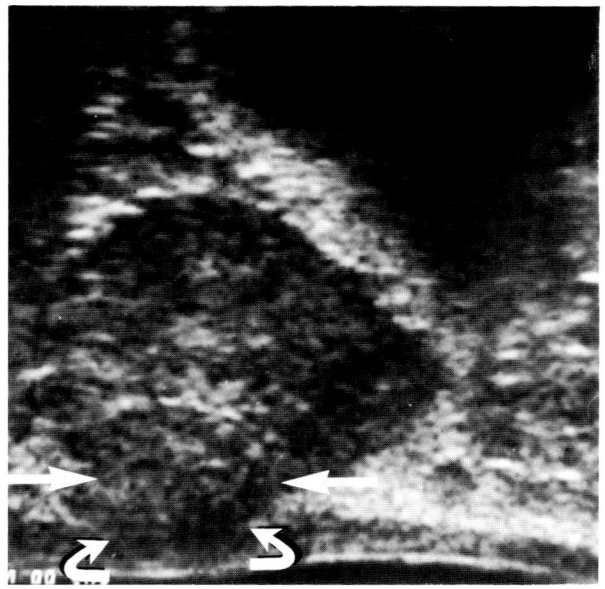

FIG. 7.7. Isoechoic lesions. Two longitudinally oriented endorectal sonograms of the prostate demonstrate isoechoic lesions (*arrows*). In one (**A**), there is thinning of the hyperechoic capsule (*curved arrows*); in the other (a different patient) (**B**), there is marked erosion (*curved arrows*) of the capsule.

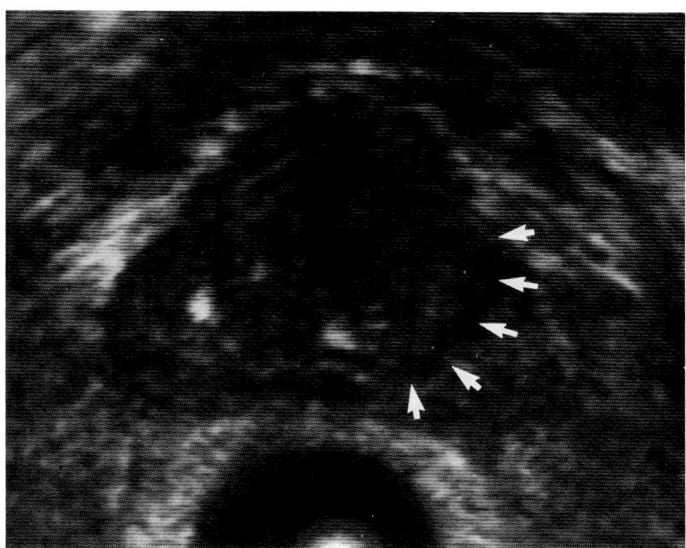

FIG. 7.8. Isoechoic lesion with "halo" sign. An axially oriented endorectal sonogram of the prostate demonstrates an enlarged periurethral area with an isoechoic lesion. A "halo" sign is clearly demarcated on the left (*arrows*). The mass has a thin, low-level echogenic area separating the abnormal area from the normal area.

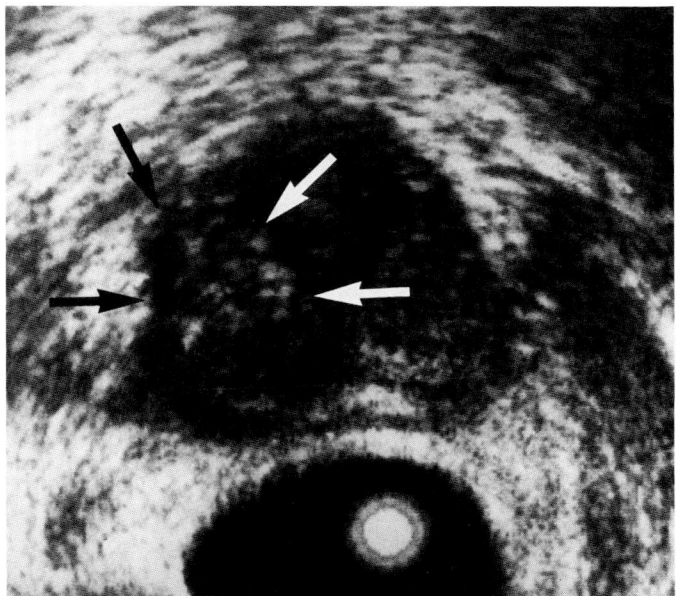

FIG. 7.9. Hyperechoic lesions. There are a variety of hyperechoic lesions. In these two patients, one studied with an axial scanner (**A**) and the other studied with a longitudinal imager (**B**), there are subtle areas of increased echogenicity (*arrows*) as compared to the normal-appearing residual tissues of the same zone.

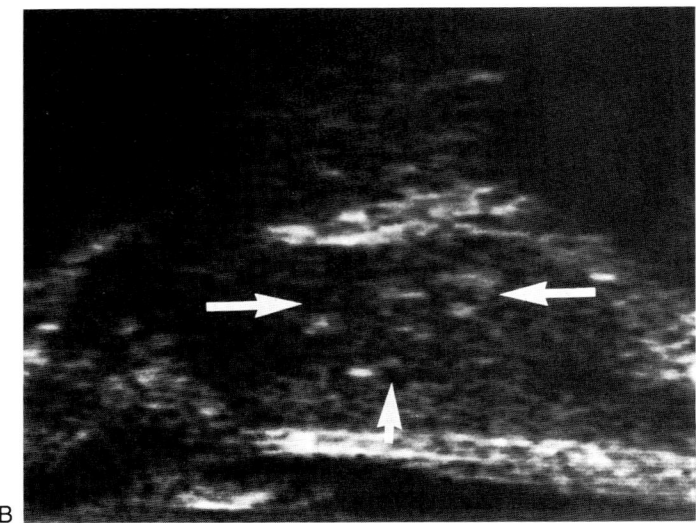

FIG. 7.9. *Continued.*

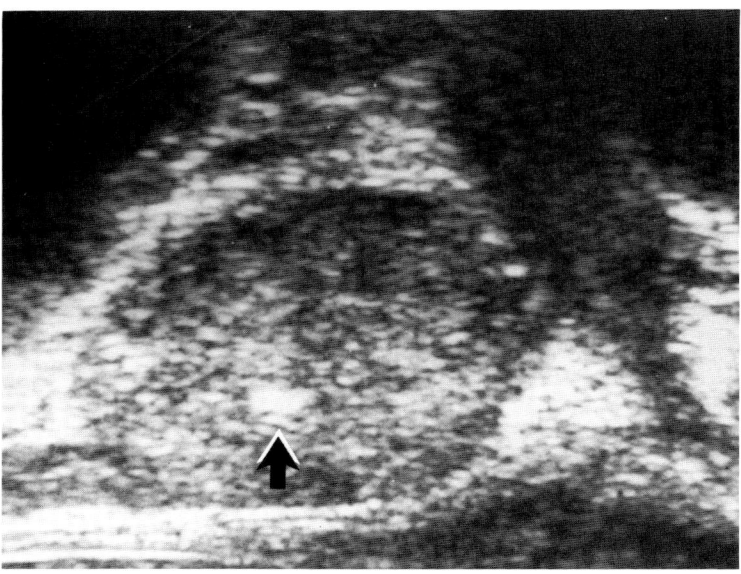

FIG. 7.10. Hyperechoic lesion. A longitudinally oriented endorectal sonographic image demonstrates a brightly echogenic area (*arrow*) without shadowing, suggesting either calculus or corpora amylacea.

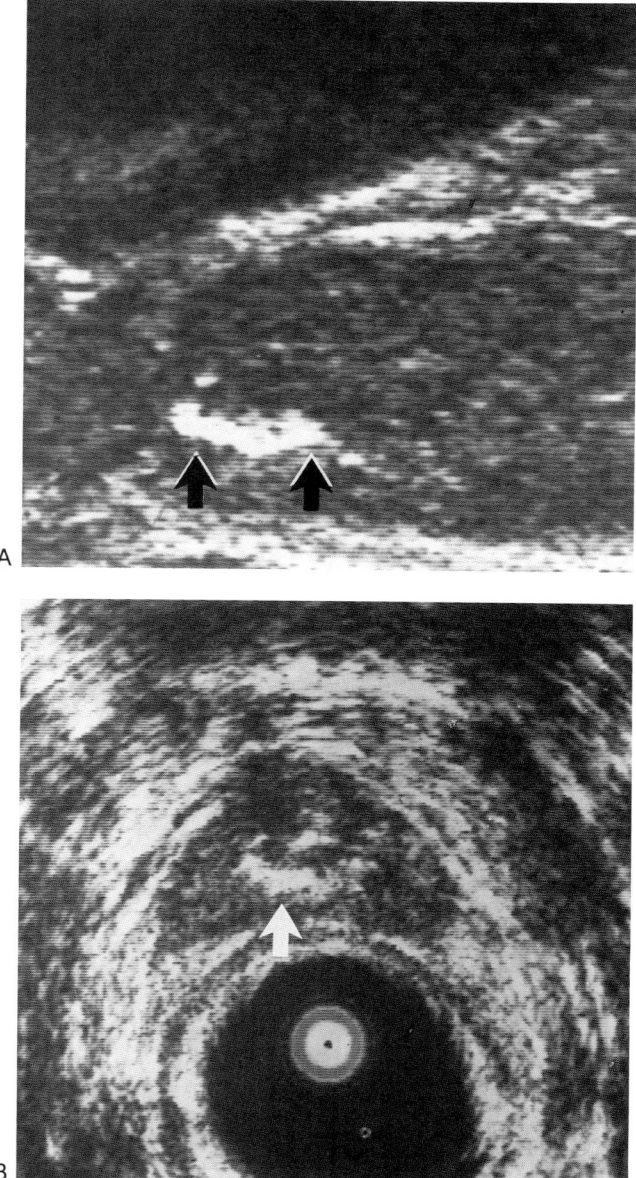

FIG. 7.11. Hyperechoic lesion. Longitudinal (**A**) and axial (**B**) images from endorectal sonograms demonstrate bright and thick echogenic areas (*arrows*). Note that these areas are more echogenic than either the residual prostate, the periprostatic fat, or the prostatic capsule.

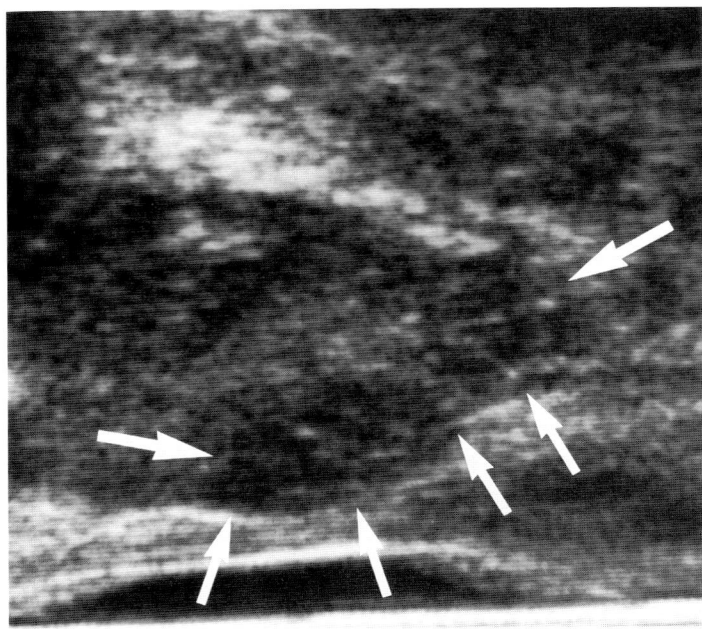

FIG. 7.12. Mixed echogenic lesion. An acoustically mixed echogenic lesion (*arrows*) is seen on this endorectal sonogram. Although there are less echogenic areas than the residual peripheral zone (where this lesion is situated), there are also scattered subtle areas of increased echogenicity, thus making this a sonographically mixed mass.

SUMMARY

Although the preceding considerations will delineate most pathologic processes within the prostate, there are obviously a certain number of abnormalities that may not or cannot be identified by sonographic evaluation. For this reason, the sonographic study, and particularly the endorectal examination, should be considered at all times as being a study that is complementary to the routine physical examination and various laboratory studies.

8 // *Biopsy Techniques*

Core-Needle Biopsy	113
Cytologic Aspiration	114
Conventional Biopsy Techniques	114
Complications	116
General Considerations of Ultrasound Guided Biopsy	117
Technique of Ultrasound Guided Biopsy: Sterile Precautions	117
Transperineal Biopsy: General Considerations	118
Transperineal Biopsy: Axial Orientation	119
Transperineal Biopsy: Sagittal Orientation	122
Transrectal Biopsy	130
Comparison of the Transperineal with the Transrectal Approach	130
Conclusions	139

The diagnosis of both the clinically palpable and the nonpalpable prostatic lesion requires tissue diagnosis. Biopsy is indicated in all patients with suspected prostatic malignancy. Biopsies are performed with either (a) a large-bore needle to extract a core of tissue for histologic evaluation or (b) a small-bore aspiration type needed for extraction of fragments of cells and a cytologic evaluation. Either of these techniques is usually adequate for diagnosis, although there are strengths and weaknesses of each technique.

A variety of different types and sizes of needles can be used for biopsy (Fig. 8.1).

CORE-NEEDLE BIOPSY

The use of a core needle (a Tru-Cut- or Vim–Silverman-type needle) yields a large piece of tissue. This is useful for the diagnosis of disease and, in cases of prostatic cancer, accurate grading of the malignancy. This may also be useful for determination of proper treatment. However, complication rates can increase with the use of the larger-sized needles. Although the Tru-Cut and Vim–Silverman needles are larger bore (i.e., 14–16 gauge), a small cutting needle usually yields a diagnostically adequate specimen.

An 18-gauge biopsy needle (Fig. 8.1) that can be used with a trigger-type device for a more ''rapid'' biopsy has recently been introduced. This needle, called a ''Biopty'' needle (by the Radiplast Corporation, Sweden) can be used freehand or can be coupled to a mechanical triggering device (''gun'') that ensures rapid, safe extraction of a core of tissue (Fig. 8.2). The use of these slightly smaller-gauge needles has helped to decrease the number of complications (i.e., hematoma) without loss of diagnostic accuracy or the ability to grade a cancer.

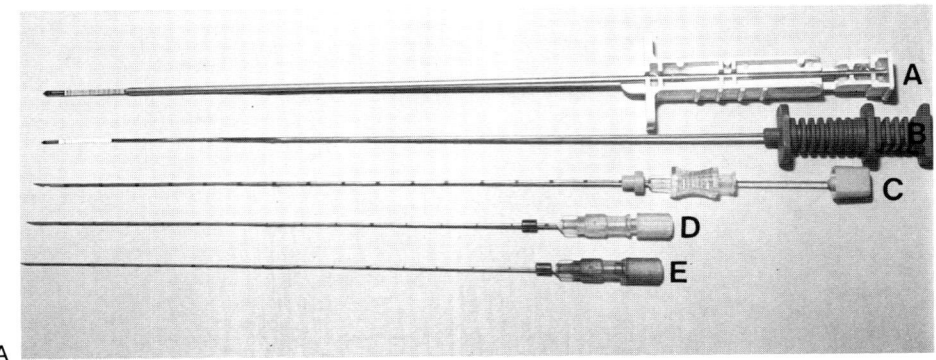

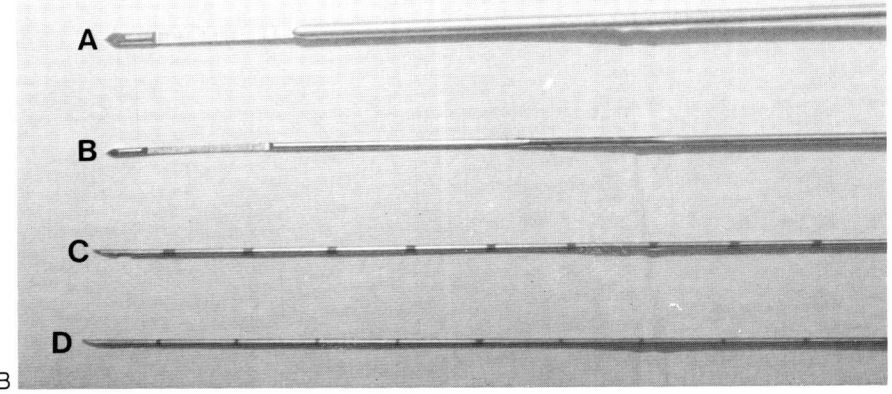

FIG. 8.1. A variety of biopsy needles in different lengths, sizes, and shapes (**A**) are shown. The tips of these needles (**B**) are different. (A) 14-gauge Tru-Cut; (B) 18-gauge Biopty; (C) 20-gauge Westcott; (D) 20-gauge spinal; (E) 22-gauge Chiba needle.

CYTOLOGIC ASPIRATION

Fine-needle aspiration for prostate biopsy has been used extensively in Europe and is now becoming more popular elsewhere (119,225,311). The diagnostic accuracy of aspiration appears to be comparable to that of a large-core biopsy (119). However, the diagnostic capabilities of the cytology are often dependent upon the pathologist, who frequently has less experience with cytologic evaluation. Additionally, while the diagnosis of malignancy is made by the microscopic analysis of a few groups of cells or even a single abnormal cell, grading is often not possible during tissue diagnosis.

CONVENTIONAL BIOPSY TECHNIQUES

Conventional techniques are usually performed with digital rectal guidance. These can be performed "transperineally" or "transrectally." The transperineal biopsy is done with a finger placed in the rectum and with a needle placed through the perineum into the area of

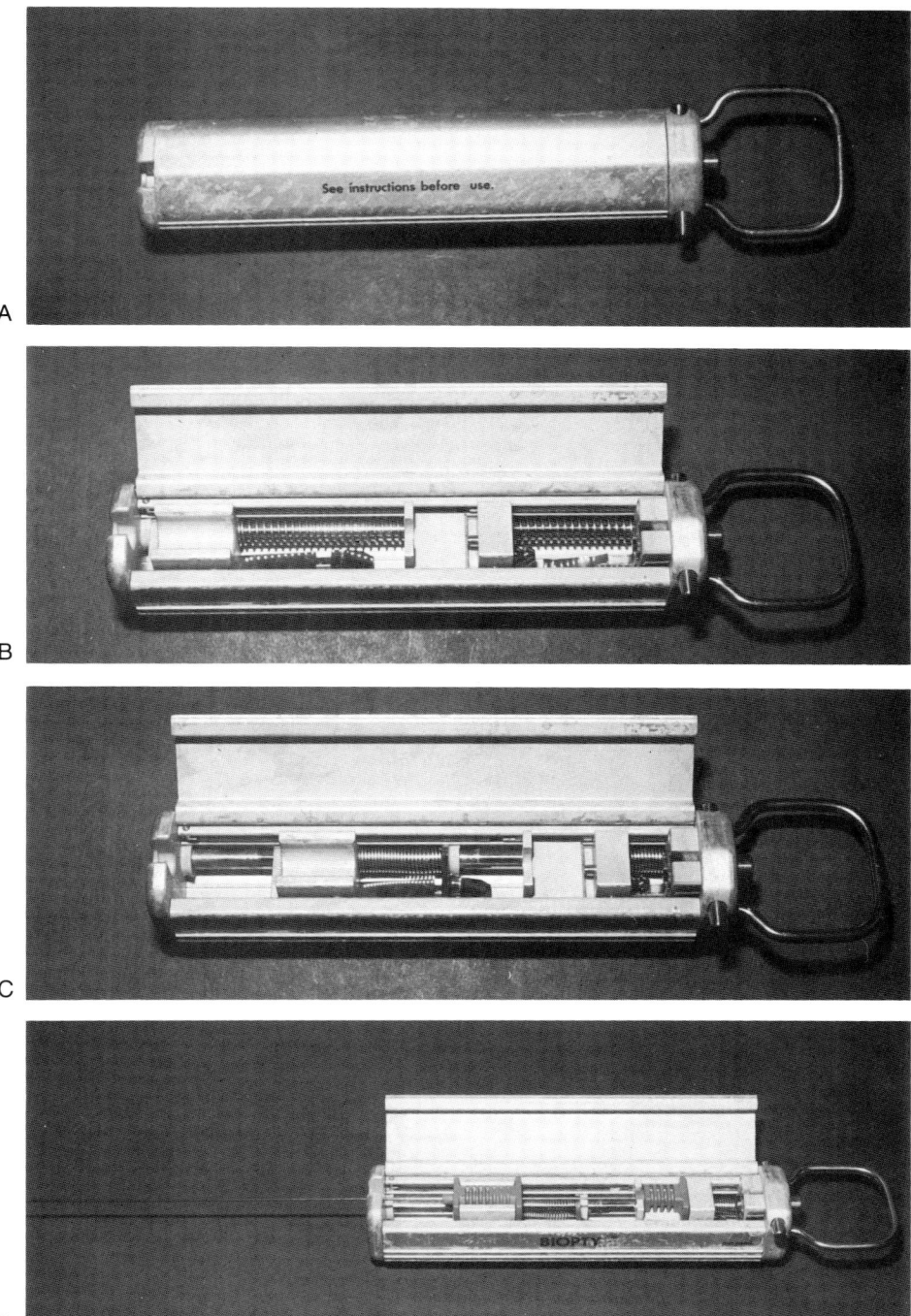

FIG. 8.2. The Biopty gun or trigger is shown in the closed (**A**) and in the open, uncocked position (**B**). When the spring mechanism is cocked, by pulling the lever on the right (**C**), the biopsy needle, when placed into the gun (**D**), is then ready for biopsy.

palpable abnormality (Fig. 8.3). Either a large-gauge biopsy core needle or a small-gauge aspiration cytologic needle can be used.

The "transrectal" biopsy utilizes a needle that is placed next to the finger or is attached to a finger tip guide placed on the rectally inserted fingertip (Fig. 8.4). With the finger palpating the area of abnormality, the biopsy needle is guided toward the area of palpable abnormality, through the rectal mucosa and into the lesion. Both core biopsy or aspiration cytology techniques can be employed with the transrectal approach.

It has been estimated that only 50% of palpable areas of abnormality on biopsy are malignant on pathologic evaluation (163). Others have slightly higher or lower yields. The false negative rate is estimated at approximately 10% (557).

COMPLICATIONS

A major complication of both the transperineal and the transrectal biopsy is hematuria, which may occur in up to 35% of all patients. Sepsis is another possible complication.

There may be an increase in certain types of complications with the transrectal, as opposed to the transperineal biopsy. Sepsis is the most common complication, and the frequency appears to be proportional to the size of the needle employed; that is, the larger the biopsy needle used, the higher the risk of sepsis. When using the transrectal approach, it has been estimated that up to 85% of patients will have positive blood cultures following biopsy (72). For this reason, it has been suggested that prophylactic antibiotic treatment be given prior to a transrectal biopsy (89,185). Others prescribe postbiopsy antibiotics prophylactically for both transperineal and transrectal biopsies. Despite the complication rate, the transrectal biopsy is usually less painful and, with the use of conventional digital guidance, may be slightly more accurate for the diagnosis of very small palpable lesions.

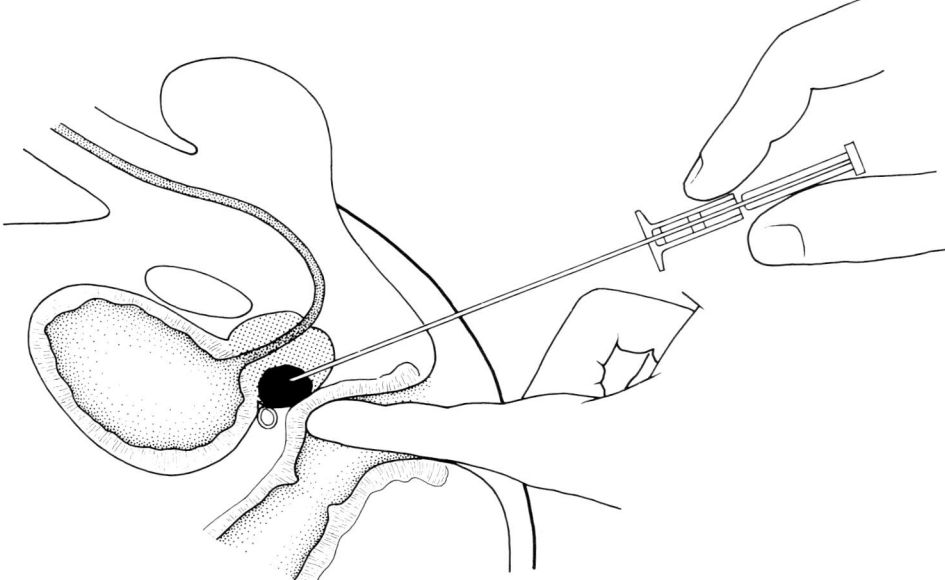

FIG. 8.3. Digitally guided biopsy—transperineal approach. This diagram demonstrates the technique for conventional digitally guided transperineal biopsy of the prostate for a palpable lesion.

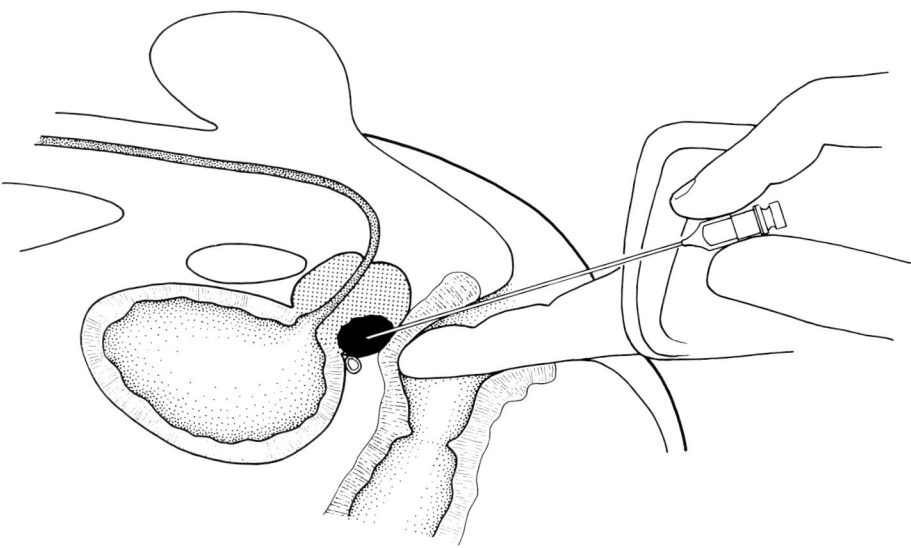

FIG. 8.4. Transrectal biopsy of the prostate with conventional guidance. This diagram demonstrates the finger and biopsy needle placed into the rectum. For biopsy of a palpable mass, the needle is placed into the area of abnormality in the prostate by digital guidance.

Needle-tract seeding along the site of biopsy with implantation of malignant cells has been estimated to be a rare occurrence in prostate biopsy (41,55), although theoretically it can occur.

GENERAL CONSIDERATIONS OF ULTRASOUND GUIDED BIOPSY

The use of digital guided biopsies can only be performed when a palpable area of abnormality is identified. However, with small lesions, this is not an accurate technique. Thus, for diagnosis of nonpalpable lesions or of small and subtly palpable ones, another means of guidance is necessary. In small, but palpable, lesions that have had a negative conventionally guided biopsy, a repeat biopsy may be indicated if these lesions are still suspect. Sonographically guided biopsy can be used accurately, safely, and quickly. There are a variety of approaches that can be utilized. All of these employ the endorectal sonogram, since the other sonographic imaging approaches are inadequately sensitive to detect these subtle lesions.

TECHNIQUE OF ULTRASOUND GUIDED BIOPSY: STERILE PRECAUTIONS

Biopsies are usually performed in either the lithotomy or the left lateral decubitus positions. Other patient positions can be utilized if clinically acceptable. Because there is no need for general anesthesia, biopsies may be performed in an outpatient setting. Following the biopsy, once the patient produces a clear voided specimen, he or she can usually return home almost immediately after the procedure.

In the majority of patients undergoing transperineal biopsy, it is not necessary to shave the perineum, but this may still be warranted in certain individuals. It is never required to shave the perineum in subjects undergoing transrectal biopsy. Cleansing of the perineum with an antiseptic solution is necessary.

The transducer and the covering latex condom are not sterile. Contamination from the transducer and gel (used for easier insertion into the rectum), to the cleansed perineum, should be avoided. Biopsy needles are usually a disposable, "one-time-use only" variety. The biopsy guides are usually autoclavable, gas sterilizable, or sterilizable in an antiseptic solution (i.e., Cidex) for an appropriate amount of time. Some are disposable.

TRANSPERINEAL BIOPSY: GENERAL CONSIDERATIONS

When performing an endorectal ultrasound guided biopsy, the biopsy needle can be guided into the prostate in two ways. When there is no direct attachment of the needle to the endorectal probe, it is called "freehand" guidance (Fig. 8.5). One can also use a biopsy guide that is attached or "fixed" to the probe (Fig. 8.6). The latter technique is useful because it simplifies the procedure. Both are equally accurate and can be used for either the axially oriented or the longitudinally oriented image guided procedure. A variety of attachments are available (Figs. 8.7–8.9).

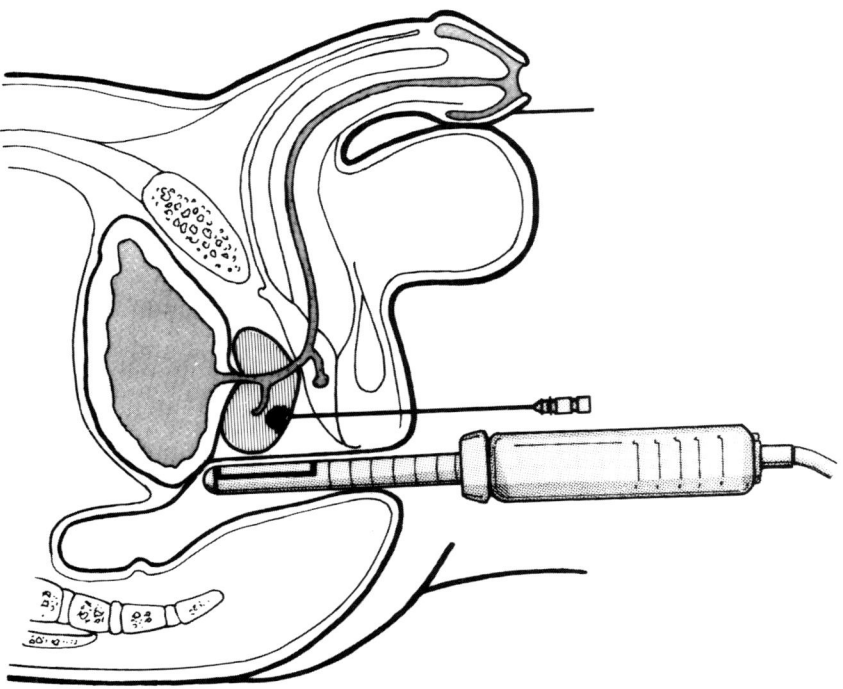

FIG. 8.5. Freehand biopsy with ultrasound guidance. With an endorectal probe placed into the rectum, a needle will be placed through the perineum, under ultrasound guidance, into the area of abnormality. The needle will be freely movable and will not be "fixed" to the endorectal probe.

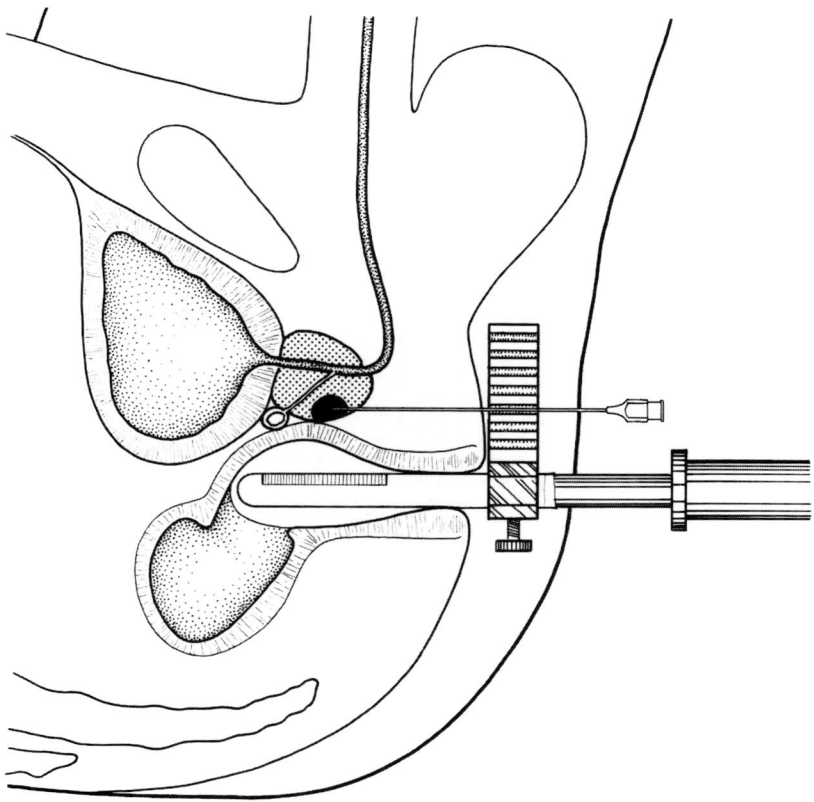

FIG. 8.6. Endorectal ultrasound guidance with guide. A guide is attached to the endorectal probe, and the biopsy needle is placed through the guide and is "fixed" to the guide–transducer complex. It is then placed under sonographic guidance into an area of abnormality.

TRANSPERINEAL BIOPSY: AXIAL ORIENTATION

The use of the axial orientation as compared to other techniques has its limitations, but it can be used effectively (189,201,202). Usually performed with the patient in the lithotomy position, the area of abnormality is ascertained on the sonogram. The transducer is then rotated so that the line of site corresponds to the area of abnormality (Fig. 8.10). The biopsy needle is placed into the perineum, either utilizing a biopsy guide or freehand guidance. The needle tip is then advanced slowly until the tip is defined as an acoustic reflection on the ultrasound image (Fig. 8.11). If the tip is placed in an inappropriate position, immediate remanipulation of the needle is possible. The needle must be totally removed and then reinserted. If not removed, the direction of needle placement (i.e., the needle tract) may not change.

There is a major limitation of the axial orientation. While the needle tip can be seen entering the area of abnormality, the actual biopsy site may not be delineated. This may result in the tissue being obtained from an area that is actually more cephalad or more caudad

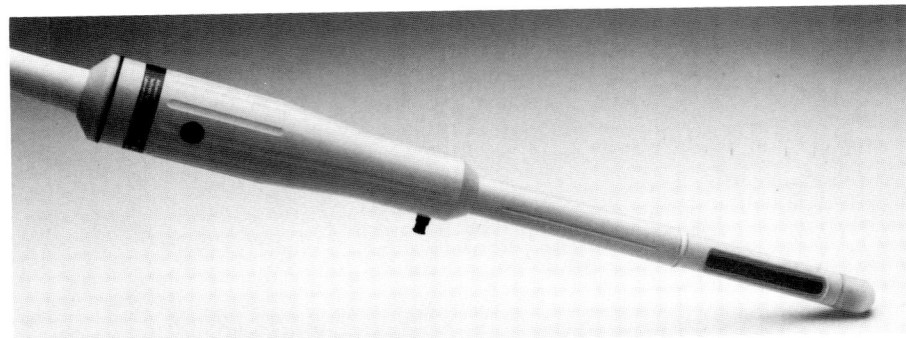
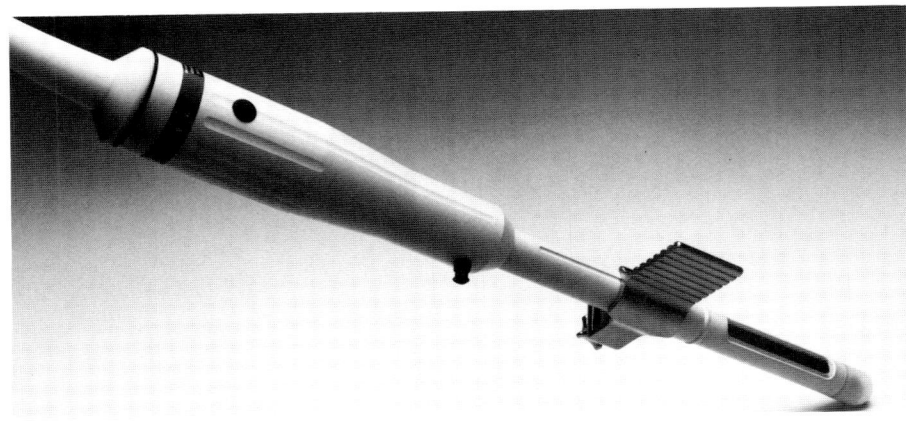

FIG. 8.7. Biplane transducer with guide. A biplane transducer (**A**) with both a linear-array longitudinally oriented transducer and a sector-scan axially oriented transducer is shown. It is also seen with the guide attached for transperineal biopsy (**B**). The guide has multiple slots for needle placement in various areas of the prostate. (Courtesy of Advanced Technology Laboratories, Bothel, Washington.)

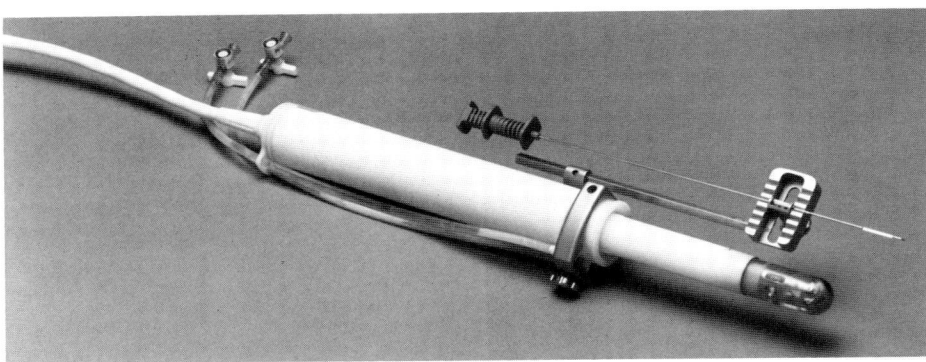

FIG. 8.8. Biplane probe transperineal guide. A biplane transducer with two sector-oriented transducers at the tips is demonstrated with the attached transperineal biopsy guide and a needle in position.

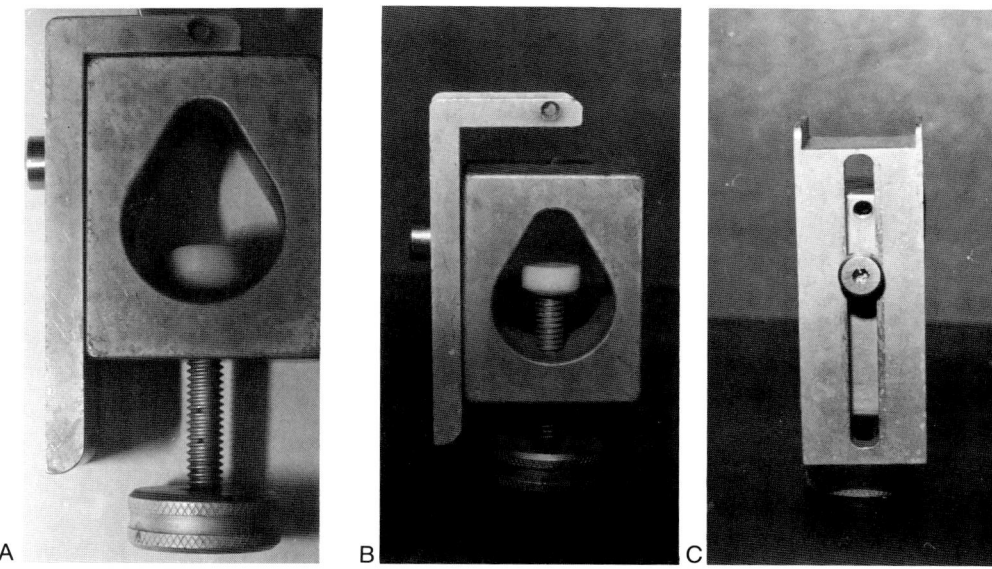

FIG. 8.9. Transrectal biopsy guide. A guide for transperineal biopsy with endorectal sonographic guidance has been produced that can be adapted to multiple different-sized transducers. It is shown in position for a posteriorly positioned lesion (**A**). Now the guide can be positioned for a more anterior lesion (**B**). A side view (**C**) demonstrates the guide with anterior and posterior "lip", with holes for securing the biopsy needle in both the front and back of the device.

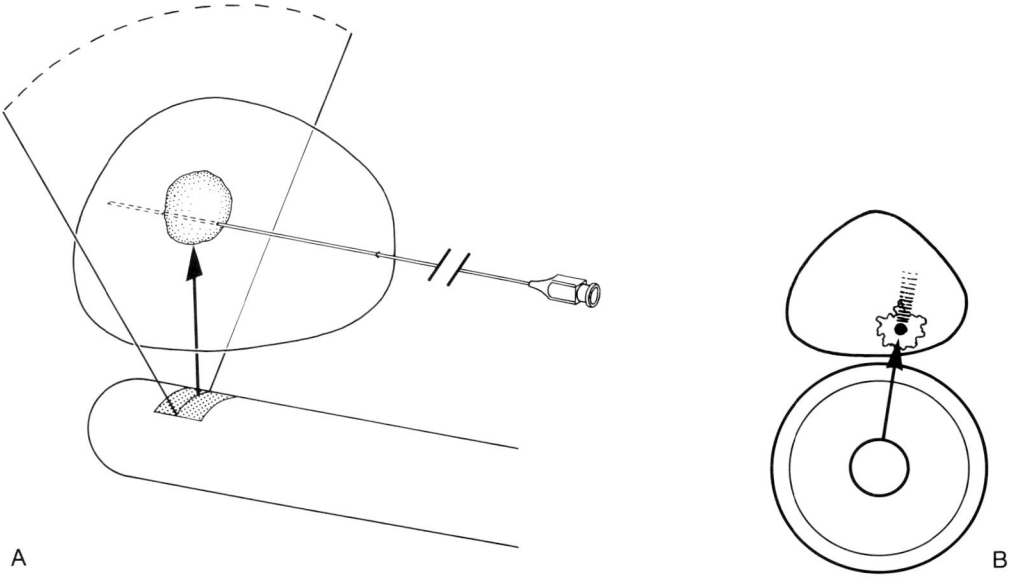

FIG. 8.10. Biopsy guidance with axially oriented ultrasound transducer. Biopsy with an axially oriented endorectal ultrasound examination will show the prostate and the area of abnormality (**A**). By rotating the transducer slightly (**B**), the lesion will be identified, and exact positioning for needle placement into the area of abnormality will be possible.

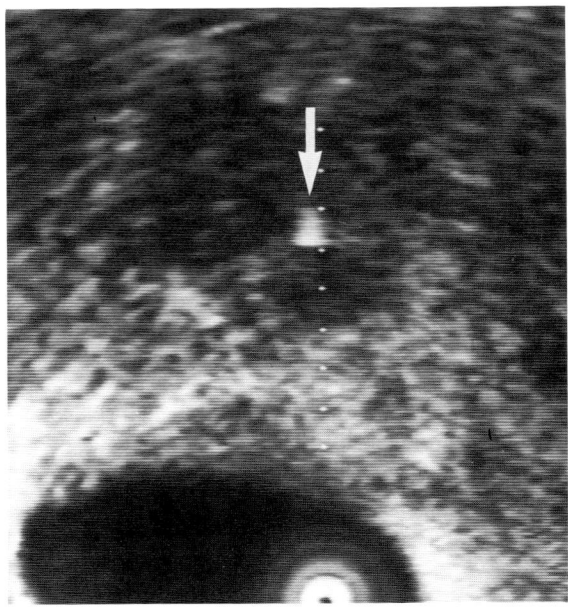

FIG. 8.11. Transperineal guided biopsy with axially oriented sonogram. As the needle tip (*arrow*) is placed into the lesion, an echogenic focus will appear on the axially oriented image of the prostate. (Courtesy of Dr. Hans Henrik Holm.)

to that of the sonographic area of abnormality. This can occur because the exact tissue being biopsied is not identified at the exact time of tissue extraction.

TRANSPERINEAL BIOPSY: SAGITTAL ORIENTATION

The use of the sagittally oriented endorectal sonogram appears to be very accurate and sensitive for biopsying lesions (128,254,395,396,425,426). With the patient in the lithotomy position (or occasionally in the decubitus position), the transducer is placed in the rectum. The needle is placed either freehand (Fig. 8.5) or with a biopsy guide (Fig. 8.6) into the area of sonographic abnormality. The entire needle, including the needle tip, can be visualized. The exact tissue being biopsied is clearly identified (Figs. 8.12–8.15).

The use of a guide theoretically simplifies the biopsy procedure by "fixing" the needle in the direction of biopsy. This allows more flexibility for the physician performing the biopsy. The guides should have either multiple slots (Figs. 8.7 and 8.8) or a movable slot (Fig. 8.9) so that lesions in different areas can be biopsied.

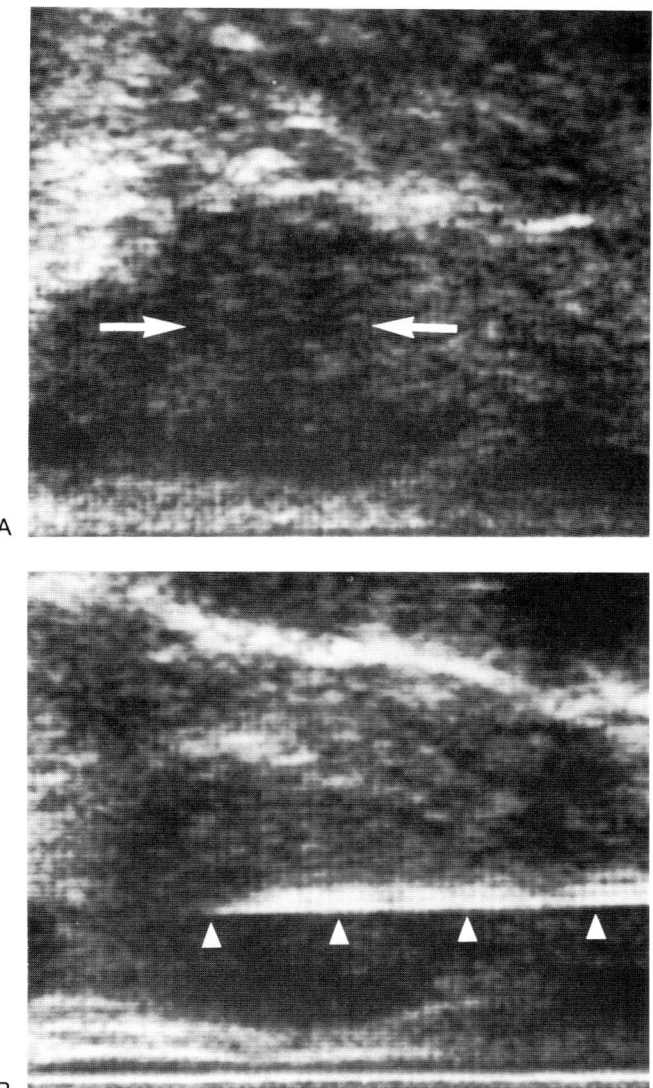

FIG. 8.12. Longitudinally oriented ultrasound guided biopsy. Transperineal biopsy of an echogenically inhomogeneous left lobe of the prostate (*arrows*) (**A**). Placement of the needle (*arrowheads*) into the area of abnormality through the perineum is then performed (**B**).

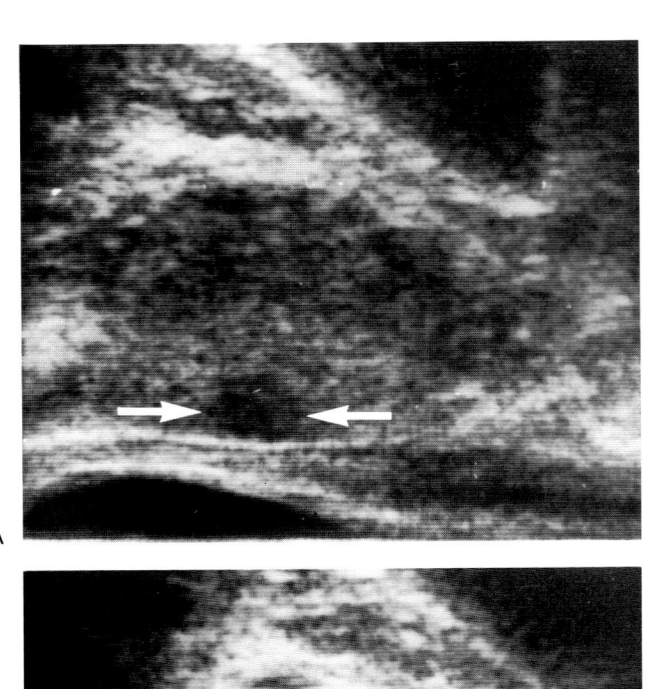
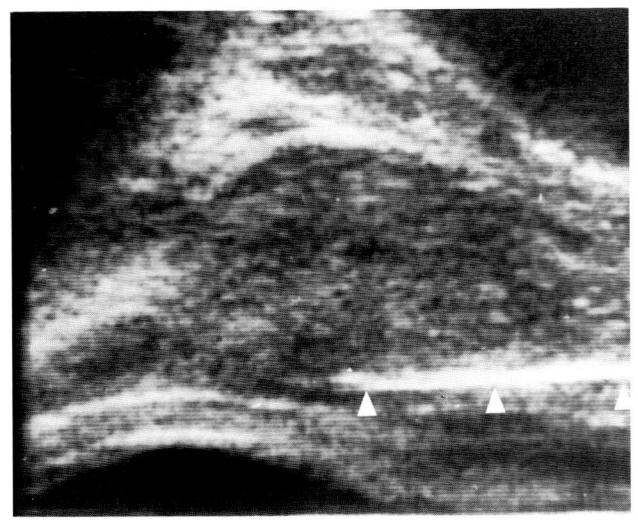
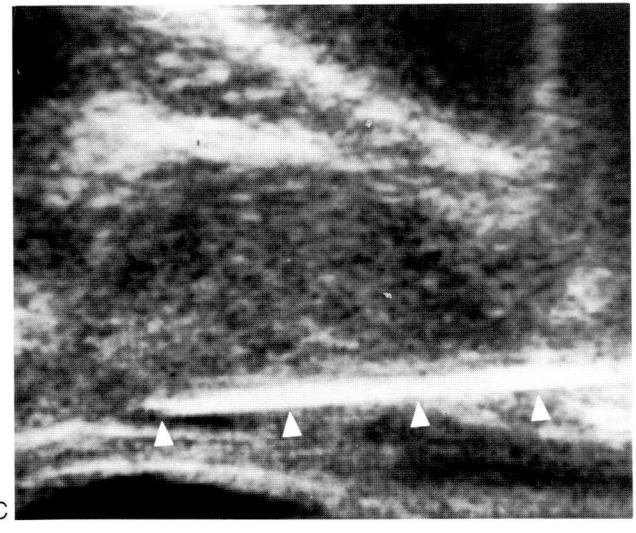

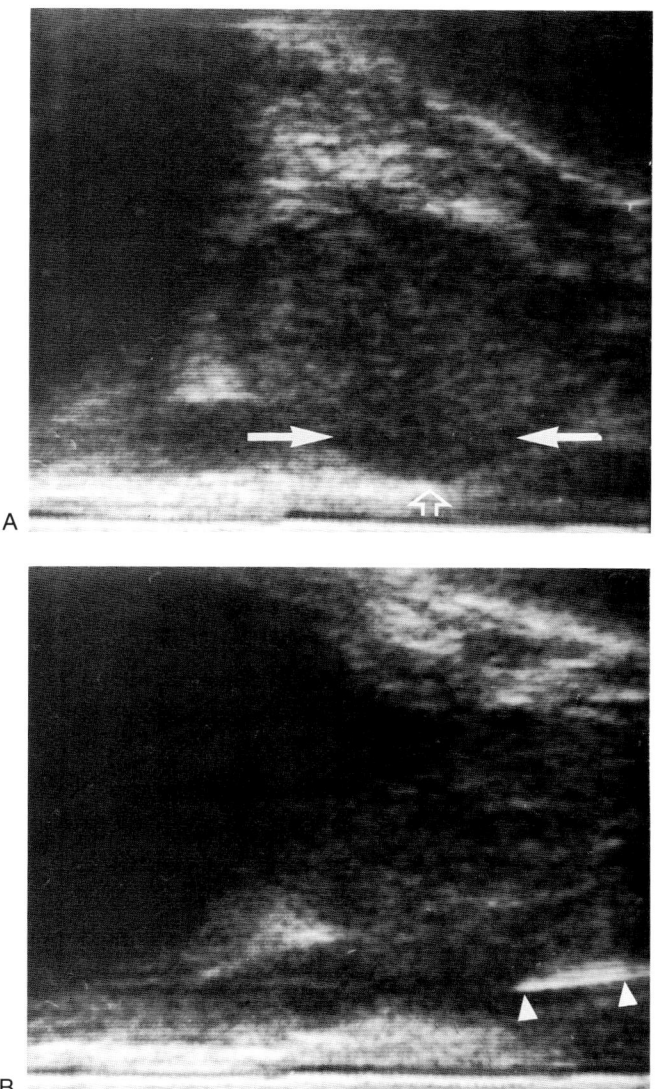

FIG. 8.14. Transperineal biopsy of isoechoic cancer. Endorectal ultrasound demonstrates a poorly defined isoechoic lesion (*arrows*) but with capsular distortion (*open arrow*) (**A**). Transperineal ultrasound guided biopsy demonstrates the biopsy needle (*arrowheads*) within the lesion (**B**).

FIG. 8.13. Transperineal biopsy of prostate cancer. A preliminary longitudinally oriented endorectal sonogram (**A**) demonstrates an 8-mm hypoechoic area (*arrows*) in the posterior portion of the prostate. Sequential images (**B** and **C**) show the biopsy needle (*arrowheads*) placed through the perineum and sequentially positioned into the lesion.

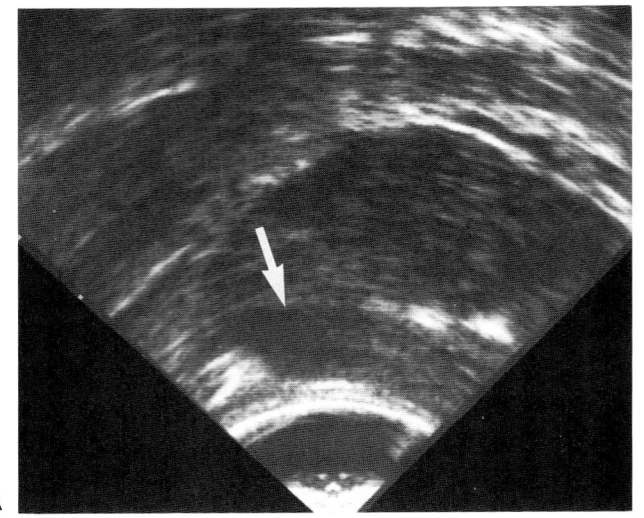

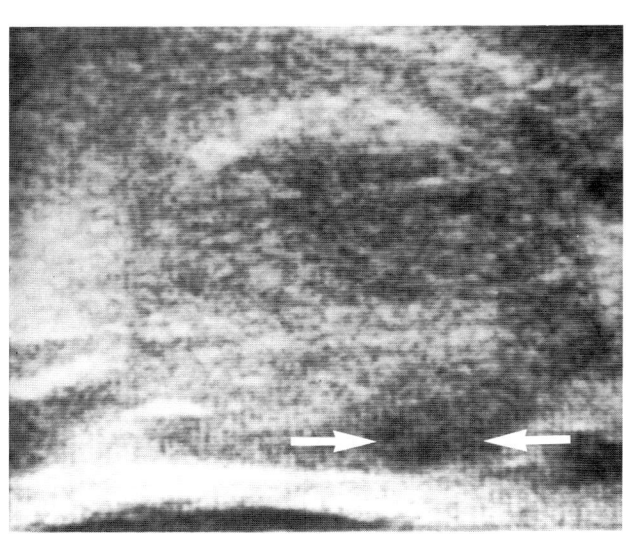

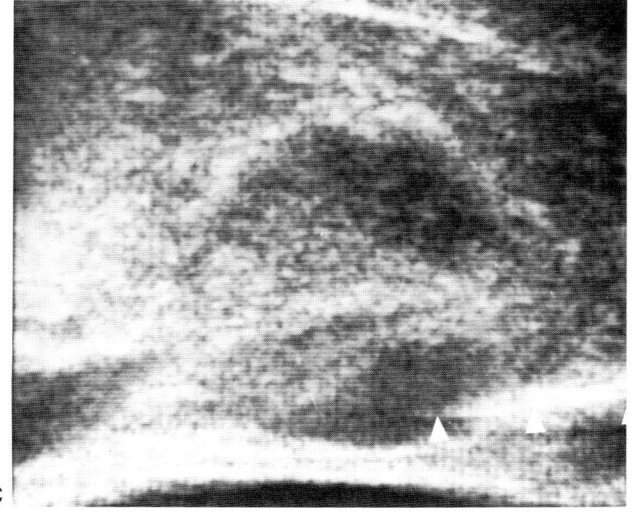

In general, the biopsy can be performed as follows:

1. A lesion is identified on a preliminary diagnostic endorectal sonogram.
2. The probe is removed.
3. The patient is evaluated to exclude a bleeding diathesis. The patient should not have ingested aspirin or other salicylates for 10 days prior to the biopsy. There should be no history of a bleeding diathesis.
4. Informed consent is obtained.
5. The patient is placed in lithotomy (or decubitus) position.
6. Antiseptic solution (i.e., Betadine) is applied to the perineal area.
7. Local anesthesia (1% lidocaine) is applied to the skin and subcutaneous tissues.
8. The transducer (with or without guide attached) is placed once again into the rectum.
9. The probe is rotated clockwise or counterclockwise to re-identify the lesion and is then fixed in that position. [For those biopsies utilizing a guide, the guide is fixed in position so that the probe is parallel to the mid-portion of the visualized section (i.e., a midline of the probe).]
10. A 22-gauge spinal needle is placed through the guide (or if the freehand technique is used, along the probe's parallel axis) into the already anesthetized subcutaneous tissues, and then anesthesia is given to the deeper soft tissues to the prostatic capsule.
11. With the lesion identified by ultrasound, the aspiration or biopsy needle is placed through the guide and into the prostate. (For freehand biopsies, the needle is placed in the perineum parallel to the crystals on the longitudinally oriented probe. One hand holds the probe, the other hand holds the needle.) When in the ultrasound image's field of view, the needle should be identified at all times.
12. For an aspiration cytology biopsy, the needle is then placed into the most caudad area of the lesion. Suction (from a tightly attached 20-cc syringe) is applied, and the needle is carefully moved gently in an in-out and side-to-side fashion without relieving suction. When completed, the suction should be released very slowly, and the needle should be removed. The material obtained should be expressed immediately onto a slide, and smears should be made. The remainder of the aspirate should be preserved for a cell block.
13. For a core biopsy, the needle should be placed just caudad to the lesion (as described in step 12); then, under conventional sonographic guidance, the biopsy is performed. The material obtained by biopsy should be "fixed" in formalin.

The sagittal orientation allows identification of the exact site of tissue extraction so that even small areas of sonographic abnormality can be clearly identified and biopsied (Figs. 8.13–8.15). Both larger (less than 22-gauge) and smaller (i.e., 22-gauge) needles can clearly and consistently be identified.

The use of a biplane probe permits rapid sweeping back and forth to identify the lesion and confirm the position of the biopsy needle in both planes (Fig. 8.16).

While freehand biopsy with core devices have been utilized, new devices (Fig. 8.12) have been utilized with trigger action plungers so that a core can be obtained in a "flash". This equipment has allowed transperineal biopsies to be performed on an outpatient basis with

FIG. 8.15. Transperineal biopsy of peripherally oriented prostatic cancer. Axially oriented sonogram (**A**) demonstrates a hypoechoic cancer in the right peripheral region (*arrow*). The lesion is also identified (*arrows*) in the longitudinally oriented sonogram (**B**). Transperineal biopsy demonstrates the needle (*arrowhead*) within the lesion during biopsy (**C**).

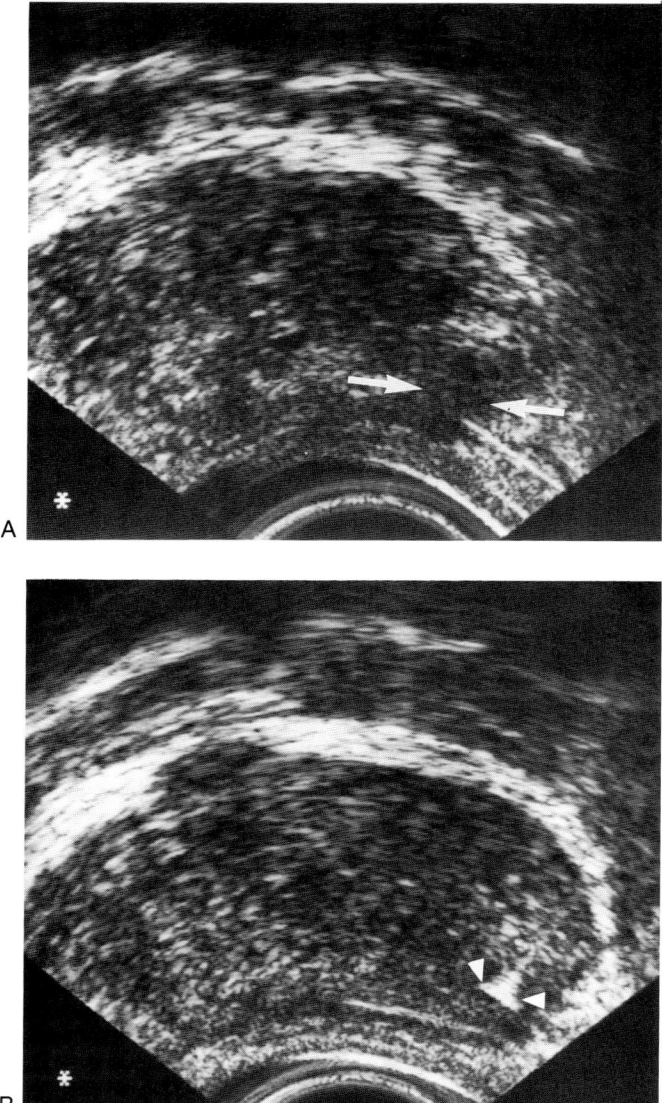

FIG. 8.16. Transperineal biopsy performed using a biplane transducer. Axially oriented ultrasound examination (**A**) demonstrates a relatively hypoechoic asymmetrically oriented lesion (*arrows*) in the left lateral aspect of the prostate. Biopsy needle (*arrowheads*) is placed into the lesion, and the needle with reverberations is seen in the axial orientation (**B**).

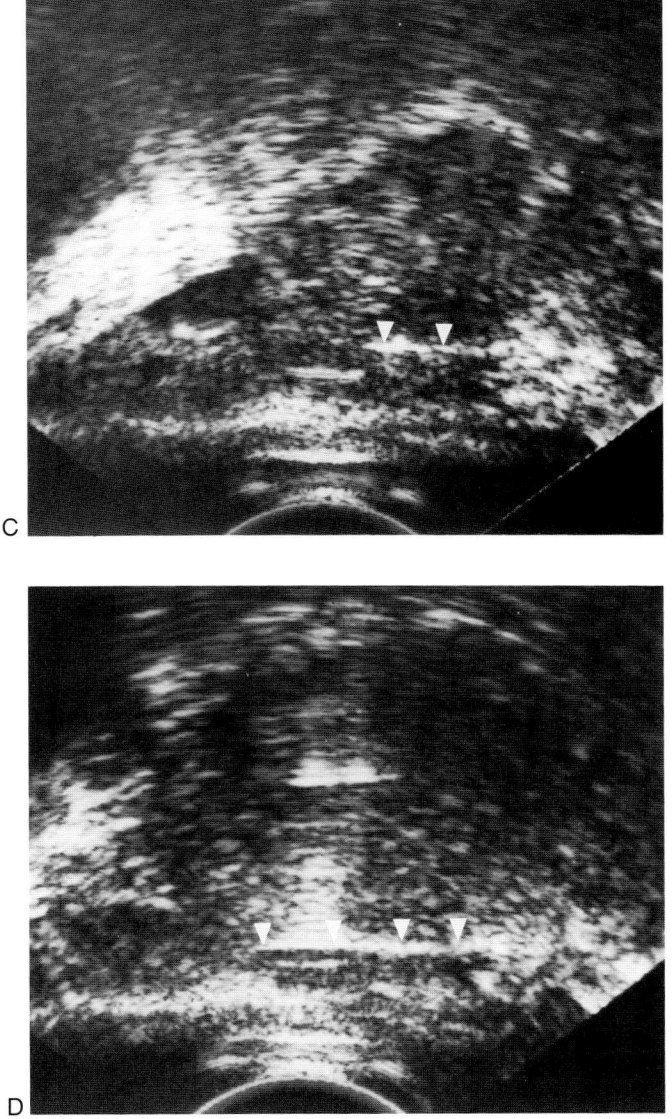

FIG. 8.16. *Continued.* The biopsy needle (*arrowheads*) is seen sequentially entering the lesion in the longitudinally oriented sector scan image (**C** and **D**). (Courtesy of Dr. Peter Cooperberg.)

no sedation or general anesthesia and with only a minimal amount of local anesthesia applied to the perineum. Major benefits, besides accuracy, include:

1. The ability to perform the biopsy easily and more accurately without the need for assistance. This eliminates the need for the occasional "third hand".
2. Significant reduction in the amount of time needed for the biopsy. The core biopsy needle is usually positioned in the patient for only a few seconds.

TRANSRECTAL BIOPSY

The transrectal approach using ultrasound guidance can also be performed (Fig. 8.17) (257,260,261). Specially produced instruments that can be placed over the endorectal probe (Figs. 8.18–8.20) and guide the biopsy needle have been made and are available for the sagittally oriented endorectal probes. Probes have also been developed with a biopsy hole placed into the instrument (Fig. 8.21). A complex arrangement of sterile preparation of the equipment is necessary, and each device has different requirements. This technique has been shown to be highly successful for biopsying the small, peripherally oriented lesion.

The biopsy is performed as follows:

1. The patient is given prebiopsy antibotics and a cleaning enema.
2. A preliminary sonogram is performed to demonstrate the lesion.
3. The endorectal probe is prepared with the biopsy guide.
4. The patient is placed in either the lithotomy or the decubitus position.
5. The probe is placed in the rectum.
6. The probe is angled until the line of sight of needle insertion is visualized on the screen and is appropriate to biopsy the abnormality.
7. Under sonographic guidance, the needle is placed through the guide into the lesion (Figs. 8.22–8.24).

Either core or cytology aspirate biopsies can be performed with this technique. No anesthesia is required.

A major benefit of the transrectal approach is the decrease in patient discomfort. No anesthesia is needed. The one problem of the technique is the increased risk of sepsis (reported in up to 2% of all patients biopsied) (257). However, reported results also show that the rate of complication is increased compared to the transperineal approach (257,407–411). For example, the incidence of hematuria is up to 37% of cases, the incidence of blood in bowel movement is 9.4%, and the incidence of hematospermia is about 5% (257).

COMPARISON OF THE TRANSPERINEAL WITH THE TRANSRECTAL APPROACH

Both the transperineal and the transrectal approach to endorectal sonographic guided biopsy of the prostate are accurate. However, each has benefits (Table 8.1), limitations, and complications (Table 8.2). They include the following:

1. *Accuracy.* Both techniques are equally accurate in obtaining tissue from a specific area (257).
2. *Patient positioning.* The transperineal approach is usually simpler to perform in the lithotomy position. The transrectal biopsy can be performed in either the lithotomy or the decubitus position.

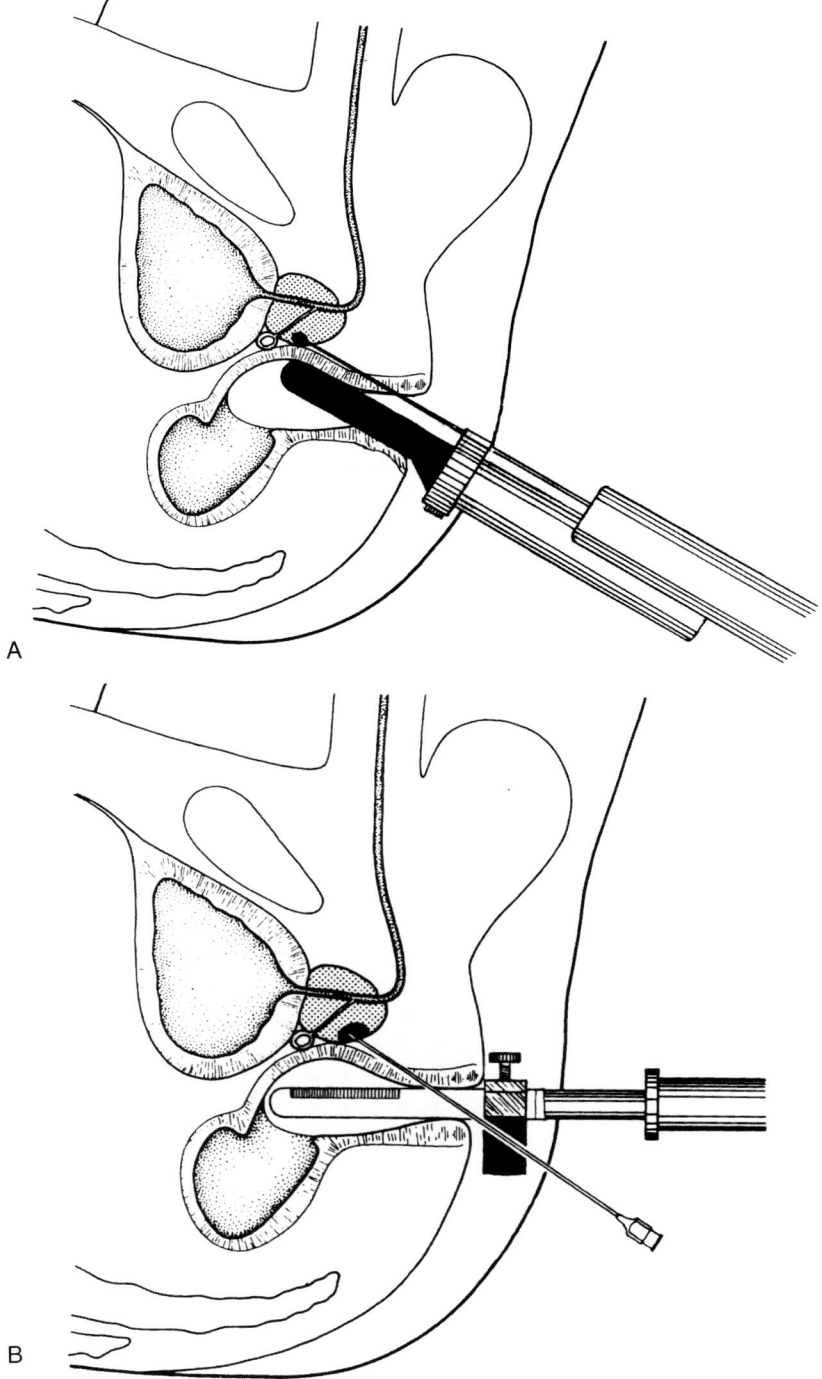

FIG. 8.17. Diagram demonstrating transrectal biopsy. Transrectal biopsies can be used with ultrasound guidance. These diagrams demonstrate different types of guidance. Devices have been developed for use with longitudinally oriented sector-scan (**A**) and linear-array (**B**) transducers.

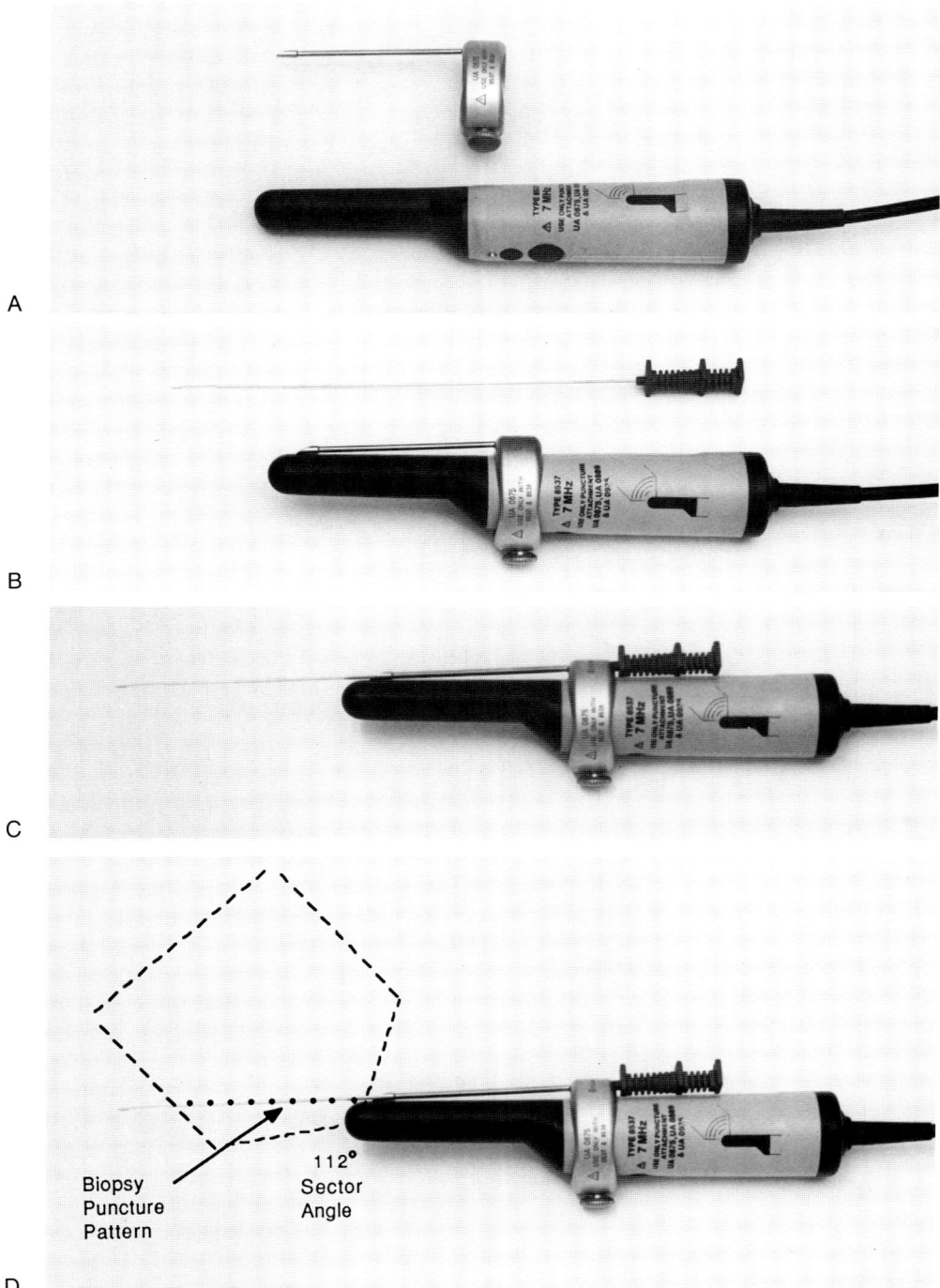

FIG. 8.18. Transrectal biopsy guide system. A specially produced transrectal biopsy guide is seen adjacent to an endorectal sector-scan transducer (**A**). The guide has been placed on the transducer, and the Biopty needle can be seen adjacent to the transducer–guide complex (**B**). The needle has been placed into the guide (**C**). The line of site, as visualized on the ultrasound image, is seen with a line-diagram overlay (**D**). (Part D, courtesy of Bruel & Kjaer, Marlborough, Massachusetts.)

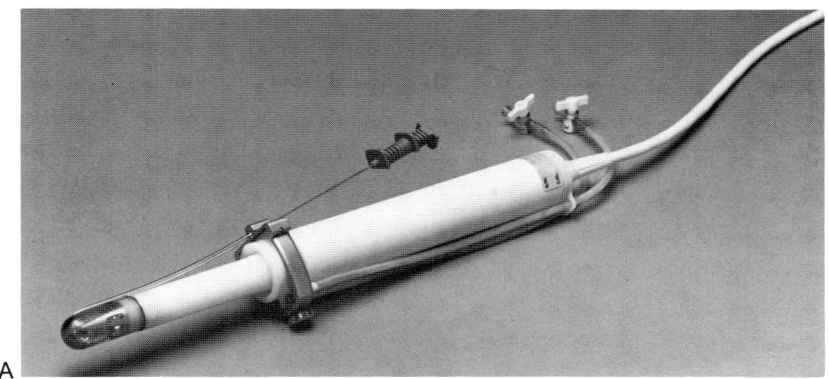

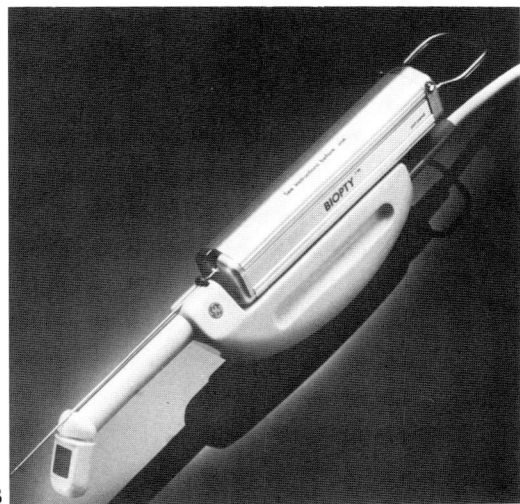

FIG. 8.19. Endorectal-ultrasound–transrectal-guide complex. **A:** A biplane endorectal ultrasound transducer with an attached transrectal biopsy guide with the Biopty needle in position. **B:** A sagittally oriented single-plane probe with an offset transducer with Biopty trigger device and needle in place. (Part A, courtesy of Teknar, Inc., Fenton, Missouri; part B, courtesy of General Electric, Milwaukee, Wisconsin.)

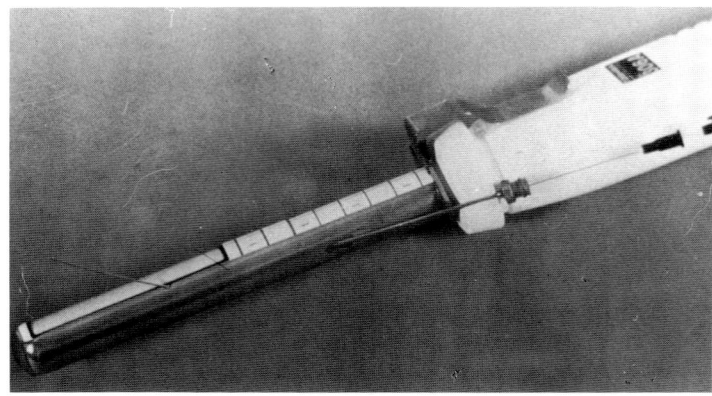

FIG. 8.20. Transrectal aspiration biopsy. A specially produced guide has been manufactured to be placed over a longitudinally oriented linear-array transducer. It has been produced so that a flexible needle (20-gauge or smaller) can be placed through the guide and will curve so that a transrectal biopsy of the prostate can be performed.

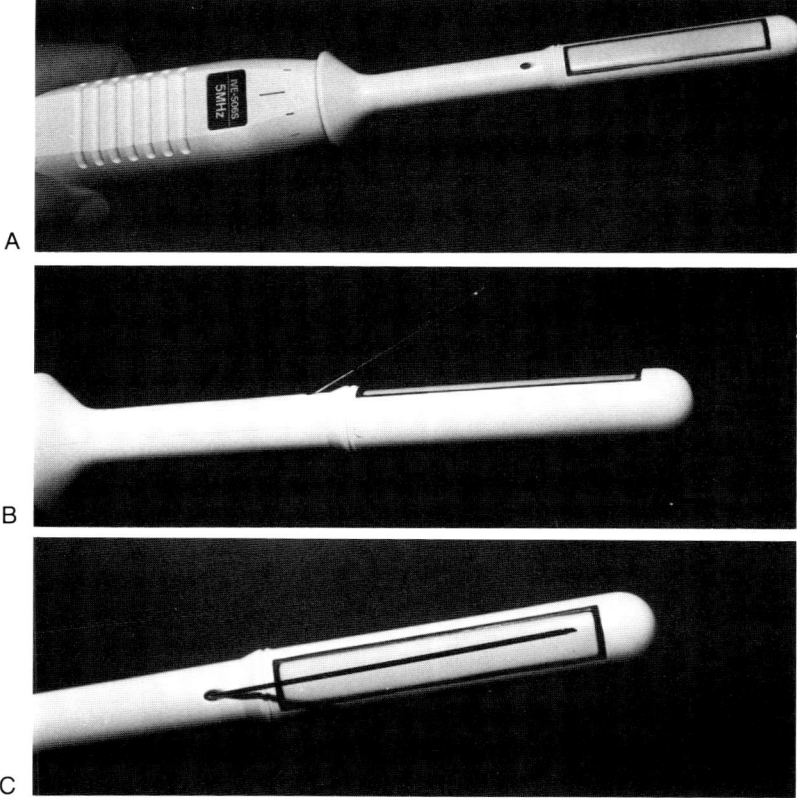

FIG. 8.21. Transrectal biopsy performed using a linear-array transducer. A longitudinally oriented linear-array transducer has been manufactured with a hole situated within the probe, proximal to the transducer crystals (**A**). The needle can be placed through the probe (**B**) and will enter the prostate obliquely oriented but parallel to the midline of the beam width of the transducers (**C**).

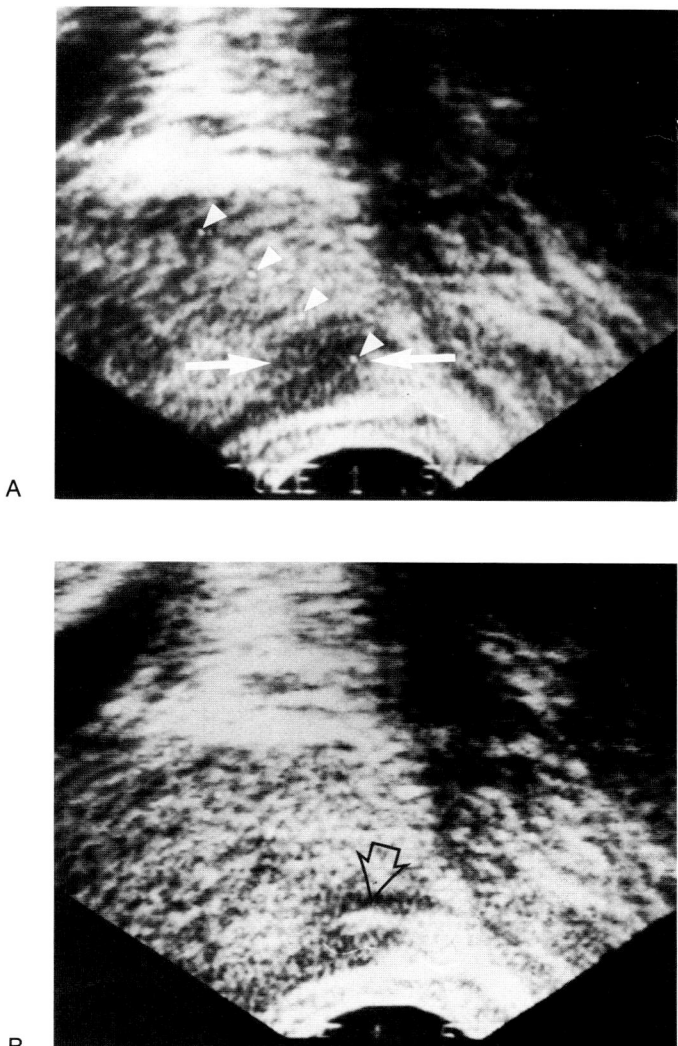

FIG. 8.22. Transrectal biopsy. Endorectal ultrasound with a longitudinally oriented sector scan demonstrates a hypoechoic lesion (*arrows*) in the apex of the prostate. The line of site of the biopsy needle placement (*arrowheads*) is identified (**A**). The biopsy needle (*open arrowhead*) is then identified during the biopsy (**B**).

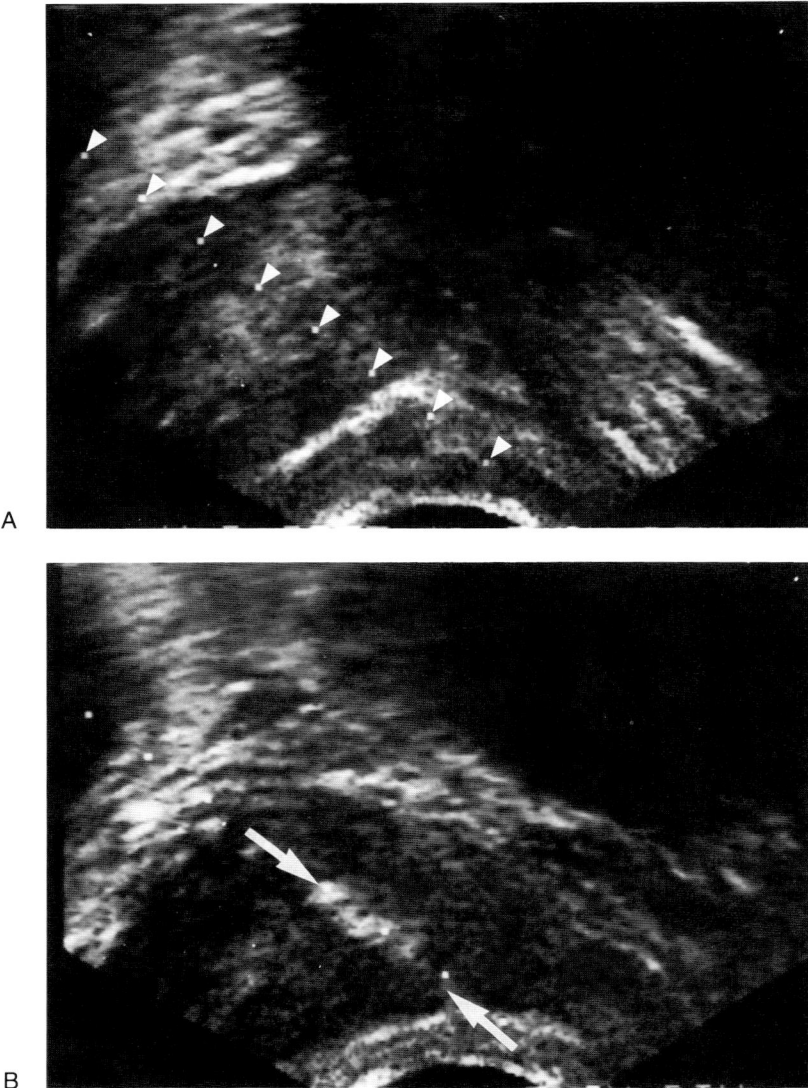

FIG. 8.23. Transrectal biopsy. Longitudinally oriented sector-scan image of the prostate demonstrates the line of site (*arrowheads*) that the biopsy needle will follow (**A**). The biopsy needle (*arrows*) is identified during biopsy (**B**).

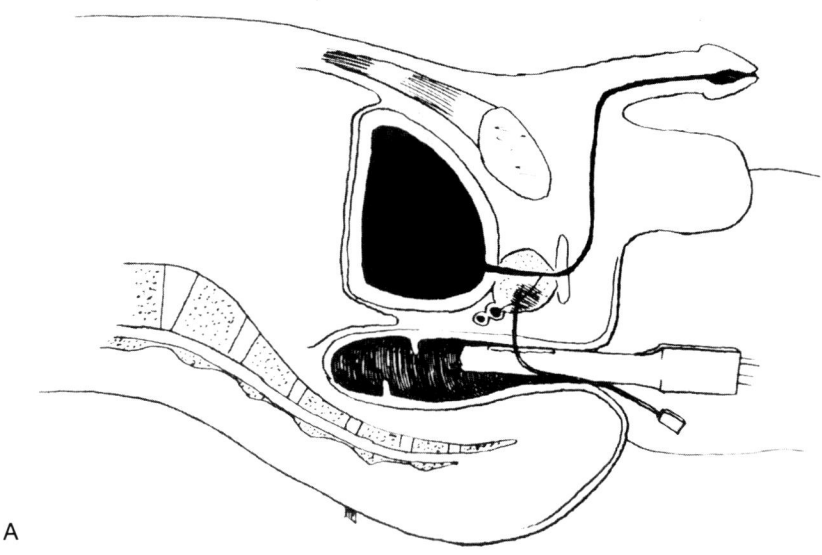

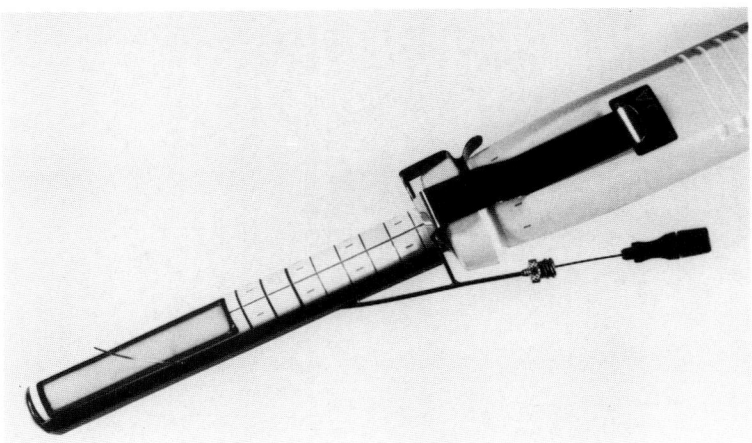

FIG. 8.24. Transrectal biopsy. **A:** Diagram of the transrectal biopsy using a curvable needle. **B:** The biopsy needle placed through the guide is identified. **C** and **D:** Sequential scans obtained during biopsy show the biopsy needle (*arrowheads*) positioned into the lesion to be biopsied (*arrows*). (Parts C and D, courtesy of Dr. Rainer Otto.)

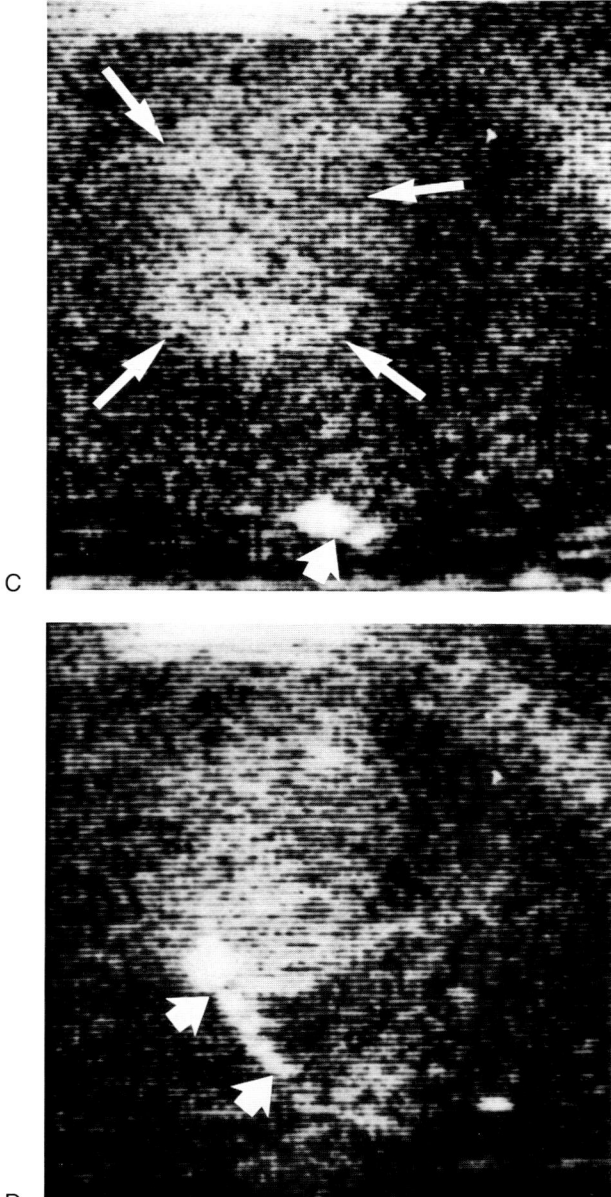

FIG. 8.24. Continued.

Table 8.1. Comparison of the benefits of transrectal versus transperineal sonographic guided biopsy[a]

Transrectal approach	Transperineal approach
No anesthesia required	Local anesthesia required; minimal patient discomfort may be experienced
Accurate biopsy	Accurate biopsy
Multiple sites can be biopsied at one sitting	Requires more anesthesia to biopsy multiple sites

[a]Data from refs. 257 and 407–411.

Table 8.2. Comparison of complications of transrectal and transperineal sonographic guided biopsy

Complication	Incidence (%) in transrectal approach[a]	Incidence (%) in transperineal approach[b]
Hematuria	37	2
Blood in bowel movement	9.4	0
Blood in ejaculate	5.0	0
Sepsis	2.0	0
Vasovagal reaction	Complication not reported	1

[a]Data from ref. 257.
[b]Data from refs. 407–411.

3. *Complications* (Table 8.2). The transurethral approach appears to have a significantly higher incidence of hematuria, blood in bowel and ejaculate, and sepsis. The transperineal approach has a minimally increased risk for a vasovagal reaction. Except for sepsis, these are usually not clinically significant complications.

CONCLUSIONS

Sonographically guided biopsy is not necessarily indicated for palpable lesions (391). However, when a palpable mass is biopsied by conventional means, repeat biopsy with ultrasound guidance may be indicated (407–411). Also, subtly or nonpalpable lesions may have to be biopsied with endorectal sonographic control.

The type of biopsy is, in general, a matter of preference. Both the transperineal and transrectal approaches appear to be equally accurate. Although the number of complications increases with the transrectal approach, these may not be clinically significant. The approach used should be according the individual's preference.

9 // Prostate Cancer: General Considerations

General Statistics 141
Pathogenesis 144
  Age
  Genetic, Racial, and National Predisposition
  Hormonal Influence
  Effects of Benign Prostatic Hyperplasia
  Environmental Factors
  Infectious Agents
Anatomy of Cancer Development 146
Prostate Cancer Classification 146
Grading Systems 146
Staging 148
  Whitmore-Jewett Staging System
  TNM Staging System
  Updated TNM Staging System
  Revised TNM Staging System
Patterns of Dissemination 154
Significant Versus Insignificant (Incidental) Carcinoma 155
Prostate Cancer Growth and Metastatic Potential 155
Conclusion 155

GENERAL STATISTICS

Prostate cancer is a pervasive disease, particularly in the United States and other western countries. The death rate varies from country to country, with the highest age-adjusted rates found in Sweden, Norway, Australia, United States, and Canada (Fig. 9.1) (72).

In the United States alone, the number of newly diagnosed cancers has increased dramatically. For example, in 1984, 75,000 new cases were reported; in 1985, 76,000 new cases; in 1986, 90,000 new cases; and in 1987, 96,000 new cases (Fig. 9.2) (451–461). The absolute number of men with prostate cancer probably has not increased. However, detection has improved. The mortality rate has also increased, although not proportionally. In 1983, there were 24,100 deaths in the United States from prostate cancer; in 1985, 25,000 deaths were reported; in 1986, 26,000; and in 1987, 27,000 (Fig. 9.2). Thus, one must realize that the number of deaths has not risen as rapidly as has the increased detection rate. It is obvious that there are many cancers that may affect an individual but will not cause a significant risk to his life.

Cancer of the prostate may also have some racial predilection. The age-adjusted mortality rate for the Negro male population in the United States has been estimated to be 50% higher than that for Caucasians (Fig. 9.3) (72,88). Other studies have shown similar results in that both the incidence and mortality in Negroes is twice that of Caucasian males (72).

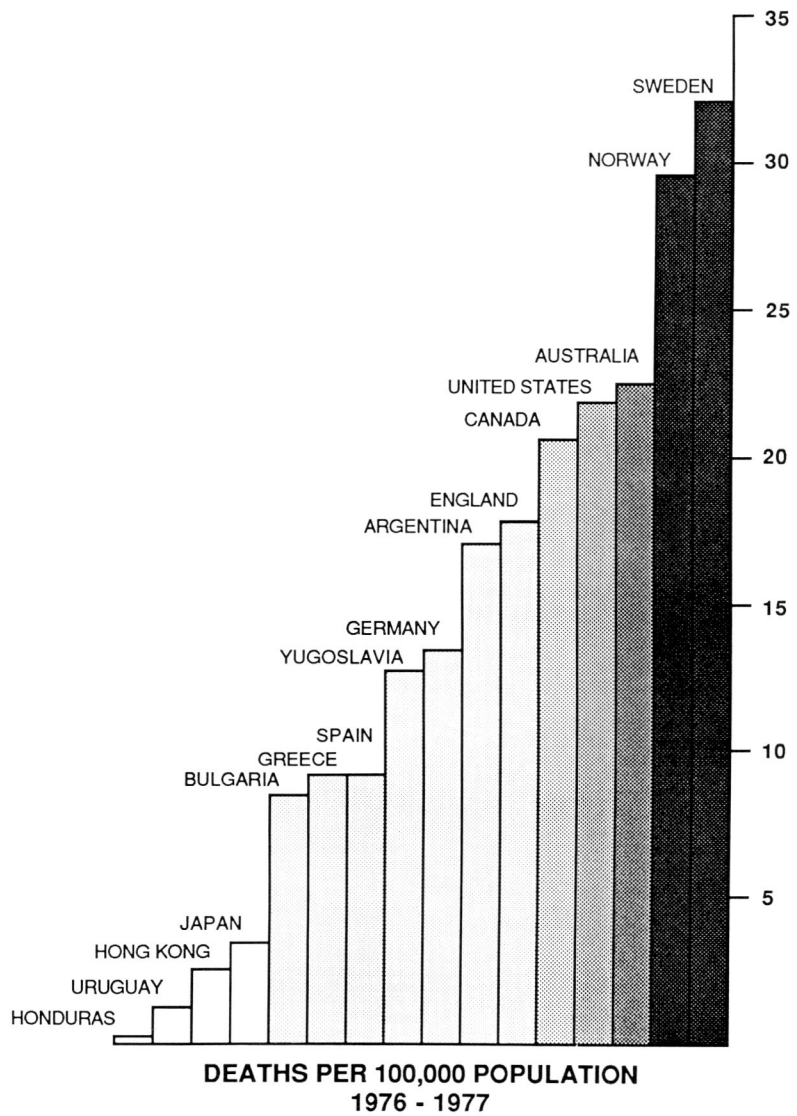

FIG. 9.1. Age-adjusted death rates due to prostatic cancer. This chart demonstrates the age-adjusted death rate per 100,000 males from prostatic cancer. (Adapted from ref. 72.)

When discussing the statistics of cancer, one must be aware of certain terms:

1. *Prevalence.* The prevalence of cancer is the number of existing cases at any one time. In the United States, the prevalence of prostatic cancer is not clearly known.

2. *Incidence.* The incidence of cancer is the total number of new cases reported per year per 100,000 population. In the United States, it was calculated at 69 cases per 100,000 males per year in 1981 (554). Although the incidence has probably not increased, the clinical diagnosis has dramatically increased.

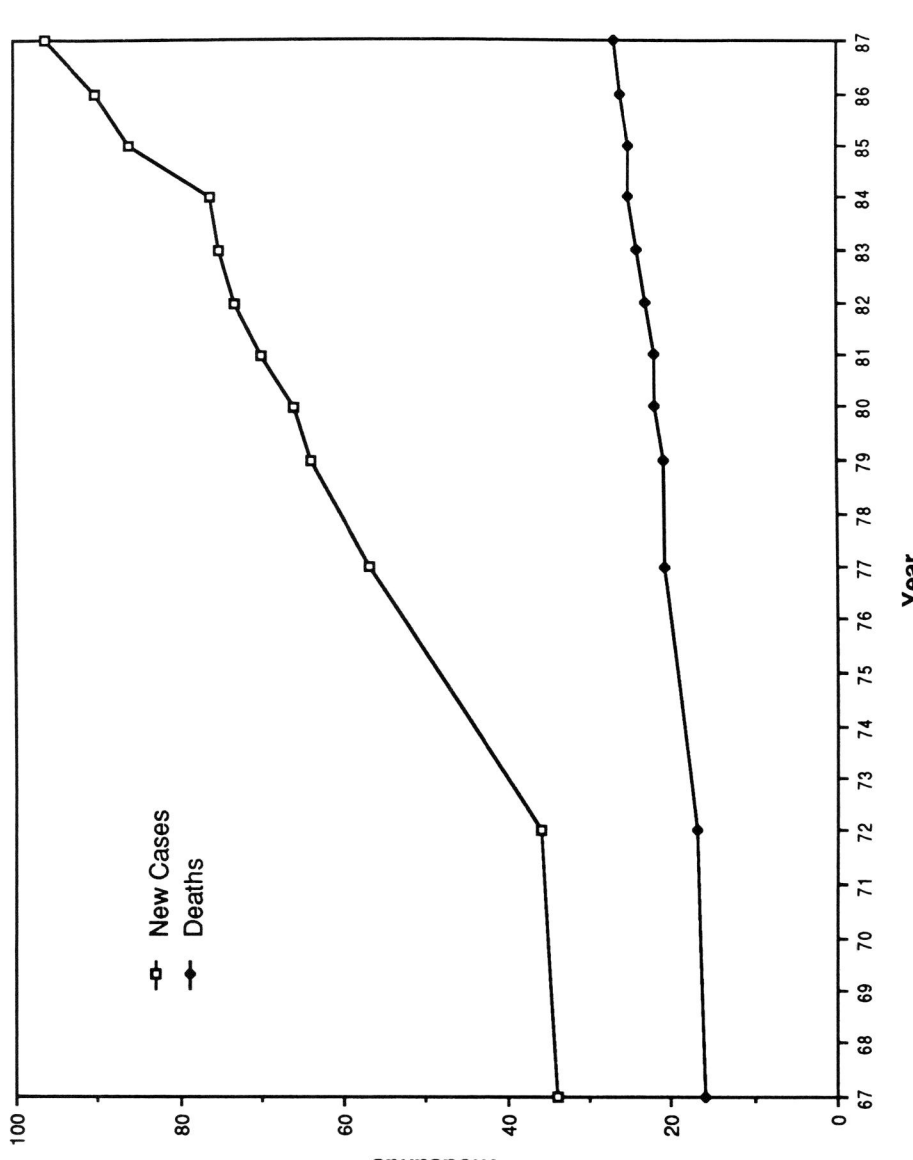

FIG. 9.2. Diagnosed cases versus deaths due to prostatic cancer. This chart demonstrates the increasing number of newly diagnosed cases of prostate cancer per year between 1967 and 1987 in the United States and the number of deaths in the United States attributed to prostate cancer. (Adapted from refs. 451–461.)

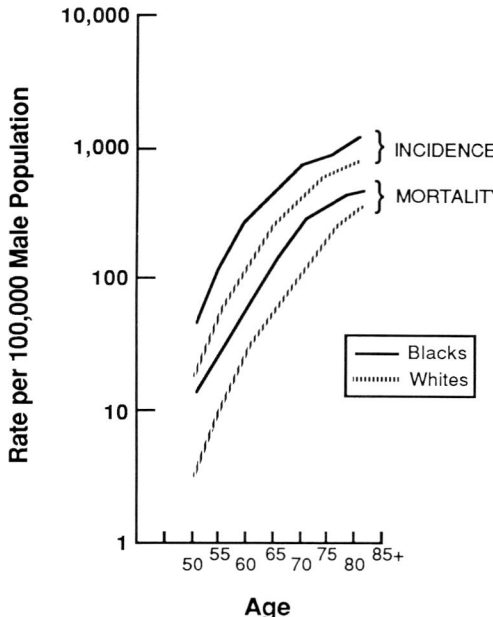

FIG. 9.3. Mortality of prostate cancer by race. This chart demonstrates the incidence and mortality per 100,000 men for Negro and Caucasian males in the United States. (Adapted from ref. 72.)

3. *Mortality.* The mortality rate is the number of deaths due to cancer per year per 100,000 population. In the United States, it was reported in 1981 to be 18.8 deaths per 100,000 males.

PATHOGENESIS

There have been a variety of suggested causes for prostate cancer, none of which is completely clear or accurate. These include: (a) age; (b) genetic, racial, or national predisposition; (c) hormonal influence; (d) effects of benign prostatic hyperplasia; (e) environmental exposure; and (f) infectious agents.

Age

The increased incidence of prostate cancer is associated with aging. It is an uncommon malignancy in young men, particularly in those under 50 years. It is quite common in the elderly male population.

Some autopsy studies have shown that as many as 30% to 40% of all men over 60 years of age harbor a prostate cancer (58,208,326,442). Many of these are only obvious on microscopic analysis.

Genetic, Racial, and National Predisposition

The incidence of clinically obvious cancer varies greatly. Some studies have suggested that Orientals are the least affected race (52,553). Others have demonstrated that the incidence is similar in all races and that clinically obvious cancer is less common, but the occult lesion is more common, in Orientals (215).

While the exact incidence is unclear, the age-adjusted incidence of mortality for the American black male is significantly higher than for the American white male (43).

Hormonal Influence

The importance, but not the exact extent, of endogenous hormonal influence appears to be relatively strong. The following documented facts to support this hypothesis include:

1. Most prostate cancers are androgen-dependent.
2. Eunuchs do not develop prostate cancer.
3. Cancer can be induced in rats if hormones (estrogen and androgen) are administered for a long period of time.
4. Cancer is associated with sclerotic prostatic atrophy (317).

Effects of Benign Prostatic Hyperplasia

There have been studies to suggest that benign prostatic hyperplasia is an inciting factor for malignancy (18). Other studies have shown the opposite (170). In general, prostate cancer is a disease of the elderly. Benign prostatic hyperplasia is also a disease of the older male population (see Chapter 12). Thus, although there may be a large percentage of patients with both processes, there does not appear to be a significant increased risk for developing prostate cancer in the presence of benign prostatic hyperplasia.

Environmental Factors

There appears to be some inciting environmental factors for the development of prostate cancer. Although there have been minor variations within various regions in the United States (43), this is not the most compelling evidence. The most important studies have shown that while prostate cancer is unusual in Japanese individuals living in Japan, males of Oriental descent living in the United States have cancer risks equivalent to the native American population (109). Similar findings have shown an increased risk for European immigrants (475).

The exact etiology of these environmental studies has not been clearly delineated, although exposure to environmental contaminants (e.g., air pollution, cadamine fertilizer, etc.) (548), cigarette smoking (552), and a high-fat diet (43) have been implicated.

Infectious Agents

Conflicting evidence has been demonstrated with regard to possible venereal causes of prostate cancer. Sexual precocity has been implicated as a cause of increased risk for prostate cancer (441,476). The converse has also been shown, i.e., that there is no increased risk with decreased sexual activity (420). Studies (441) have shown increased risks for the unmarried man, while other studies (552) have shown a higher risk of developing cancer in those men having fathered several children. One study (419) has shown that Catholic priests develop prostate cancer with a slightly higher incidence than similar age-controlled groups. Thus it seems that there is little consistent evidence; in fact, there are contradictory data which suggest that sexual activity, or possibly venereal disease processes, can not be adequately implicated in the development of prostate cancer.

Prostatitis and development of prostatic calculi have also been implicated in the development of prostate cancer (552), although many men have similar clinical and pathologic findings without the presence of malignancy.

ANATOMY OF CANCER DEVELOPMENT

There has been a great deal of controversy regarding the exact site of prostate cancer development. Prior to the late 1960s it was assumed that most cancers originated in the posterior portion of the prostate. This was suggested because it was the only area of possible palpation.

Anatomical research has refined this concept, and much of the newer and accepted ideas stem from McNeal's research (296–306). The origin of cancer is often related to the histology of the prostate. Cancer often originates selectively in the peripheral zone of the acinar tissues, but it can also arise (although less frequently) from the central zone of the acinar tissues and the transition zone. This has been broken down by McNeal as follows:

1. 70% of cancers originate *de novo* in the peripheral zone;
2. 10% of cancers originate *de novo* in the central zone;
3. 20% of cancers originate *de novo* in the transition zone (308).

Of those cancers developing in the peripheral zone, the anterior lateral and lateral cancers (originating in the anterolateral and lateral aspects of the peripheral zone) are almost as common as the posterior tumors.

Cancers arising medially are from the transition zone and often develop from areas also involved by benign prostatic hyperplasia.

PROSTATE CANCER CLASSIFICATION

The majority of prostate cancers are epithelial-type adenocarcinomas and account for over 95% of malignant tumors. In addition to the epithelial tumors, there are also nonepithelial tumors, including rhabdomyosarcoma, leiomyosarcoma, and a variety of others (i.e., carcinoid tumors, carcinosarcoma, and malignant melanoma). A small subgroup of other malignancies can also affect the prostate (Table 9.1).

GRADING SYSTEMS

The grading systems used for evaluation of prostate cancer are usually dependent upon the degree of cellular differentiation and/or anaplasia. The type of glandular pattern (151,500), the differentiation of nuclear anaplasia (320,321), and the clarity of cell borders (117) are independent variables. All correlate, to varying degrees, with the risk of death due to cancer. There are various types of grading systems that try to evaluate the variables involved in determining the invasiveness and the prognosis for individuals with prostate cancer.

The Gleason system (152) takes into consideration the degree of glandular differentiation and dedifferentiation as well as the relationship of the glandular tissue to prostatic stroma as seen under a low-powered magnification. Histologically, there are five distinct grades. Tumor grading ranges from 1 through 5. These calculations are based on the number ''1'' being assigned to well-differentiated tumors, with the number ''5'' being assigned to an

Table 9.1. World Health Organization histologic classification of malignant prostate tumors[a]

Epithelial
    Adenocarcinoma
        Small acinar
        Large acinar
        Cribiform
        Solid/trabecular
        Other
    Transitional-cell carcinoma
    Squamous-cell carcinoma
    Undifferentiated carcinoma
Nonepithelial
    Rhabdomyosarcoma
    Leiomyosarcoma
Miscellaneous
    Carcinoid
    Carcinosarcoma
    Malignant melanoma
    Phyllode tumor

[a]Adapted from ref. 72.

anaplastic lesion (Fig. 9.4). Intermediate numbers are assigned to moderately differentiated tumors. A Gleason score is calculated by adding a first or primary grade (which is the predominant degree of anaplasia) to a secondary grade (which is the less representative area of differentiation). Thus, Gleason grading can range from scores of 2 to 10. Some utilize the Gleason system by further adding the tumor stage of the tumor (see the following section, entitled "Staging") for a grading "sum" or total for a "final" Gleason score. Stage A tumors receive a grade of 1, stage B tumors receive a grade of 2, stage C tumors receive a grade of 3, and stage D tumors receive a grade of 5.

The Mostofi system (320,321) considers cellular anaplasia, the glandular pattern, and the relationship of the stroma to the glandular tissue. Grade I tumors show slight nuclear anaplasia and well-defined tumor glands. Grade II tumors also have well-defined tumor glands but only a moderate amount of nuclear anaplasia. The grade III tumors (the most severe tumors) have no glandular formation, and there is marked nuclear anaplasia.

The Gaeta (140) grading system considers the same characteristics as the Mostofi system. However, within this system there are four grades, but only the most severe elements or more severely involved areas are categorized if present in at least one-third of the specimen.

The Mayo Clinic grading system (500) considers a variety of factors, including the acinar structure, nuclear characteristics, presence of nucleoli, the characteristics of the cytoplasm, mitotic activity, and invasiveness. Tumors are graded from 1 (the mildest) to 4 (the most severe).

The MD Anderson Hospital grading system (MDA) (51) evaluates tumors in accordance with the percentage of tumor glandular formation. There are three major categories in this group. Grade I tumors are the best differentiated, and grade III tumors are the most anaplastic histologically.

The Diamond system (102) uses computerized analysis, and grading is dependent upon nuclear roundness.

A limitation of all grading systems is the size of the core of the biopsy. The biopsy may be indicative of only a small section of the tumor and not of the entire cancer.

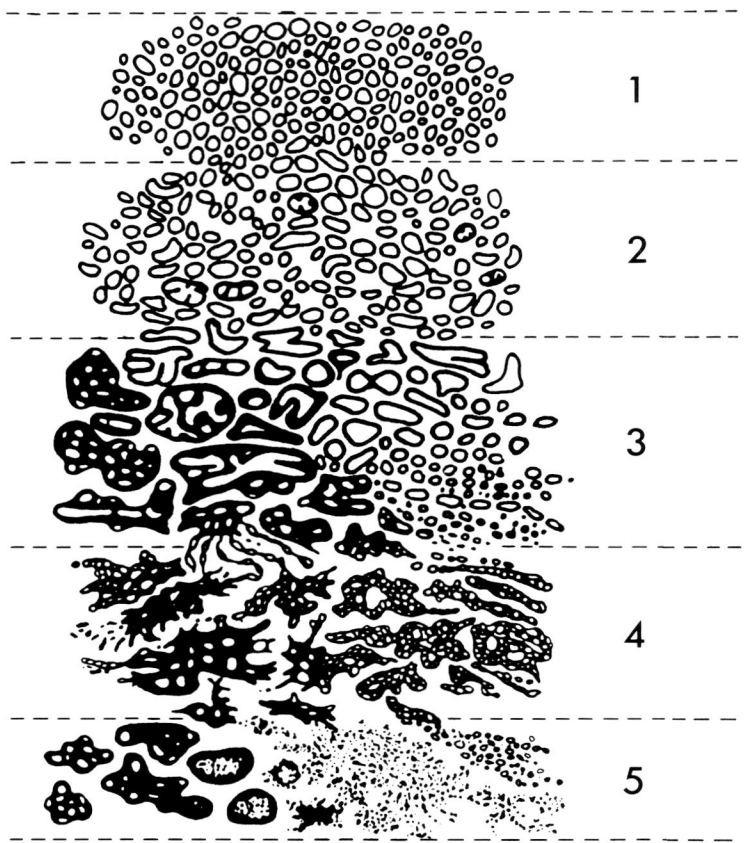

FIG. 9.4. Gleason grading system. This diagram demonstrates typical histological appearances for well-differentiated (Gleason grade 1) to anaplastic (Gleason grade 5) prostatic cancer. (Adapted from ref. 72.)

Aspiration biopsies can certainly diagnose cancer accurately. While some good results have been reported in grading the tumor with cytology (119), the grading of the tumor may be less accurate (275) than the core biopsy.

STAGING

Although many staging systems have been devised, the one most commonly used in the United States is the Jewett-modified Whitmore system (220), also known as the Whitmore-Jewett staging system. The other frequently used system is a TNM system which has been adopted by the American Joint Committee for Cancer Staging and End Results Reporting (510).

Whitmore-Jewett Staging System

In the Whitmore-Jewett staging system, tumors are classified according to four stages (A through D) (Fig. 9.5). There are many variations of this system and only the most commonly used will be discussed.

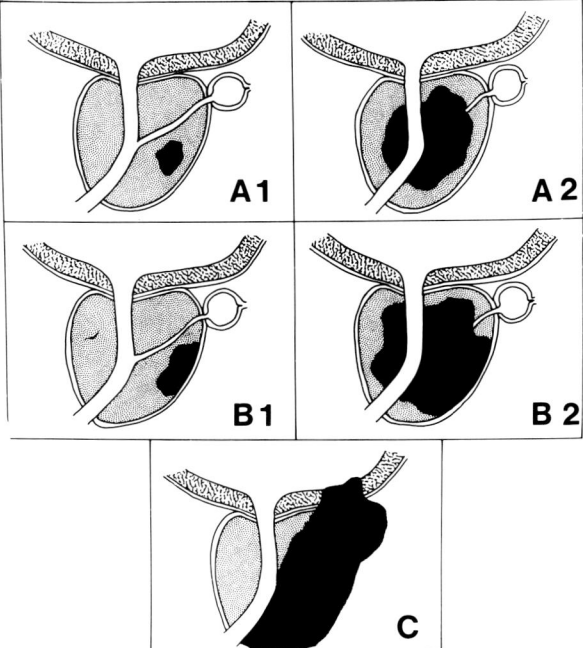

FIG. 9.5. Stages of prostate cancer. The diagram delineates stages of prostate cancer. The cancers (*black areas*) are broken down into stage A (nonpalpable), stage B (palpable but not through the capsule), and stage C (invasion through the capsule and/or into seminal vesicles) lesions.

Stage A tumors are clinically nonpalpable and clinically unsuspected. These tumors are divided into focal lesions (stage A1) and diffuse disease (stage A2) and are usually diagnosed on specimens obtained by a transurethral resection. The stage A1 lesions have only a few chips (less than 5%) of specimen with cancer. Additionally, these are histologically well-differentiated. If anaplastic, they are staged as A2 lesions. Where there is a more substantial amount (greater than 5% of the specimen) of tumor, regardless of cellular differentiation, these cancers are staged as A2 tumors. A subset of researchers feel that a stage A1 lesion may be a nondiffuse lesion that can be larger than a few chips of cancer. They have divided the focal (A1) lesions into two groups: One has a small, single focus of cancer (stage A1F); the other is larger and has cancer involving only one segment of the prostate (stage A1). In general, the stage A tumors may theoretically be cancers that originate in the transition zone.

Stage B tumors are palpable on digital rectal examination and are confined to the prostate without extension through the capsule. These have also been divided into (a) focal involvement less than 2 cm in size and involving one side of the gland (stage B1) and (b) diffuse involvement (stage B2). Some feel that the focal lesion can be subdivided into a single focal lesion less than 1 cm in size (stage B1N) or a more irregular (and perhaps larger) focus involving one side of the prostate (stage B1).

Stage C tumors are palpable and have extended beyond the prostatic capsule, but there are no distant metastases. These may be subclassified into stage C1 (minimal extracapsular involvement) and stage C2 (more extensive extracapsular tumor, perhaps producing bladder outlet obstruction or ureteral dilatation due to obstruction). The C2 stage can also involve the seminal vesicles.

Stage D tumors have metastasized to distant areas; this category has various subclassifications. Stage D0 tumors are found in those patients who have normal bone scans but have persistently elevated serum acid phosphatase levels. Stage D1 tumors are found in those patients who have been previously staged clinically as stage A, B, or C but who, following either an operation or aspiration biopsy, have metastatic pelvic lymph-node involvement. Stage D2 tumors are diagnosed in patients having clinical evidence of distant metastases to bone, lymph nodes, or elsewhere prior to initial surgical exploration. Occasionally a stage D3 subcategory is included. These are found in patients who have had a previously staged and treated D2 lesion but have relapsed following hormonal treatment.

TNM Staging System

In the TNM staging system, T evaluation refers to tumor stage, N refers to lymph-node involvement, and M is used to categorize distant metastases. Tumor stages are as follows:

1. Stage T0a are clinically nonpalpable occult tumors, focally situated.
2. Stage T0b are nonpalpable tumors with diffuse involvement of the prostate.
3. Stage T1a is a palpable nodule, less than 1 cm in size, confined to the prostate.
4. Stage T1b tumors demonstrate a palpable nodule, greater than 1 cm in size, in one lobe of the prostate.
5. Stage T1c is a palpable tumor, diffusely involving the prostate but not involving the capsule.
6. Stage T2 is a tumor that has invaded into, but not through, the prostatic capsule.
7. Stage T3 is a tumor that has extended beyond the prostatic capsule, perhaps involving the seminal vesicles.
8. Stage T4 is a tumor that has grown outside the prostate with fixation to periprostatic tissue, adjacent viscera, or other organs.

Lymph-node involvement is defined below:

1. N0 has no lymph-node involvement.
2. N1 is a tumor with a single ipsilateral lymph-node metastasis.
3. N2 has multiple or contralateral lymph-node metastasis.
4. N3 has large, bulky, fixed, involved lymph nodes.
5. N4 has widespread lymph-node involvement.

The metastasis portion of the system is categorized as follows:

1. MX implies inadequate data to assess possible distant metastatic involvement.
2. M0 has no distant metastasis.
3. M1 has distant metastasis present.

Figure 9.6 grossly compares the Whitemore-Jewett to the TNM staging system.

Updated TNM Staging System

At a June 1986 meeting of the Task Force on urologic sites of the American Joint Commission on Cancer, a revised system was proposed by Dr. G.M. Farrow (161). It is as follows:

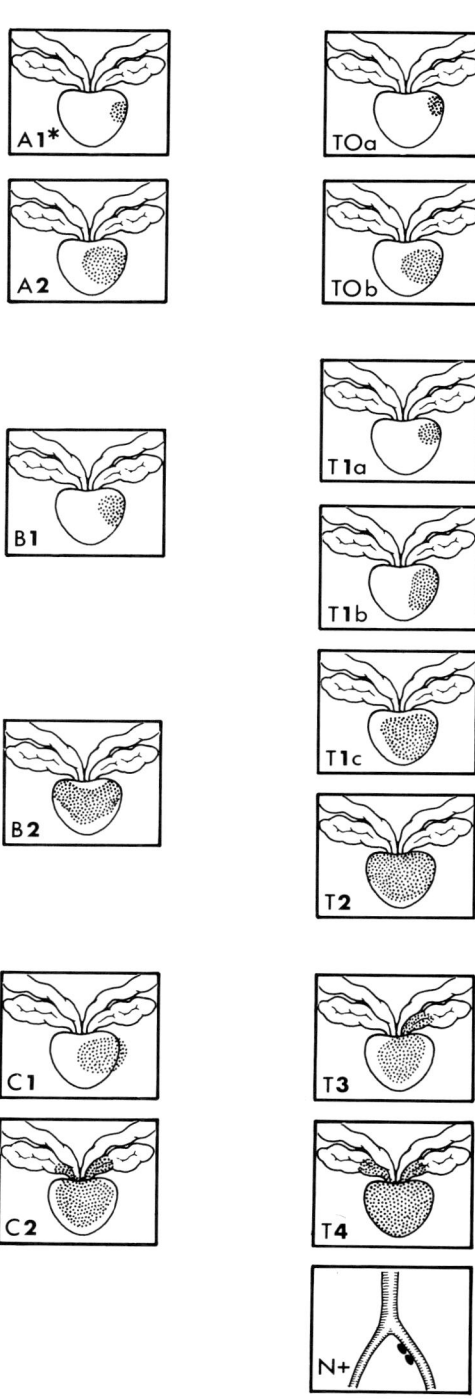

FIG. 9.6. Correlation of Whitmore-Jewett and TNM staging systems. A diagrammatic correlation of the different stages of prostate cancer according to the Whitmore-Jewett (*left*) and the nonmodified TNM (*right*) staging systems is shown.

T: Primary tumor.
- TX: Primary tumor cannot be assessed.
- T0: No evidence of primary tumor.
- T1: Tumor is an incidental histological finding on a specimen from a transurethral resection of the prostate (TURP).
    - i. T1a: Not more than three miscroscopic foci have cancer.
    - ii. T1b: More than three microscopic foci have cancer.
- T2: Palpable tumor grossly limited to the gland without capsule invasion.
    - i. T2a: Tumor less than 1.5 cm in greatest diameter; normal tissue present on at least three sides of the cancer.
    - ii. T2b: Tumor greater than 1.5 cm in greatest diameter or present in both sides of the gland.
- T3: Tumor is not fixed to periprostatic tissues but invades beyond the prostatic capsule or into the bladder neck or seminal vesicles.
- T4: Tumor is fixed and invades structures not listed in T3, adjacent to the prostate.

G: Histological grading.
- GX: Grade of cellular differentiation cannot be assessed.
- G1: Well-differentiated tumor with slight anaplasia.
- G2: Moderately differentiated tumor with slight anaplasia.
- G3: More severely differentiated with severe anaplasia.
- G4: The most poorly differentiated with maximum anaplasia.

N: Lymph-node involvement.
- N0: No lymph-node involvement.
- N1: Tumor with single ipsilateral lymph-node metastasis.
- N2: Scattered, involved pelvic lymph nodes.
- N3: Large, bulky, fixed pelvic lymph nodes.
- N4: Widespread lymph-node involvement.

M: Distant metastases.
- M0: No distinct metastasis.
- M1: Distant metastasis present.

The final stage is then determined as follows:

Stage 0	T1a	N0	M0	G1
	T2a	N0	M0	G1
Stage I	T1a	N0	M0	G2–4
	T2a	N0	M0	G2–4
Stage II	T1b	N0	M0	Any G
	T2b	N0	M0	Any G
Stage III	T3	N0	M0	Any G
Stage IV	T4	N0	M0	Any G
	Any T	N1–3	M0	Any G
	Any T	Any N	M1	Any G

One example of this system is as follows:

A patient presents with three microscopic foci of tumor on a transurethral resection of the prostate specimen (a T1a tumor) that is well-differentiated (a G1 tumor), with no distant metastasis (an M0 tumor) but a single lymph node infiltrated with tumor (an N1 tumor).

The last factor, an N1 tumor, would dictate the overall stage; thus, this patient has a stage IV cancer.

A second patient has an anaplastic cancer (G4) without metastasis (M0) or lymph-node involvement (N0). His tumor is palpable but is less than 1.5 cm in size (a T2A tumor). The overall stage would be stage I.

Table 9.2 demonstrates equivalent stages in the Whitmore-Jewett system, the TNM system, and this proposed updated TNM system.

Revised TNM Staging System

A fourth system, also a modification of the TNM stages, has also been recently proposed and is used to describe histologically proven tumors of the prostate (517). This proposal was made to consider imaging studies as an integral part of the staging procedure. The digital examination is used to determine the T category. The N group can be assigned by clinical (c) (i.e., imaging) studies or by histology (h) (i.e., lymph-node sampling). The M category is obtained by the chest X-ray, the radionuclide bone scan, and at least two serum acid phosphatase levels.

The system is as follows:

T category.
  Tx: Anatomical relationships undetermined.
  TA: Normal digital examination.
    TA1: 5% or less of the total surgical specimen is tumor, and histology is low or medium grade.
    TA2: More than 5% of the total surgical specimen is tumor, and/or histology is high grade.
    TAX: Implies TA, but stratification into A1 or A2 category is not possible.
  TB: Palpable tumor without capsular extension.
    TB1: Less than one-half of one lobe in size.
    TB2: Tumor no more than one lobe in size.
    TB3: Tumor greater than one lobe in size, or multiple palpable tumors.
    TBX: Palpable tumor that is not otherwise characterized.
  TC Tumor: Palpable tumor with extension beyond the capsule.
    TC0: Possible (equivocal) extension beyond the capsule at apex, the lateral sulcus, and/or the seminal vesicle(s).

Table 9.2. Comparison of staging systems

Modified Whitmore-Jewett	UICC (TNM)	Farrow-modified UICC (TNM)
A1	T0a	0 or I
A2	T0b	II
B1	T1a	0 or I
	T1b	
B2	T1c	II
	T2	
C1	T3	III or IV
C2	T4	IV
D1	N+	IV
D2	M+	IV

TC1: Definite unilateral extension.
TC2: Definite bilateral extension.
TC3: Definite extension with involvement of bladder base and/or rectum and/or levator muscle(s) and/or pelvic side wall(s).
TCX: Capsule extension but not otherwise characterized.

Lymph-node status (N).
N: Pelvic lymph-node involvement below the aortic bifurcation by imaging studies (C) and/or histology confirmation (H). The clinical imaging modality(s) should be specified.
N0(C and/or H): No regional lymph-node metastasis.
N1(H): Microscopic regional lymph-node metastasis.
N2(C and/or H): Gross regional lymph-node metastasis.
N3(C and/or H): Extraregional lymph-node metastasis (including inguinal, periaortic, supraclavicular, or axillary nodes, etc.).
NX: Minimal requirements have not been met.

Distant metastasis status (M).
M: Distant metastasis (excluding lymph nodes).
M0: No evidence of metastasis.
M1: Elevated acid phosphatase only (serum study repeated and elevated at last on two additional occasions; i.e., total of three elevations).
M2(V and/or B): Visceral (V) and/or bone (B) metastasis.
Mx: Minimal requirements have not been met.

A deficiency of all of these staging systems is the knowledge that cancer may be multifocal in origin. Thus, even a tumor staged as a focal lesion may, on an in-depth analysis, be more widespread. Many of these incidental findings are only detected on surgical or autopsy material.

The endorectal sonogram findings may conflict with the clinical staging. These findings may then effect a change in tumor staging. The possible implications of these differences in clinical sonographic staging on clinical treatment will be discussed in Chapter 10.

PATTERNS OF DISSEMINATION

Prostate cancer can spread locally by direct invasion, or it can spread distantly through the vascular or lymphatic systems. Local invasion can cause involvement of the bladder and ureters, causing renal obstruction. The lymphatics of the prostate drain predominantly into the perivesical, hypogastric, obturator, presacral, and presciatic lymph nodes. The obturator nodes are those most commonly involved with cancer (292). Other sites of lymphatic involvement include the inguinal, common iliac, and para-aortic nodes. Rarely, tertiary involvement of the mediastinal and supraclavicular nodes will occur.

Hematogenous or vascular spread most commonly involves the osseous system. These include, most often, the axial skeleton and the lumbar spine. Less commonly involved in descending order of frequency are the proximal femura, pelvis, thoracic spine, ribs, sternum, skull, and humeri.

Visceral involvement can also occur. It has been estimated that 25% to 38% of lethal prostatic cancers involve the lung (14,265). Many of these are microscopic and are not always identified on chest radiographs. The liver and adrenal glands can also be involved. Central nervous system involvement is often due to direct extension of osseous involvement.

SIGNIFICANT VERSUS INSIGNIFICANT (INCIDENTAL) CARCINOMA

The exact significance of each individual cancer is not definitely known. It has long been thought that cancers grow and may, after a period of time, become clinically significant lesions. However, the data are not yet conclusive. Many cancers grow, whereas others do not. Extensive data suggest (see next section) that early diagnosis generally has a better prognosis.

PROSTATE CANCER GROWTH AND METASTATIC POTENTIAL

Although the exact metastatic potential of prostate cancer is not known, strong evidence suggests that the larger cancers have a greater metastatic potential. It has been suggested that the size of the cancer and the degree of differentiation are often correlative (307,308).

Prostate cancer originates as a small focus. It has been suggested that those cancers that originate in the peripheral zone are well-differentiated when small. Histologically, as the tumor enlarges in size and volume, it dedifferentiates. Additionally, as the tumor enlarges, it can grow along three tissue planes: (a) along the prostatic capsule; (b) internally into the more central tissues; and (c) through the prostatic capsule into periprostatic fat and surrounding structures. For example, the smaller cancers are usually relatively well-differentiated. As the cancer enlarges in size, it will either spread along the prostatic capsule, become extracapsular, or invaginate into the central aspects of the gland. A combination of these methods of spread is possible.

As tumors enlarge, they can metastasize. It has been contemplated that this sequence is often related to the size of the cancer. McNeal has suggested that the incidence or possibility of tumor extending beyond the prostate increases drastically with tumor volume larger than 1.42 cc. This size of tumor has been termed the *window of curability* (307,308).

Once a cancer has reached this certain size, invasion through the capsule occurs. It is felt that invasion into the periprostatic tissues with lymphatic involvement and secondary and hematogenous embolization occurs at this time. However, the actual sequence has not been definitively demonstrated.

There are small cancers that have great malignant potential, and there are large cancers that do not cause death. Thus, many questions about the spread, invasiveness, and clinical importance of prostate cancer have yet to be answered.

CONCLUSION

Although some theories have suggested the pathogenesis and spread of prostatic cancers, these are not necessarily unanimously accepted. For example, some researchers feel that: (a) some cancers are anaplastic from inception; (b) metastasis may occur with tumors smaller than 1.42 cc; and (c) not all larger cancers have metastasized.

Regardless, the presented theories have, at least in part, been accepted into clinical practice. Obviously there are, and will be, exceptions to the rule. Only as more research is performed will more definitive answers be realized.

10 // Prostate Cancer: Sonographic Characteristics

Historical Perspective	157
Sonographic Determination of Small Prostate Cancers: The Hypoechoic Cancer	163
The Isoechoic Lesion	165
The Mixed Echogenic Cancer	169
The Hyperechoic Cancer	169
Transition Zone Cancer	177
Tumor Extension	177
Capsular Invasion	179
Staging Tumors with Ultrasound	181
Accuracy of Sonography in Determining the Presence of Prostate Cancer	184
Cancer in the Presence of Benign Prostatic Hypertrophy	184
Conclusion	184

HISTORICAL PERSPECTIVE

There was great expectation that early diagnosis of prostate cancer would be possible with the advent and development of diagnostic ultrasound.

Although early studies did suggest that conventional ultrasound would permit early diagnosis of prostatic cancer (4,167,168), more recent studies have shown the opposite findings, with one exception—the ability to detect bulky extension of invasive prostate cancer (386,397). The transabdominal and transperineal approaches are unable to detect and/or delineate small cancers. The conventional approaches can detect calculi and corpora amylacea but cannot demonstrate textural differences that are seen in prostate cancer. Only the large bulky masses, which may or may not have changes in echogenicity from normal, may be seen as a result of their large size and extension from the prostate into the periprostatic tissue (Fig. 10.1).

Because of the inadequacy of conventional ultrasound, most of the interest in prostate sonography has been centered around the intraluminal, endorectal approach. Even with this technique, there has not been unanimous acceptance in the ability of this approach.

There has been much controversy within the past 20 years regarding the sonographic appearance of prostate cancer with the endorectal approach. With the advent of this technique during the 1960s, certain criteria were developed to detect and delineate prostate cancer. These characteristics were used both to define the lesions on the ultrasound and to differentiate cancer from benign prostatic changes. With the development of higher-resolution equipment, with varying focal characteristics, better lateral and axial resolution, and an improvement in beam width, the detection of smaller lesions and better definition of the cancers became possible.

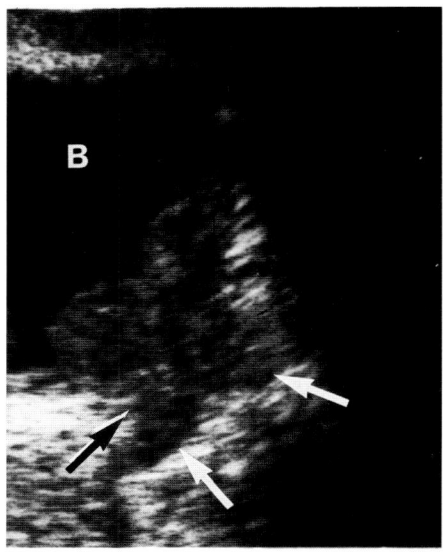

FIG. 10.1. Transabdominal scan showing extensive infiltrating prostatic carcinoma. A longitudinally oriented transabdominal ultrasound demonstrates a massive prostatic cancer (*white arrows*) with infiltration and extension (*black arrow*) into the urinary bladder (*white arrows*). (B) Bladder.

A review of the original sonographic characteristics described in the 1970s would suggest that prostate cancer has the following characteristics (385–390,444,521–525,529):

1. It involves an irregularly deformed area of the prostate.
2. The anterior-posterior dimension of the gland becomes elongated (with some exceptions).
3. The superior-inferior diameter will occasionally be elongated and will be irregular and asymmetric.
4. Symmetry will not be present.
5. There will be a marked change in the normal homogeneous echogenicity.
6. Capsular echoes will be irregular, discontinuous, and uneven.
7. The internal echopattern will be disorderly, occasionally absent, and will have some subtle areas of increased echogenicity.

These changes were in comparison to prostatic hypertrophy and prostatitis, which had more symmetrical abnormalities or had areas of greater increase in echogenicity.

These studies, performed in the late 1970s and early 1980s, showed that most prostate cancers appeared slightly hyperechoic but that others had a slightly hypoechogenic finding on the sonogram (385–390,397,444,521–525,529).

The more recent studies using newer generation equipment with more sophisticated machinery have shown an even different appearance of cancer. Utilizing ultrasound units with 5-, 6-, and 7.5-MHz transducers with a more sharply focused near-field, these latter studies have demonstrated that prostate cancer is mostly hypoechoic in comparison to residual prostatic tissue (91,135,252–254,405).

Why has there been this continuing controversy both in the literature and in the minds of those who perform these studies on a routine basis?

Most likely, this is secondary to a number of factors, which include:

1. modification and improvement in equipment;
2. the stage and size of the cancer at initial diagnosis; and
3. the manner in which proof was obtained.

With regard to equipment, the newer machinery has been able to resolve smaller, peripherally oriented lesions. Additionally, the focal zone has been placed to have a much sharper near-field, so that axial and lateral resolution has been improved in the areas where prostate cancer is frequently present (i.e., the peripheral zone in the posterior portion of the prostate).

With regard to the stage (or size) of carcinoma, it is obviously more difficult to detect very subtle and small lesions with lower-resolution equipment than with the newer and slightly higher-resolution machinery. For this reason, the older scans were not able to detect as many stage A and stage B lesions as clearly and consistently as have the scans in more recent studies.

Correlation with tissue diagnosis is probably the most important aspect in studying the differences in appearance of prostate cancer. For example, the only truly accurate technique and "gold standard" to delineate the exact extent and sonographic appearance of prostate cancer is to obtain a radical prostatectomy specimen immediately following the sonographic examination. Only by comparing whole mount slides of the gross pathology to the sonograms can an exact correlation be made. Realistically, it is quite difficult to obtain the exact correlation because most patients with prostate cancer do not undergo radical prostatectomy. Most studies have used other methods of correlation.

The second most accurate technique in determining the sonographic characteristics of prostate cancer is by utilizing ultrasound guided biopsy of the prostate. This will allow correlation of the sonographic characteristics of a small core of tissue with histology. However, a more definite overall evaluation of the prostate may still not be possible.

The least acceptable and most misleading technique includes correlation of (a) digitally palpated conventional biopsies of the prostate for palpable lesions with an ultrasound examination and (b) transurethral resection specimens in patients demonstrating the presence of prostate cancer with an after-the-fact correlation with the sonogram.

These results can be particularly misleading. For example, if an abnormality is present on the ultrasound study and the patient has a known prostate cancer (i.e., from previous biopsy or on a transurethral resection specimen), one may inappropriately assume that the abnormality on the sonogram is the cancer. Additionally, if a patient has an abnormality on an ultrasound study and a digitally palpable abnormality on the rectal examination, and a conventional nonsonographically guided biopsy is performed, one could assume (perhaps incorrectly) that the sonographic area of abnormality conforms to the biopsied area of carcinoma. Again, this is not necessarily accurate, since the biopsy of the prostate may not actually be the area of the sonographic abnormality. It is because of these two correlative fallacies that such misleading information still exists regarding the sonographic characteristics of prostate cancer.

Another problem occurs when attempting to compare one study to another. There may be difficulty when two individuals do not agree on the definition of echogenicity (see Chapter 7). This is most important when evaluating the isoechoic, hyperechoic, and acoustically mixed lesions (see below).

Newer studies have shown that the earliest and smallest prostate cancers generally appear slightly hypoechoic in nature (Figs. 10.2 and 10.3) (91,253,405). It is essential that a basis of comparison is determined. For example, peripheral zone lesions should be compared to the remaining normal-appearing peripheral zone; centrally placed lesions should be compared to the central area.

Hypoechoic lesions range from anechoic (cystic and noncystic) (Figs. 10.4–10.6) to slightly more echogenic in appearance. They must all be less echogenic in relation to the residual normal prostate to be termed hypoechoic. The anechoic lesion will have no internal

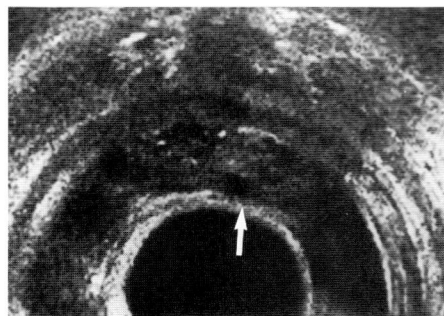

FIG. 10.2. Endorectal axial sonogram showing small prostatic cancer. Endorectal ultrasound of the prostate in axial orientation demonstrates a small hypoechoic area (*arrow*) in the posterior portion of the prostate to the left of midline.

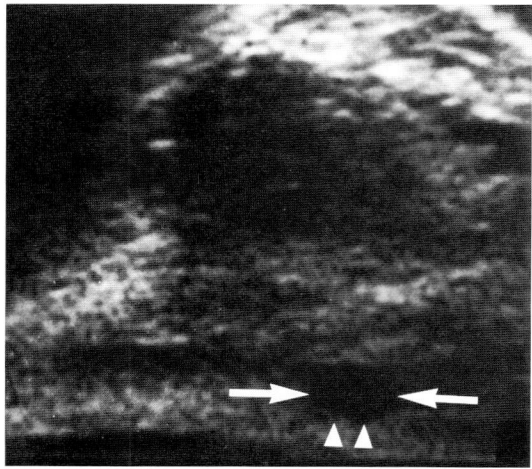

FIG. 10.3. Endorectal longitudinal sonogram showing small prostatic cancer. A longitudinally oriented sonogram demonstrates a small, hypoechoic cancer (*arrows*) with slight bulging of the posterior aspect of the capsule (*arrowheads*). The margins of the lesion are relatively poorly defined.

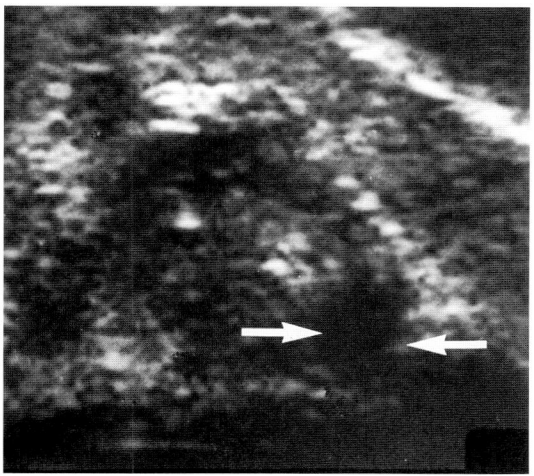

FIG. 10.4. Endorectal longitudinal sonogram showing prostatic cancer. Endorectal ultrasound of the prostate in longitudinal orientation demonstrates a poorly defined, but hypoechoic (*arrows*), lesion (a prostatic carcinoma in the apex of the gland).

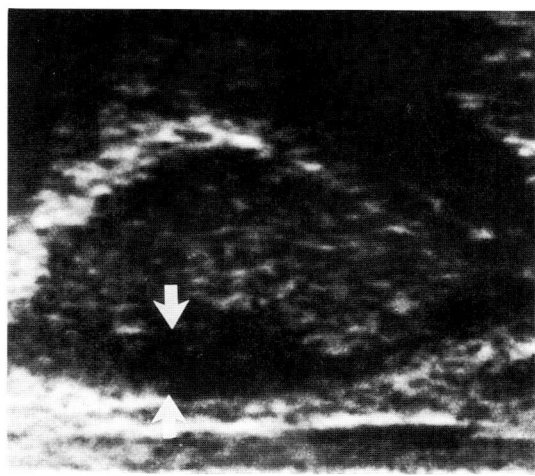

FIG. 10.5. Endorectal longitudinal sonogram showing prostatic cancer. Endorectal ultrasound of the prostate demonstrates an irregularly marginated hypoechoic lesion (compared to the residual peripheral zone) in the mid-portion of the peripheral zone, posteriorly situated. The margins of the superior portion (*arrows*) of the tumor are very poorly delineated.

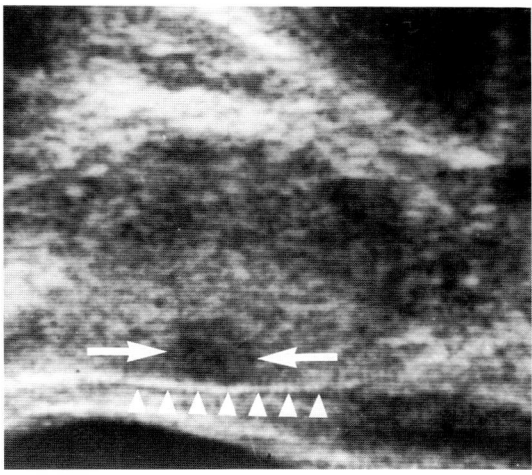

FIG. 10.6. Endorectal sagittal sonogram showing prostatic cancer. A longitudinally oriented endorectal ultrasound demonstrates a poorly marginated, hypoechoic tumor (*arrows*). Although this lesion is less echogenic than the normal peripheral zone, it is more echogenic than cancers in Figs. 10.2–10.5. The capsule, denoted by a relatively well-defined echogenic band (*arrowheads*), is clearly marginated and not infiltrated.

echoes and will not have the sharp walls and good through-transmission as seen in simple cysts (also an anechoic lesion). Most early cancers that are detected by ultrasound will be seen in the peripheral zone.

A large percentage of the early lesions detected by ultrasound will be apically placed or will be in the posterior portion of the prostate. Others will be in the lateral and anterolateral aspects of the peripheral zone of the prostate. Lesions as small as a few millimeters have been detected and are best seen when they are hypoechoic as compared to the more echogenic normal peripheral zone. The smaller lesions, when hypoechoic, can have accurate sonographically guided biopsy (see Chapter 8) performed, allowing early diagnoses.

There are other cancers that may not have the same sonographic characteristics as the smaller (and more hypoechoic) lesions (56,91,405,429). If the cancer has a sonographic reflectivity similar to that of the remainder of the prostate, these lesions are termed *isoechoic* (Fig. 10.7). The exact number of cancers that have this sonographic appearance has not yet been determined. However, one project (using high-resolution equipment) has shown that in a study of 52 patients with clinical stage A and B carcinomas who underwent radical

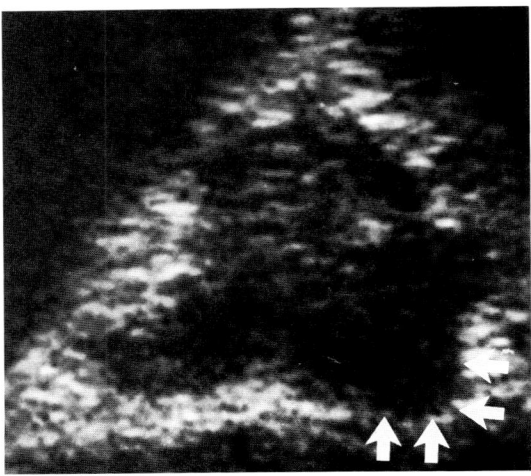

FIG. 10.7. Endorectal sagittal sonogram showing isoechoic prostatic cancer. Endorectal ultrasound in longitudinal orientation demonstrates a bulge in the posterior portion of the prostate, distorting the capsule (*arrows*). The lesion, which proved to be a malignancy, does not have clearly different sonographic characteristics as compared to the remainder of the normal gland.

prostatectomy, 24% had an isoechoic appearance and could not be identified by the sonogram (91).

The mixed echogenic lesion, with areas of subtle hypoechogenicity and subtle hyperechogenicity, may also be present (Fig. 10.8) (56,405,430). These have been variably determined as hypoechoic lesions, hyperechoic lesions or lesions with mixed echogenicity by different researchers (56,405).

The hyperechoic lesion is probably the most poorly understood of all the sonographic appearances of prostate cancer. This is a lesion that has never been defined as brightly and thickly echogenic, although many individuals who have reviewed the literature and are performing the sonogram of the prostate have misinterpreted its appearance. The hyperechoic

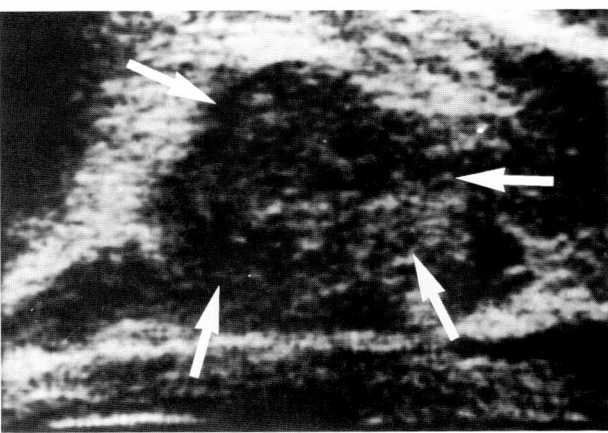

FIG. 10.8. Sagittal endorectal sonogram showing prostatic cancer with mixed echogenicity. The entire lateral aspect of the prostate seen on a longitudinally oriented linear-array endorectal sonogram with the probe rotated clockwise to the lateral aspect of the gland demonstrates diffuse inhomogeneous echogenicity (*arrows*). Although the gland appears to be slightly hypoechoic, there are subtle scattered echoes throughout. The entire gland, on multiple biopsies, was shown to be infiltrated with malignancy.

lesion has always been a very subtle lesion with poor definition of the margins and just barely perceptible areas of increased echogenicity with echoes that are very thin and punctate (56,397,405,429). This is in comparison to what appears to be residual normal-appearing prostatic tissue. The exact cause of these areas of echogenic changes is unclear. It may be a reflection of the malignancy itself, but more likely it is related to a number of other factors, perhaps infiltration of noncancerous tissue with malignancy. This can set up a number of factors, namely: (a) an intermixing of benign prostatic hyperplastic disease (which may have subtle areas of increased echogenicity) with cancer; (b) increased numbers of interfaces caused by the intermixing of normal and abnormal tissues; or (c) perhaps even a desmoplastic-type reaction. The cancer itself may not be hyperechoic. The increased echogenicity may actually be due to changes in benign tissue. Since the only appearance of the malignancy is increased acoustic reflectivity, the tumor must be considered to have a minimal hyperechoic appearance; that is, the overall appearance of the lesion is slightly hyperflective. Regardless of the cause of echogenicity, the cancer may present as an acoustically reflective lesion.

Why do these differences in appearance of prostate cancer exist? It has been suggested that these differences may be due to a change in size and/or cellular differentiation of the malignancy. It has also been suggsted that, in general, as prostate cancers enlarge, the cellular differentiation becomes more anaplastic; that is, the larger cancers are usually more anaplastic histologically than the smaller cancers, which are often better differentiated (307,308).

A study of the ultrasonogram and radical prostatectomy specimens was undertaken using some of the newer equipment. This study (Table 10.1) has shown that the well-differentiated cancer (which implies, in general, a smaller lesion) is generally more hypoechoic than (a) the moderately well-differentiated lesion (which implies the medium-sized lesion), which is more isoechoic in nature, and (b) the anaplastic (i.e., the poorly differentiated) lesions (which suggests the larger lesions), which are more hyperechoic or have more mixed echogenicity than the better differentiated tumors (429).

SONOGRAPHIC DETERMINATION OF SMALL PROSTATE CANCERS: THE HYPOECHOIC CANCER

Small prostate cancers, which are oriented in the peripheral zone (the large majority) are generally less echogenic (i.e., hypoechoic) than the residual peripheral zone. These lesions will not have the characteristics of a simple cyst but may actually appear anechoic with no internal echoes (Fig.10.3 and 10.4). Their margins, although perhaps well-defined in certain areas of the tumor, will have some segments that are ill-defined with discontinuity (Fig. 10.9 and 10.10). There will be no enhanced or good sound through-transmission. These will be in the peripheral zone, and a capsular bulge may be seen (Fig. 10.11). The capsule and

TABLE 10.1. Tumor echogenicity versus histologic differentiation[a]

Tumor histology	Hypoechoic tumor	Isoechoic tumor	Mixed echogenicity or hyperechoic
Well-differentiated ($N = 5$)	3	2	0
Moderately differentiated ($N = 10$)	5	3	2
Poorly differentiated ($N = 5$)	0	1	4
Total:	8 (40%)	6 (30%)	6 (30%)

[a] Data taken from ref. 405.

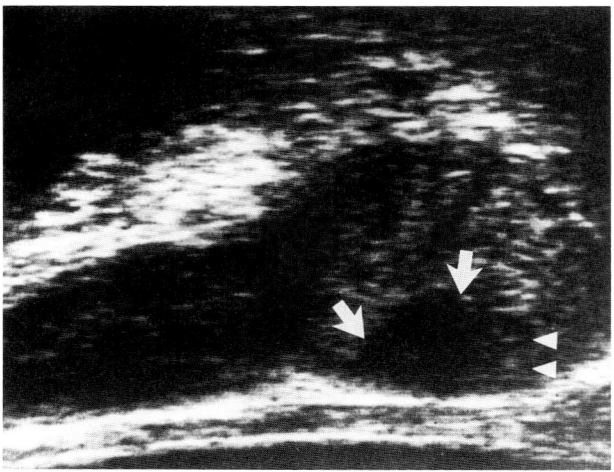

FIG. 10.9. Sagittal endorectal sonogram showing prostatic cancer. Endorectal ultrasound of the prostate demonstrates a 1-cm hypoechoic cancer. Although the anterior and superior (*arrows*) margins are relatively well-defined, the inferior portion of the tumor (*arrowhead*) is not clearly delineated from the remainder of the gland.

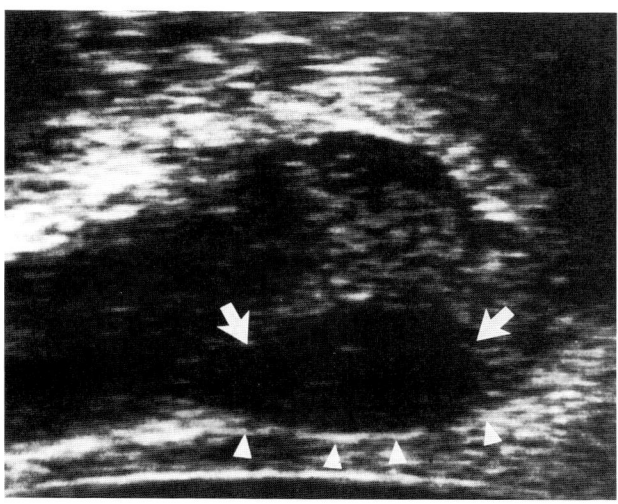

FIG. 10.10. Endorectal sagittal sonogram showing prostatic cancer. Endorectal ultrasound with a longitudinally oriented scanner demonstrates a hypoechoic lobulated mass (*arrows*). The prostatic capsule (*arrowheads*) is clearly defined and not infiltrated by this cancer.

pericapsular fat, seen as a brightly echogenic area, will be intact if the tumor has not invaded through; however, if there is erosion of the capsule by tumor, then poor definition or thinning of the capsule echogenicity will be seen (Fig. 10.12).

As the lesions enlarge, they may extend into the capsule, causing a more pronounced bulge. As they progress, they may continue to spread along the capsule so that they appear more elongated than rounded (Fig. 10.13). Additionally, they may infiltrate into the central portions of the prostate (Fig. 10.14). Regardless of the manner of growth and extension, a close evaluation of the peripheral zone with comparison of the right versus the left side is quite important (Fig. 10.15). Some of the more subtle lesions may be seen only by a close comparison of right and left sides.

Some lesions are so subtle that a careful examination with changes in gain and TGC controls, as well as in contrast (Figs. 10.16–10.18), are essential to show the abnormalities.

It is important that the surrounding venous structures that are usually present in the lateral and anterolateral (Santorini's plexus) portions of the prostate (Fig. 10.19) are not misconstrued and misinterpreted as infiltrating hypoechoic lesions of the peripheral zone of the gland.

THE ISOECHOIC LESION

As cancers enlarge, they may appear more isoechoic or equally echogenic as compared to the remainder of the peripheral zone or the normal central zone (see Chapter 12) (405,429).

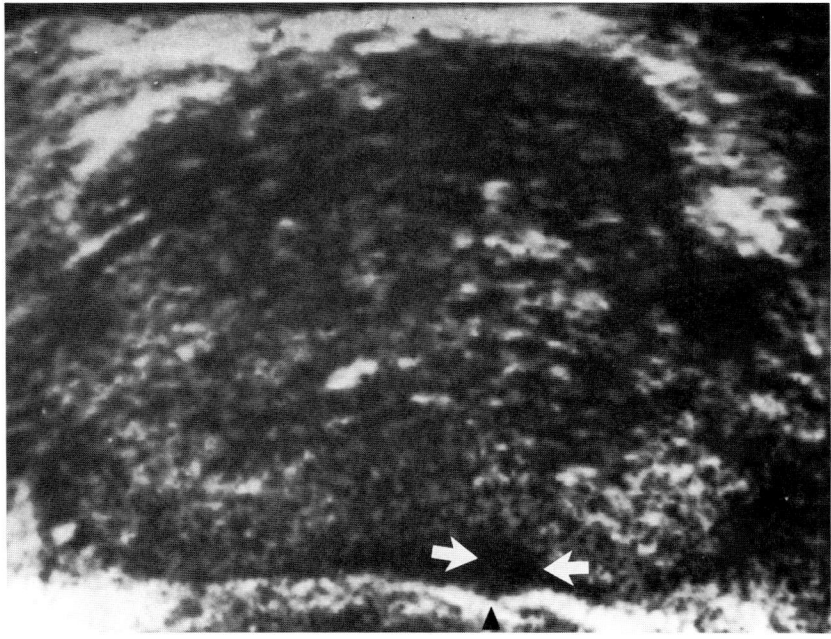

FIG. 10.11. Endorectal axial sonogram showing small cancer with capsular bulge. A small, peripherally oriented hypoechoic lesion (*arrows*) with capsular bulge (*arrowhead*), but no evidence of capsular disruption, is seen. There is no thinning of the hyperechoic capsular echoes.

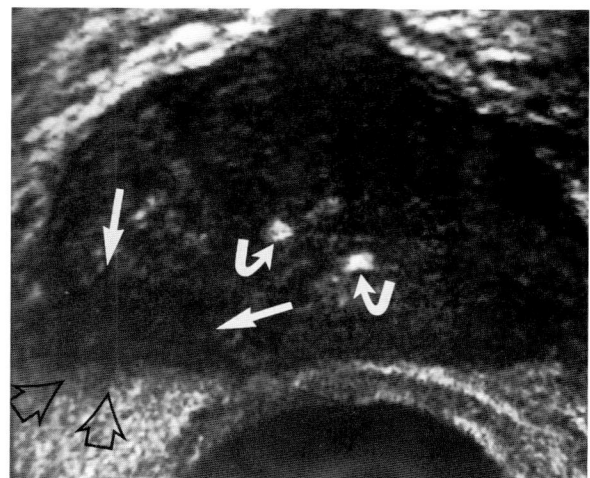

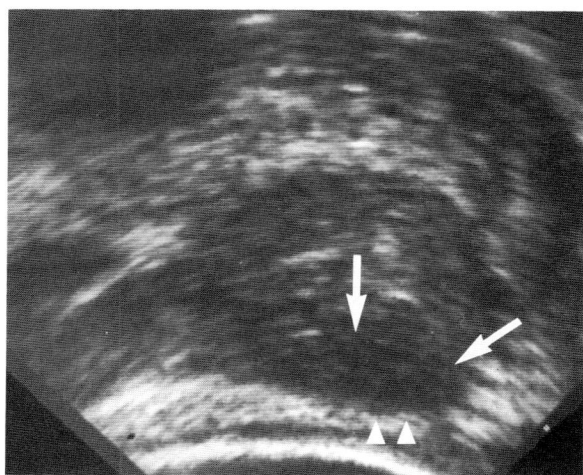

FIG. 10.12. Endorectal sonograms showing capsular thinning. Endorectal ultrasound of the prostate in axial (**A**) and longitudinal (**B**) orientation demonstrates a subtle, but relatively hypoechoic, lesion (*arrows*) in the right posterolateral peripheral portion of the gland. The longitudinal scan demonstrates some thinning (*arrowheads*) of the capsule-pericapsular fat complex. However, on the axial image, marked capsular disruption (*open arrowheads*) is seen. Scattered calculi (*curved arrows*) are also seen.

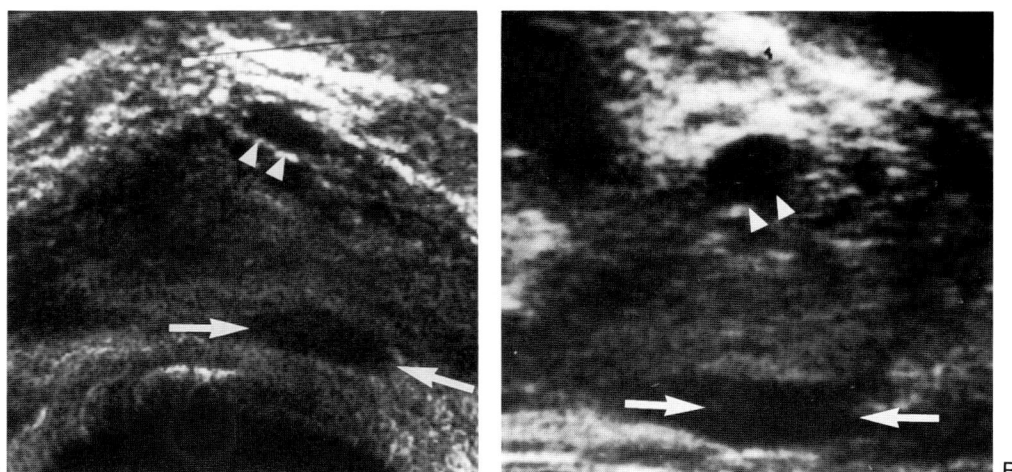

FIG. 10.13. Endorectal sonograms showing prostatic cancer. A prostatic cancer (*arrows*) is seen spreading (elongating) along the prostatic capsular margin in both the axially (**A**) and longitudinally (**B**) oriented images. Anteriorly seen on both scans are periprostatic vessels (*arrowheads*).

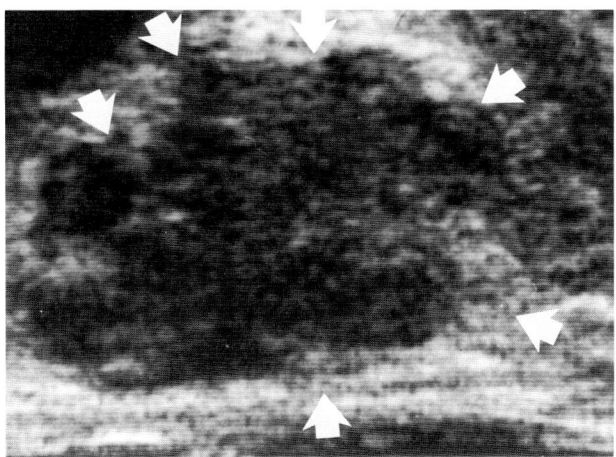

FIG. 10.14. Endorectal sagittal sonogram showing infiltrative malignancy of the prostate. Endorectal ultrasound in longitudinal orientation demonstrates diffuse lobularity of the lateral aspect of the prostate. The margins of the capsule appear to be irregular (*arrowheads*) and destroyed. The entire gland's inhomogeneous echogenicity, in addition to the capsular margins, is highly suggestive of infiltrating (stage C) prostatic cancer.

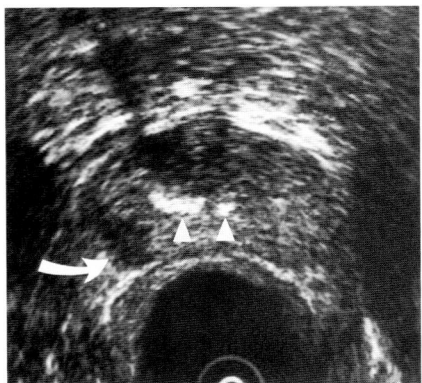

FIG. 10.15. Axial endorectal sonogram showing asymmetrical echogenicity. Axial sonogram demonstrates the right prostatic posterolateral margin to be irregularly hypoechoic (*arrow*) compared to the left side, which has homogeneous echogenicity similar to the remainder of the normal peripheral zone. Additionally noted are two calculi (*arrowheads*) with acoustic shadowing.

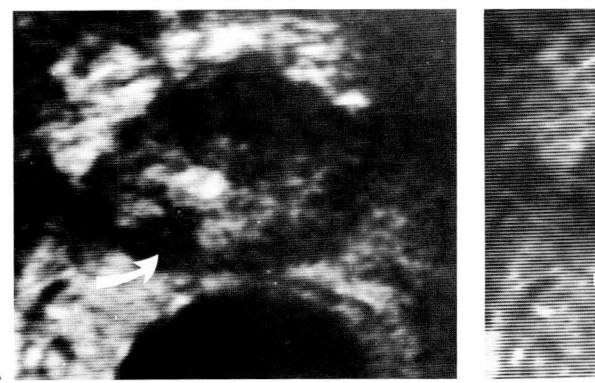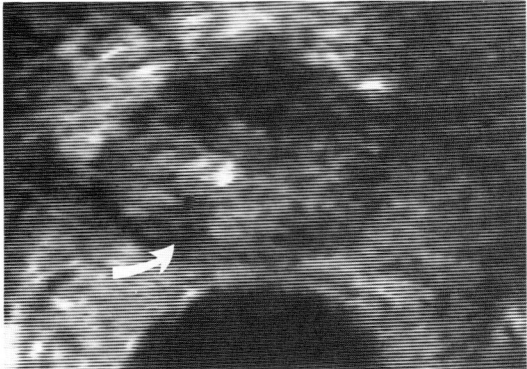

FIG. 10.16. Prostatic cancer—differences with contrast changes. Axial images of the prostate are seen with two different contrast levels. The hypoechoic cancer in the right posterior margin of the prostate (*arrows*) is poorly seen with low contrast (**A**); however, by increasing the contrast (**B**), the lesion becomes much more obvious.

These lesions will usually not be seen clearly by themselves, but their secondary sonographic characteristics may be present. An isoechoic lesion, by definition, will only be seen if there are either secondary characteristics or a surrounding abnormal echogenic area (either hyper- or hypoechoic) that will offset the lesion from the normal tissues. These areas have been termed "halos" and are generally not seen with malignancies.

The majority of isoechoic lesions, if seen by ultrasound, will only be identified because of capsular bulge (Fig. 10.20), capsular distortion (Fig. 10.21), or asymmetry in the size and shape of the prostate (Fig. 10.22). Whereas benign lesions may bulge the capsule, only

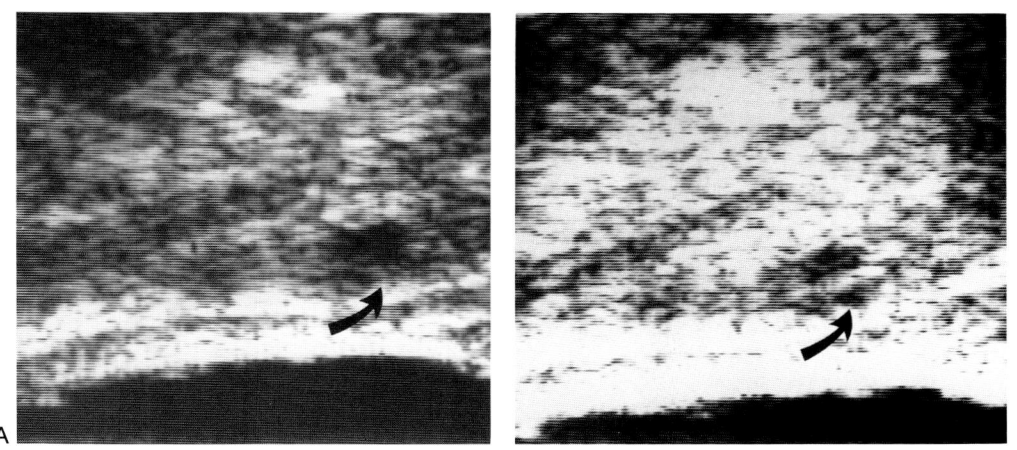

FIG. 10.17. Prostatic cancer—differences with gain changes. A highly magnified view of a 6-mm prostate cancer (*arrows*) in longitudinal orientation demonstrates the malignancy to be subtle with normal gain settings (**A**). By increasing the overall gain (**B**), the tumor becomes more obvious.

malignant tumors will infiltrate through the capsule. If they have not extended into or beyond the capsule, they may bulge (i.e., distort) the contour of the capsule, similar to some cases of benign prostatic hyperplasia. A close comparison for symmetrical capsular bulge and/or distortion is important to define these lesions.

THE MIXED ECHOGENIC CANCER

The mixed echogenic lesion may be incompletely identified and/or misconstrued as a benign tumor. The mixed lesion is usually a larger tumor than the smaller and more hypoechoic cancer (429). Its exact borders may be difficult to identify unless distortion and/or asymmetry of the peripheral zone is identified (Figs. 10.23 and 10.24). Additionally, the mixed lesion may occur in those neoplasms that originate in the nonperipheral zone acinar tissues. Although these tumors are unusual, sonographic definition of the lesion may be difficult to ascertain.

These cancers may also cause capsular bulge and/or distortion; once again, an evaluation for symmetrical or asymmetrical involvement of the prostate is essential.

THE HYPERECHOIC CANCER

The hyperechoic lesion is usually identified only with the larger and/or more invasive tumors. These may be difficult to identify on the sonogram, and their sonographic characteristics may be largely related to the mixing of normal, benign, and malignant tissues (Figs. 10.25–10.28). These tumors may have sonographic characteristics which are related mostly to benign hyperplastic changes with tumor infiltration. The tumor itself may not be clearly seen.

The larger lesions are probably more difficult to accurately map for volumetric calculations because their margins and definition of extension are not clearly seen.

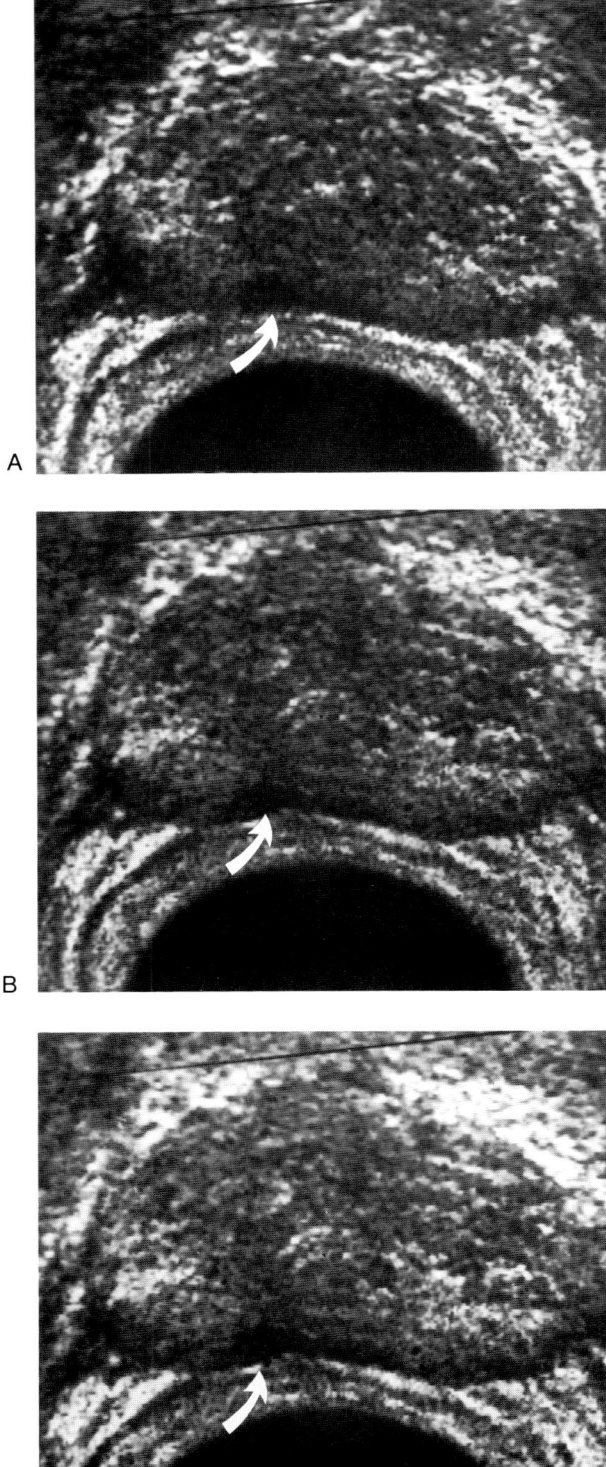

FIG. 10.18. Prostatic cancer—differences with power output change. Three axially oriented images of the prostate at the same position demonstrate a subtle prostatic cancer (*arrows*) which becomes progressively more obvious (**A–C**) as the overall power output is increased.

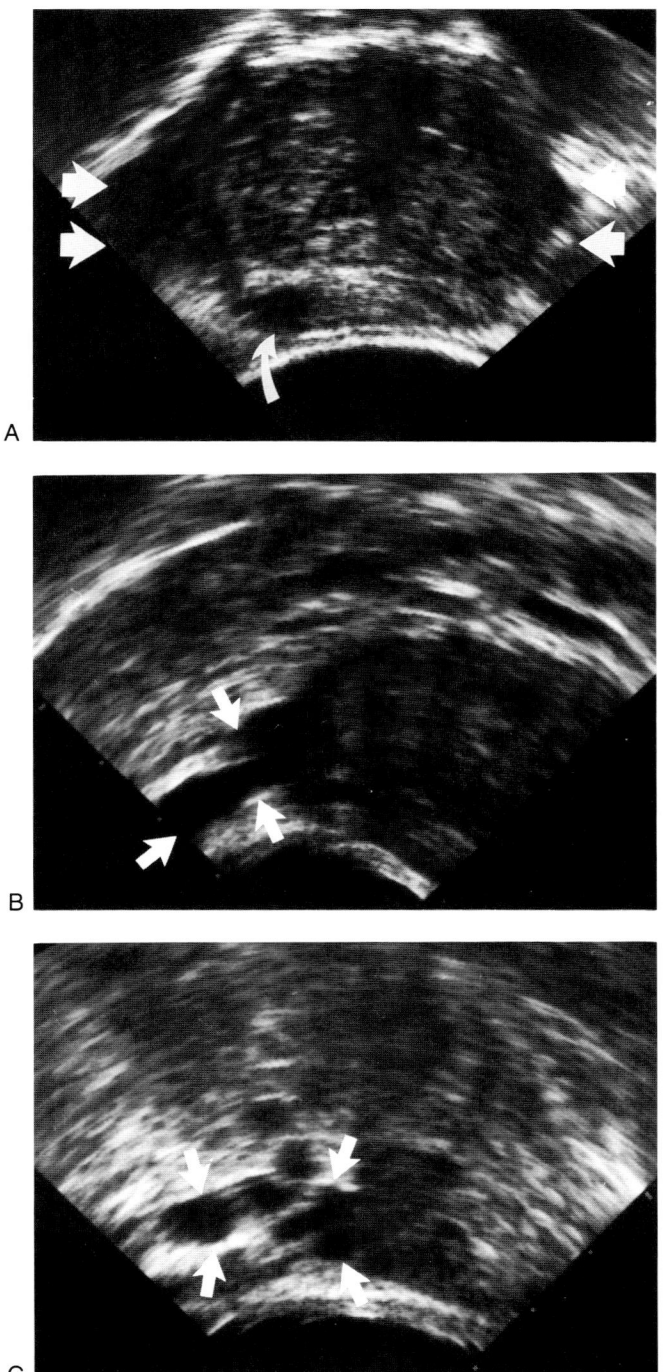

FIG. 10.19. Endorectal sonograms showing prostatic cancer and venous plexi. Axially oriented image (**A**) of the prostate demonstrates a cancer (*curved arrow*) in the right posterolateral margin of the gland. There is poor delineation of the prostatic capsule directly lateral on both sides (*arrowheads*), not due to capsular infiltration but caused by the adjacent periprostatic venous plexus. A second patient viewed in axial (**B**) and sagittal (**C**) orientations demonstrates very prominent veins (*arrows*) on the left sides.

172   *PROSTATE CANCER: SONOGRAPHIC CHARACTERISTICS*

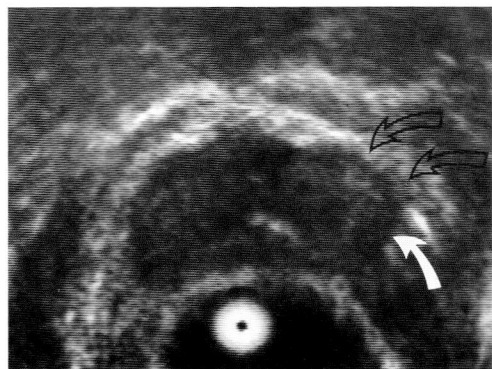

FIG. 10.20. Axial endorectal sonogram showing isoechoic cancer. Axially oriented scan demonstrates a bulge (*arrows*) from the left lateral aspect of the prostate. The capsule is also slightly distorted at this level (*open arrows*), suggesting tumor infiltration. The lesion itself has sonographic characteristics identical to those of the remainder of the gland and would not be seen if the capsule bulge was not present.

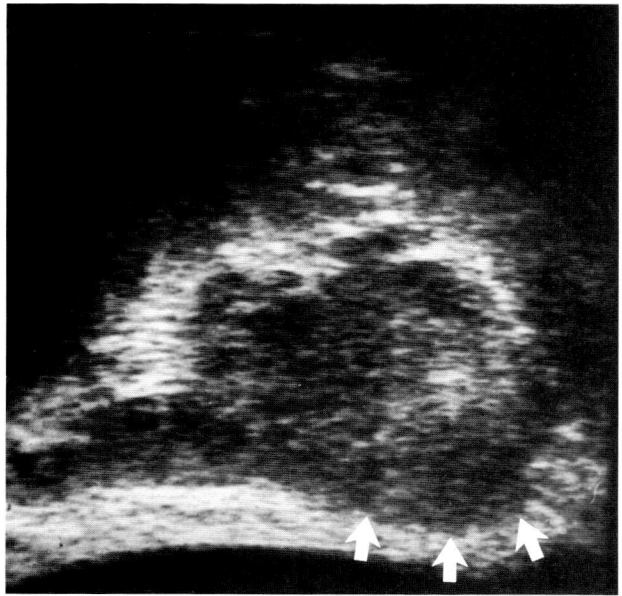

FIG. 10.21. Longitudinal endorectal sonograms showing isoechoic cancer. Sagittal endorectal sonograms of the prostate on the left (**A**) and right (**B**) sides demonstrate an isoechoic prostate cancer (*arrows*) with thinning of the capsule on the left (**A**) side. There is no abnormal or asymmetric echogenicity from the tumor.

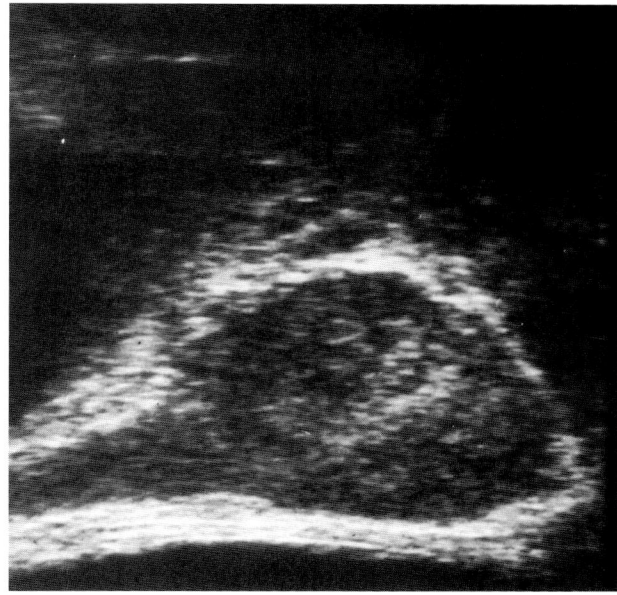

FIG. 10.21. Continued.

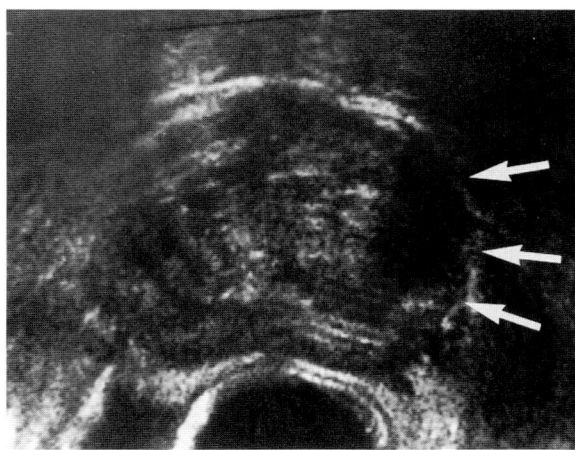

FIG. 10.22. Axial endorectal sonogram showing asymmetry of the echogenicity of the prostate. Asymmetrical echogenicity is discerned on the left (arrows) as compared to the right side of the gland. Close comparisons of the two lateral aspects will demonstrate these findings.

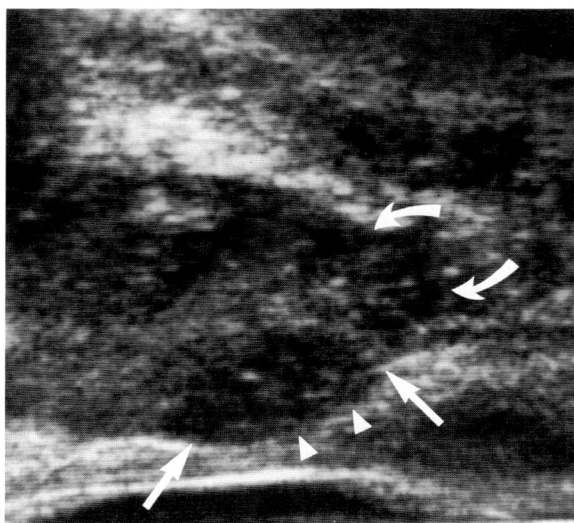

FIG. 10.23. Sagittal endorectal sonogram showing a mixed echogenic lesion. A longitudinally oriented sonogram of the prostate demonstrates a poorly defined, irregularly marginated mass (*straight arrows*) in the posterior apical portion of the gland. A second lesion (*curved arrows*) is seen in the more anterior apical portion of the gland. Although the lesion is predominantly hypoechoic (compared to the residual peripheral zone), there are subtle scattered acoustic reflectors throughout the entire lesion. This signifies that this is a cancer of mixed echogenicity, even though it is a predominantly hypoechoic lesion. Additionally (*arrowheads*), there is a capsular disruption and distortion, suggesting infiltration of the cancer beyond the capsule (a stage C malignancy).

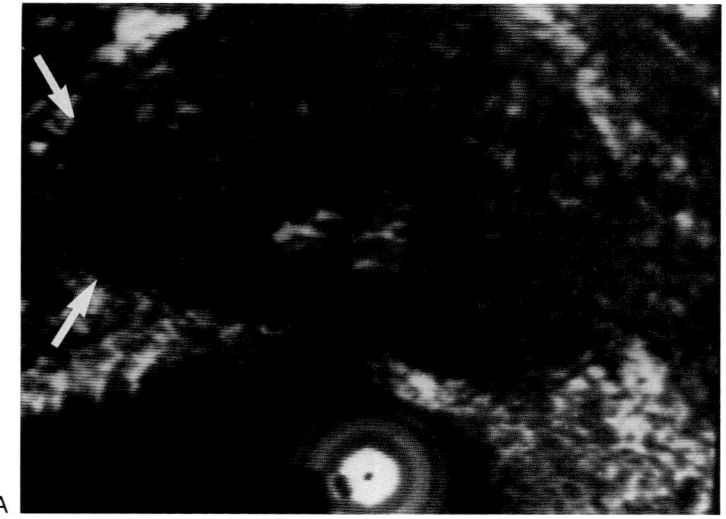

FIG. 10.24. Endorectal sonogram showing a mixed echogenic lesion.

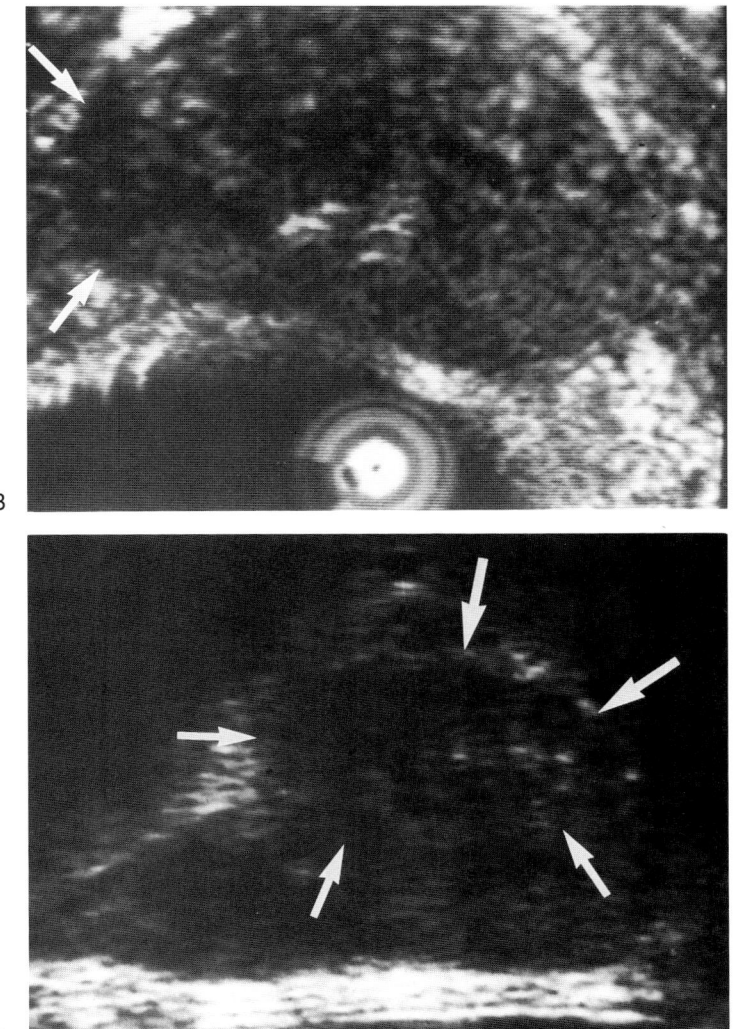

FIG. 10.24. *Continued.* Axial endorectal sonograms of the prostate with low (**A**) and high (**B**) gain settings, along with a longitudinal image (**C**), demonstrate the left and posterior portion of the prostate's peripheral zone to be relatively intact. There is complete loss of the peripheral zone in the right lateral and anterolateral portion of the gland (*arrows*); and although there is a predominantly hypoechoic lesion, there are also scattered acoustic reflectors. Because of the marked asymmetry, this is highly suggestive of malignancy. The capsule appears to be intact.

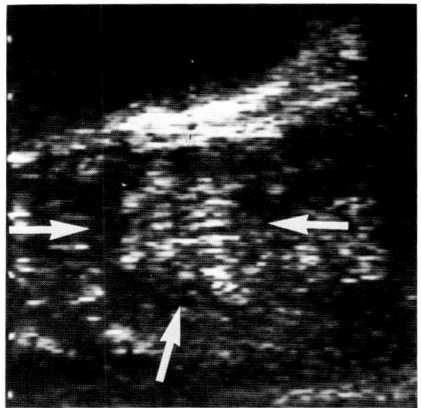

FIG. 10.25. Sagittal endorectal sonogram showing hyperechoic cancer. This longitudinal sonogram demonstrates a subtle hyperechoic lesion (*arrows*). Biopsies of the subtly echogenic areas throughout the mid-portion of the lateral aspect of the prostate showed a cancer throughout the gland. Although the malignancy itself may not be truly hypoechoic, the sonographic appearance of those biopsied areas suggests that there is some hyperacoustic reflectivity of this lesion.

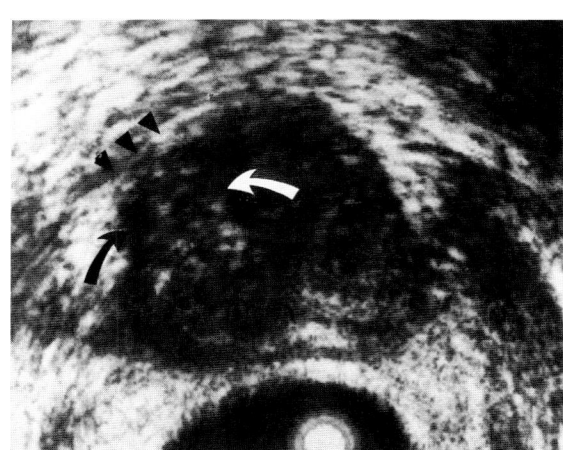

FIG. 10.26. Axial endorectal sonogram showing hyperechoic cancer. Marked asymmetry (*arrows*) and capsular distortion (*arrowheads*) in this axially oriented sonogram suggest a mass infiltrating the peripheral zone on the right side of the prostate. The left side of the posterior portion of the gland is intact.

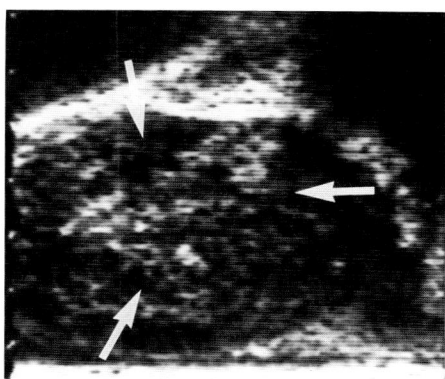

FIG. 10.27. Sagittal endorectal sonogram showing cribiform carcinoma. Subtle acoustic reflectors have infiltrated the entire gland (*arrows*), which, on radical prostatectomy, demonstrated that almost all of the prostate was involved with cribiform (stage A2) carcinoma.

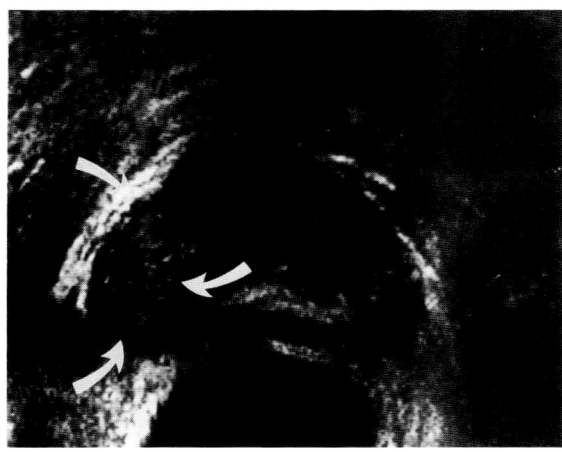

FIG. 10.28. Axial endorectal sonogram showing hyperechoic cancer with asymmetry. This axially oriented endorectal sonogram demonstrates a bulge from the right side of the prostate (*arrows*) with a subtle increase in echogenicity in the peripheral zone. These asymmetrical findings suggest (although are not necessarily diagnostic of) malignancy.

TRANSITION ZONE CANCER

There are a substantial number of cancers, estimated at about 20%, that originate in the transitional zone (308). Because this is the same area where hyperplasia develops, sonographic differentiation may be difficult. Further work and effort to attempt to distinguish these two processes must be undertaken.

TUMOR EXTENSION

Tumor extension into the capsule, the periprostatic lymph nodes, or the seminal vesicle or surrounding tissues may be demonstrated. In general, the endorectal sonogram will only define lymph nodes in the periprostatic areas (Fig. 10.29). Normal lymph nodes are not usually seen. Thus, if a lymph node is identified on the endorectal ultrasound, it must be

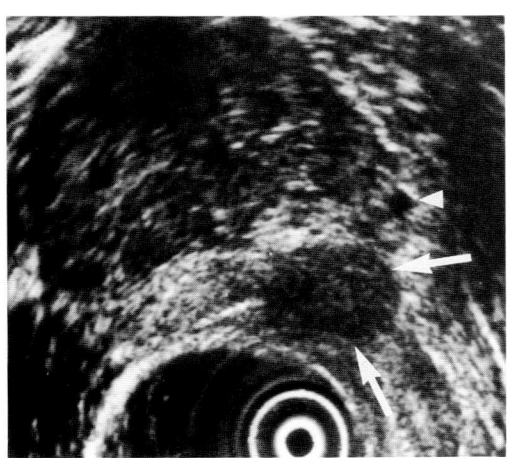

FIG. 10.29. Axial endorectal sonogram showing prostatic cancer tumor extension. Axially oriented ultrasound of the prostate demonstrates an infiltrating malignancy (*arrows*) extending from the left posterolateral aspect of the peripheral zone into the soft tissues. There is also a subcentimeter hypoechoic area (*arrowhead*) unrelated to the venous system, suggestive of lymph node.

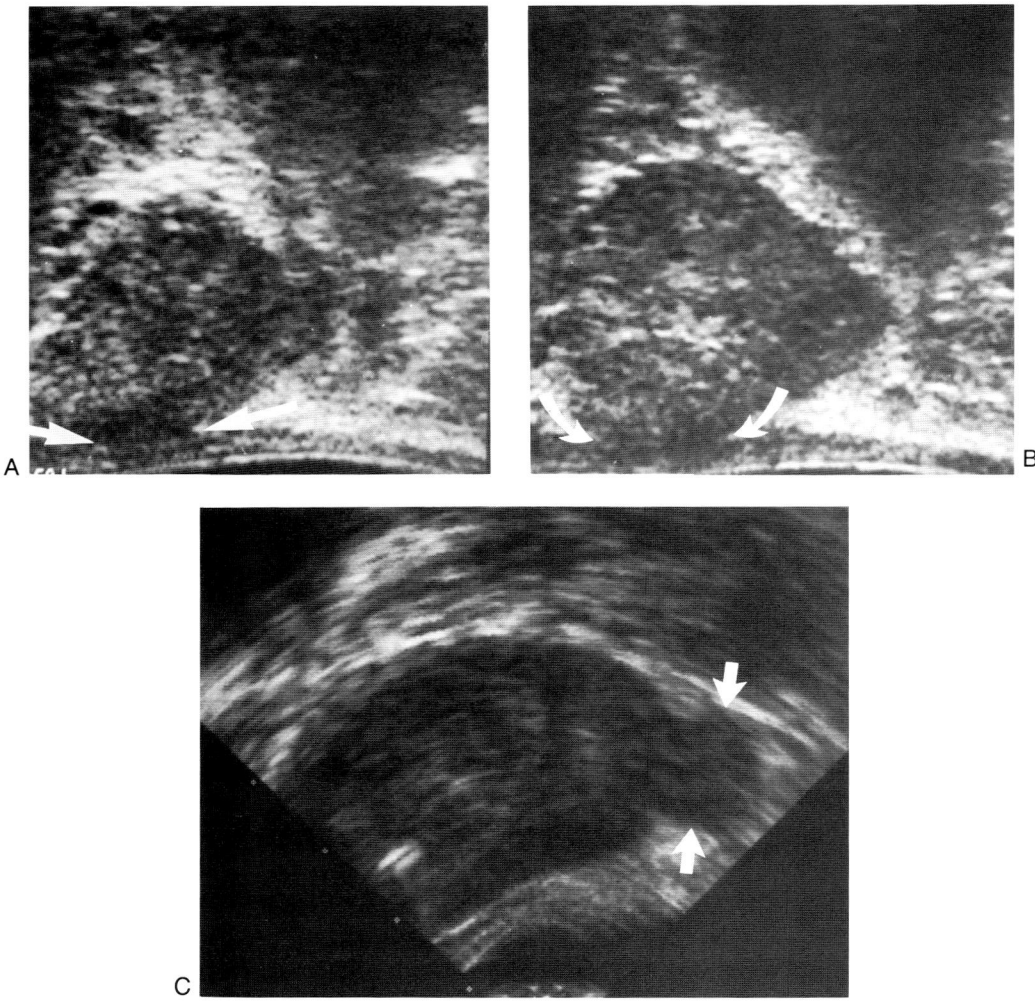

FIG. 10.30. Capsular infiltration of isoechoic cancers in different patients. The first patient (**A**) demonstrates marked thinning of the capsule (*arrow*) without distinct differentiation or delineation of the tumor. A second patient (**B**) demonstrates more obvious capsular disruption (*curved arrow*), although malignancy is not clearly identified. A third man (**C**) demonstrates loss of the periprostatic fat on the left with isoechoic tumor (*arrows*) infiltration.

assumed (although not necessarily accurately) to be involved. The deeper pelvic lymph nodes (both normal and abnormal) are not identified by the endorectal sonogram and require other imaging studies (i.e., conventional ultrasound, computed tomography, or magnetic resonance imaging).

Because of the small percentage of patients who have undergone staging pelvic lymphadenectomy and radical prostatectomy and have also had endorectal ultrasound correlation, the exact ability of the sonogram to delineate lymph-node involvement is not (to date) known.

CAPSULAR INVASION

The exact accuracy of the ability of ultrasound (in particular, endorectal ultrasound) to define capsular invasion has not, as yet, been definitively determined. A few studies, small in size, have given preliminary information. Presently, large-scale studies are underway so that these data will be more clearly calculated over the next few years. The preliminary studies have shown that there is at least a 70% ability to determine capsular invasion (77).

As previously described, the determination of capsular invasion is dependent upon identification of infiltration into, as well as erosion and/or break through of, the relatively echogenic capsule (Figs. 10.12, 10.21, 10.23, and 10.30–10.32).

Seminal vesicle involvement seems to be detected with at least a 70% accuracy rate by endorectal ultrasound (77).

The normal seminal vesicles can have a variety of appearances ranging from moderate to moderately low-level echogenicity. The most definitive determinant of involvement is an asymmetrical appearance of the seminal vesicle. The normal seminal vesicles are fluid-filled tubules; with tumor infiltration, these tubules may be replaced with more solid material. Asymmetry in the size, shape, and echogenicity of the seminal vesicles is thus important for this determination. One criteria to determine subtle seminal vesicle involvement is the obliteration of the "nipple" sign. This may be very subtle (Fig. 10.33). Asymmetric erosion of the "nipple" has been determined to be a relatively reliable sign of tumor infiltration. Unfortunately, the presence of a nipple is not a consistent finding, and thus its absence may be inconclusive.

Another sign of tumor infiltration is the determination of the angle formed between the seminal vesicles and the prostate. This is best seen on the longitudinally oriented scan, since the angle is not clearly defined on the axial orientation. This angle is dependent upon the position of the seminal vesicles to the prostate; normally, this is very variable from one individual to another. However, the angle in each individual should be similar on both the right and left side. Asymmetry of this angle is a suggestion of subtle infiltration of tumor from the base of the prostate into the seminal vesicle (Fig. 10.34). Close comparison of the similar regions of the right versus the left seminal vesicle (e.g., the medial aspect of the right compared to the medial aspect of the left, or the more lateral aspect of the right compared to the lateral aspect of the left) should be performed to detect these subtle changes. Regardless, a comparison must be made between the right and the left side for each individual and not between different patients.

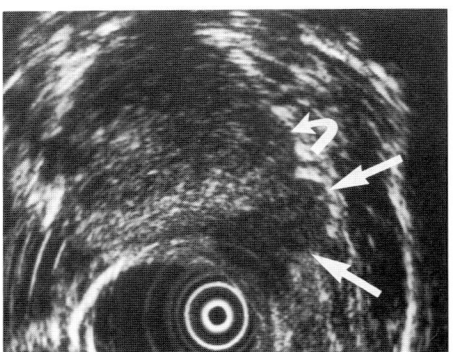

FIG. 10.31. Axial endorectal sonogram showing infiltrating cancer. Axially oriented endorectal ultrasound demonstrates, in the left lateral aspect (*arrows*), tumor infiltration through the pericapsular fat. Note that this tumor extends to the anterolateral margin, where the peripheral zone in this area is disrupted (*curved arrow*).

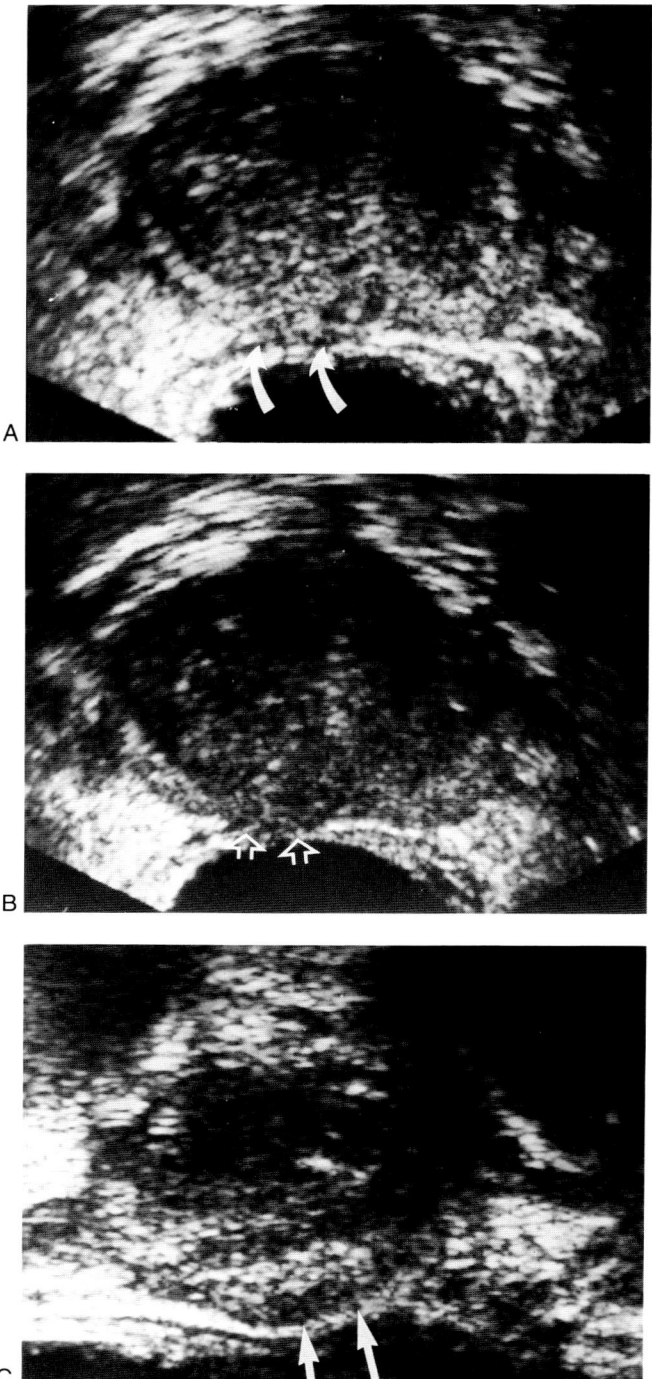

FIG. 10.32. Endorectal sonogram showing isoechoic cancer with prostatic infiltration. Axially oriented scans of the prostate demonstrate poor delineation of the tumor but show distortion (*curved arrows*) of the peripheral zone (**A**). The capsule in the axial orientation (*open arrowheads*) is clearly abnormal (**B**). A longitudinally oriented ultrasound of the left side of the prostate (**C**) demonstrates the capsule to be intact (*straight arrows*).

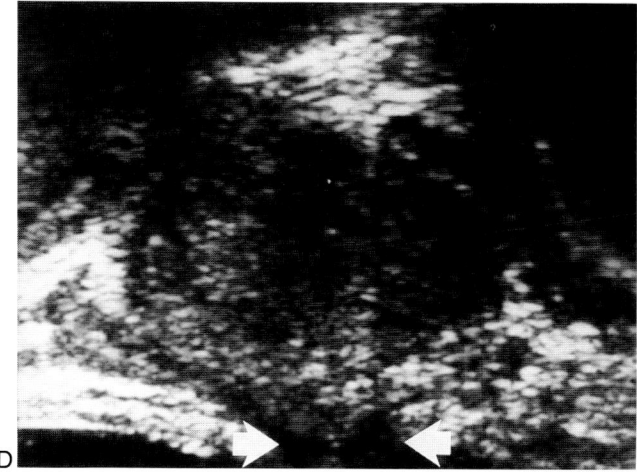

FIG. 10.32. *Continued.* A longitudinally oriented sonogram of the right side of the prostate (**D**) demonstrates the isoechoic cancer to have broken through the capsule (*large arrowheads*).

STAGING TUMORS WITH ULTRASOUND

The ability to detect some cancers that have distinctly different sonographic characteristics than normal tissue has been well described. In these instances, the clinical stage may not correlate with the sonographic findings. An ultrasound staging system has been suggested that may be used in certain cases where the ultrasound and clinical findings disagree (255,259). Some cancers, staged differently by ultrasound than by clinical means, may require a different therapeutic approach than suggested by conventional means without the use of ultrasound. A proposed ultrasound staging system is as follows (255):

1. Stage UA: Tumors confined to the prostate gland.
   a. UA1: Tumors 0–1.0 cm in size.
2. Stage UB: Tumors confined to the prostate gland.
   a. UB1: Tumors 1.0–1.5 cm in size.
   b. UB2: Tumors greater than 1.5 cm but *less* than 50% of glandular involvement.
   c. UB3: Tumors greater than 1.5 cm and *greater* than 50% of glandular involvement.
3. Stage UC: Tumors having extended beyond the prostate capsule and/or having extension into the seminal vesicles.
   a. UC1: Tumors with less than 50% of glandular involvement.
   b. UC2: Tumors having greater than 50% of glandular involvement.

The UA category in the ultrasound staging generally attempts only to evaluate the peripheral zone tumor, which may be a more significant lesion when small. The application of central zone tumors to this staging system has only been done to a minimal degree; its benefit, as yet, is not known.

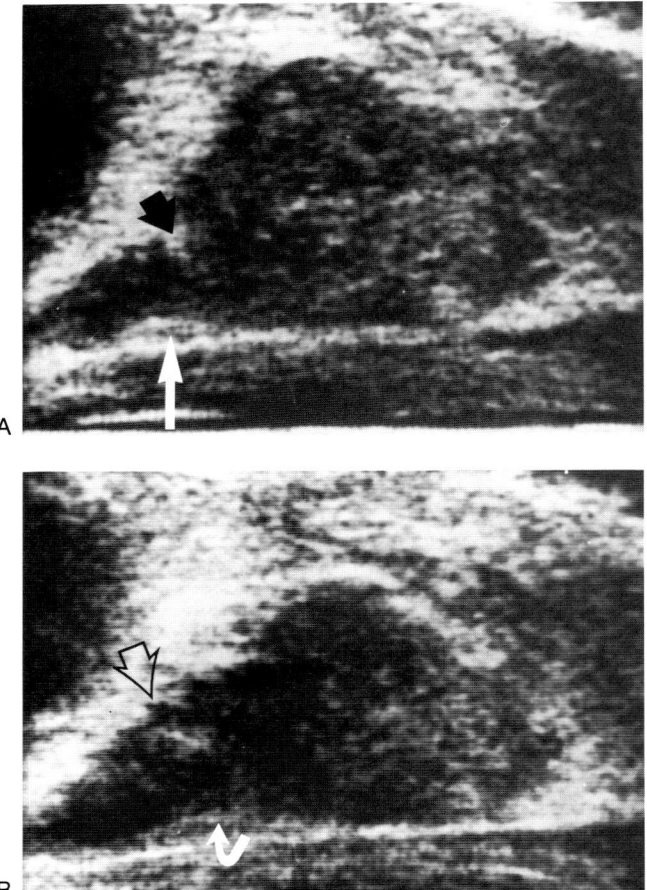

FIG. 10.33. Endorectal sonogram showing seminal vesicle infiltration ("nipple" sign). A normal seminal vesicle with a normal seminal vesicle "angle" (*arrowhead*) and a normal seminal vesicle "nipple" sign (*arrow*) is seen on this longitudinally oriented scan on the left side (**A**). On the right side (**B**), the seminal vesicle "angle" is widened (*open arrowhead*), and the lack of the "nipple" (*curved arrow*) is demonstrated. These are signs of tumor infiltration.

An example of how this staging system may change therapy is described as follows. A man has a nonpalpable cancer in the peripheral zone less than 1.0 cm in size. According to the Whitmore-Jewett system, this would represent a stage A1 tumor and may not, according to some studies, require therapy. However, according to the ultrasound staging system, this tumor would be staged as UA1. It may, therefore, be more appropriate to treat this tumor as a peripherally oriented Whitmore-Jewett stage B1 tumor. Further work is necessary to accurately evaluate the application of this system.

Table 10.2 attempts to correlate the Whitmore-Jewett staging system to the ultrasound staging system and a theoretical clinical system (yet to be clinically used).

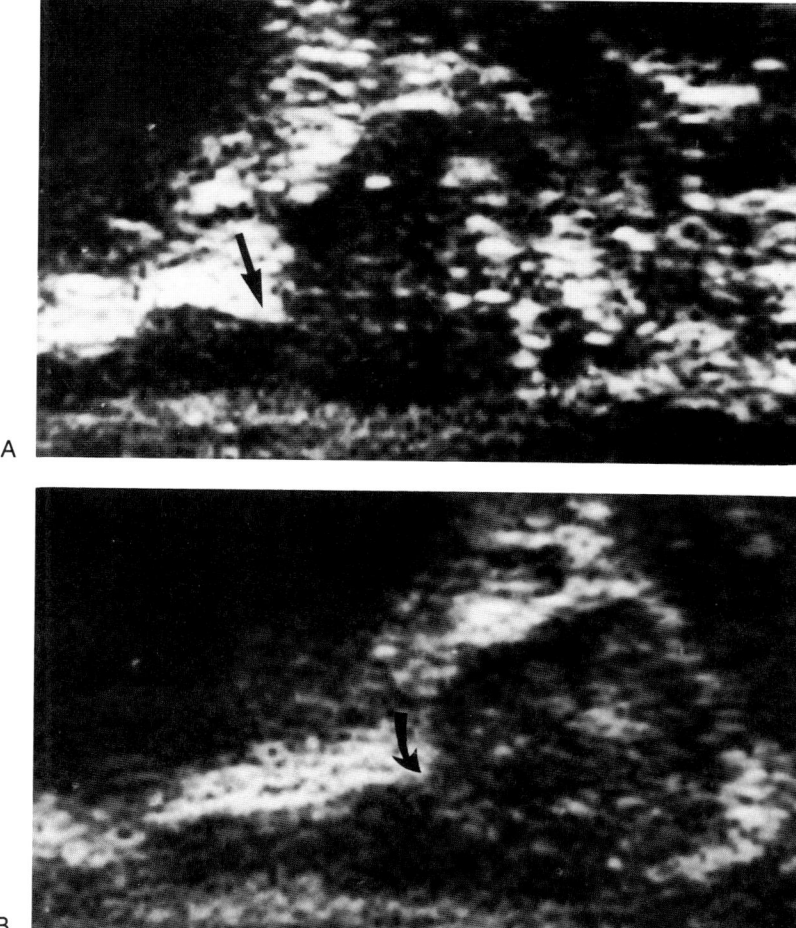

FIG. 10.34. Tumor infiltration—seminal vesicle "angle" distortion. Longitudinal ultrasound on the left side (**A**) demonstrates a normal acute "angle" (*straight arrow*). On the right side (**B**), the seminal vesicle is enlarged and the "angle" (*curved arrows*) is widened.

TABLE 10.2. Comparison of the Whitmore-Jewett, theoretical clinical, and ultrasound staging system

Whitmore-Jewett stage	Ultrasound stage	Theoretical clinical stage	Comments
A1	UA1	A1	If in transitional zone
A1	UA1	B1	If in peripheral zone
A2	UB1, UB2, UB3	A2	If in transitional zone
A2	UB1	B1	If in peripheral zone
A2	UB2 or UB3	B2	If in peripheral zone
B1	UB2	B1	When tumor is less than 50% of glandular prostate
B2	UB3	B2	When tumor is greater than 50% of glandular prostate
C1 or C2	UC1	C	Tumor less than 50% of glandular prostate
C1 or C2	UC2	C	Tumor greater than 50% of glandular prostate

ACCURACY OF SONOGRAPHY IN DETERMINING THE PRESENCE OF PROSTATE CANCER

Is there at least one sonographic characteristic that is specific for prostate cancer only? As discussed in previous sections, cancer has a variety of sonographic appearances. However, is there one sonographic appearance that can diagnose and differentiate prostate cancer from all other cancers? This is unclear at the present time for a variety of reasons. They include:

1. Poor correlation with pathology.
2. An inability to obtain a large number of radical prostatectomy specimens for a one-to-one correlation.
3. Poor correlation of digitally palpated lesions to ultrasound visualized lesions, which may be inconsistent between readers or may be poorly identified.
4. Bias of observers. This is probably the most difficult area to evaluate. If an individual observer is looking for a specific sonographic characteristic (i.e., the hypoechoic lesion or the hyperechoic lesion), only those areas will be biopsied under ultrasound guidance.

Is the small and peripherally oriented hypoechoic lesion pathognomonic for prostate cancer? Studies have shown that between 0% and 50% of these lesions may be malignant, depending upon the observer (73,253,257,291,407–411,418). The largest of these studies has shown an approximate 25% cancer rate (291). Other tissue diagnoses include prostatitis, infarct, benign prostatic hyperplasia, and what appears to be nonspecific benign prostatic tissue.

The potential to use ultrasound as a screening tool will be discussed in Chapter 16.

CANCER IN THE PRESENCE OF BENIGN PROSTATIC HYPERTROPHY

There are certain anatomic changes of the prostate that occur in men with benign prostatic hyperplasia. The peripheral zone and, to a greater degree, the central zone of the acinar tissues are compressed by benign hyperplastic changes of the periurethral tissues. This compression may be quite significant, particularly posteriorly, so that the bulk of the peripheral zone will be situated anterolaterally. Thus, an extensive search for determination of normal (although distorted) peripheral zone is important to demonstrate those tumors that arise from it. The benign changes above are further discussed in Chapter 12.

CONCLUSION

There is much known about the sonographic characteristics of prostate cancer, yet there is even more to determine in the future. Prostate ultrasound has great benefit in the evaluation of the prostate for demonstration of prostate cancer. However, as shown in this chapter, there are still limitations in various diagnoses. The clinical implication of prostatic ultrasound will be discussed in detail in Chapter 16.

11 // Percutaneous Use of Radiation Treatment and Treatment Planning

Ultrasound Guided Radioactive Seed Implantation: General Considerations	185
Planning for the Procedure	186
Procedure of Seed Implantation	186
Follow-up Studies	188
Success of Treatment	188
Ancillary Treatment	188
Complications	188
Conclusion	190

The only truly "curative" procedure for the treatment of prostatic carcinoma is radical prostatectomy (87,220). However, while absolute cures may not be possible with other treatment modalities, clinically effective results may be obtained. These successes depend upon a number of variables, which include tumor size and volume, cellular differentiation, and aggressiveness. Nonsurgical procedures can include chemotherapy, hormonal administration, radiation treatment administered by external beam, and intraoperative or percutaneous placement of radioactive implants (seeds) (21,28,85,86,101,106,113,127, 165,173,178,192,267).

The choice of treatment can depend upon a number of factors, including the size and aggressiveness of the lesion, the patient's age and general medical condition, and the individual patient's acceptance of the risks and possibilities of various side affects.

Although interstitial radiation therapy is useful because a large radioactive dose can be given to the prostate with minimal damage to the surrounding periprostatic tissues, it was necessary, until recently, to do this intraoperatively. The procedure, however, can lead to an increased risk of morbidity. Recently, percutaneous transperineal placement of radioactive seeds has been utilized with success (44,86,203,204,258,284,391,507).

ULTRASOUND GUIDED RADIOACTIVE SEED IMPLANTATION: GENERAL CONSIDERATIONS

When percutaneous placement of radioactive material is contemplated, a number of considerations must be realized. A major question arises as to what radioisotope to use. In most instances, iodine-125 has been used because of its intrinsic properties, including (a) a half-life of 60 days and (b) a half-value layer (HVL) of 1.7 cm.

Because of these characteristics, slow but persistent administration of the radioactive dose to the prostatic and periprostatic tissues is possible (44,203,258). Treatment of the malignancy without severe involvement of adjacent tissue, particularly the rectal wall, can be undertaken. Other radioactive compounds used in these procedures have included palladium-103 (with a half-life of 17 days), gold-198 (86,284), and iridium-192. Seed implanatation has been performed in a manner similar to digital guided biopsy but without the use of ultrasound (203,204,497). However, this technique has limitations because of the lack of precise accuracy which is needed in the placement and positioning of the seeds. In the early 1980s, the technique of transperineal biopsy of the prostate under endorectal ultrasound guidance was extended for treatment of prostatic carcinoma with positioning of the needles and placement of radioactive seeds under endorectal ultrasonic guidance. This approach permitted accurate placement of the seeds to various portions of the prostate as continuous ultrasound guidance was utilized. The patient did not require general anesthesia, open surgical approach, or even removal of the seeds following therapy.

Although pelvic lymphadenectomy is the "ideal" technique in staging carcinomas to exclude or confirm the presence of a stage D1 tumor, extraperitoneal pelvioscopy can also be performed to assess the possibility of local node infiltration. This technique is usually limited to patients without previously known pelvic lymph-node involvement.

PLANNING FOR THE PROCEDURE

Accurate volumetric calculations of the prostate (and, if possible, the carcinoma) must be performed prior to seed placement. Although these are not necessarily essential, accurate calculation enables assessment of the success of treatment (203). More accurate measurements and volumetric calculations are obtained by examining the patient in the same position that will be used for seed implantation. Because the procedure of seed implantation requires a relatively long (up to 1 hr) time frame, it has been found that the lithotomy position is frequently the most useful (203,204). For this reason, preliminary volumetric calculations should also be performed in the lithotomy position. The patient should be studied, and volumetric calculations should be obtained with a "stepper" device as described in Chapter 6. Following a volumetric calculation of the prostate, a computer-analyzed cylindrical model is defined so that the appropriate position of seed implantations and isotope administration can be planned.

After the initial study, isotope curves are then calculated to delineate the dose of radioactive material to be administered to the prostate and the surrounding periprostatic tissues if necessary (203).

During the volumetric and radioisotope calculation, needles are prepared and marked for dose and exact position of implantation.

PROCEDURE OF SEED IMPLANTATION

Although local anesthesia is usually adequate for biopsies, mild sedation may be useful for radiation seed implantation because of the length of the procedure (up to 1 hr). Some patients may even require spinal anesthesia.

Once anesthetized, the patient is placed in the same (the lithotomy) position as in the initial volumetric calculation study. For placement of the needle, the specially produced guidance device (the matrix) is used to place the needle into position and it can also be

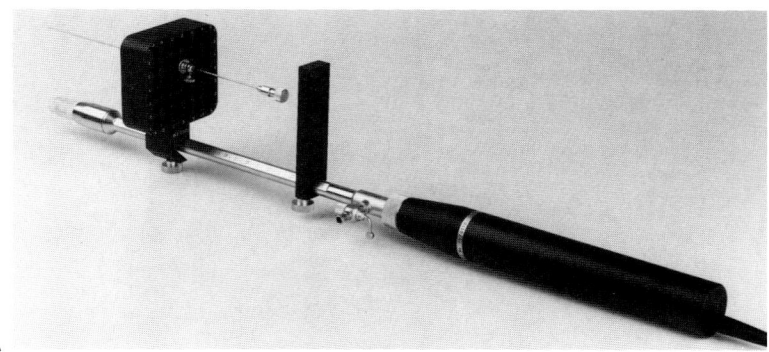

A

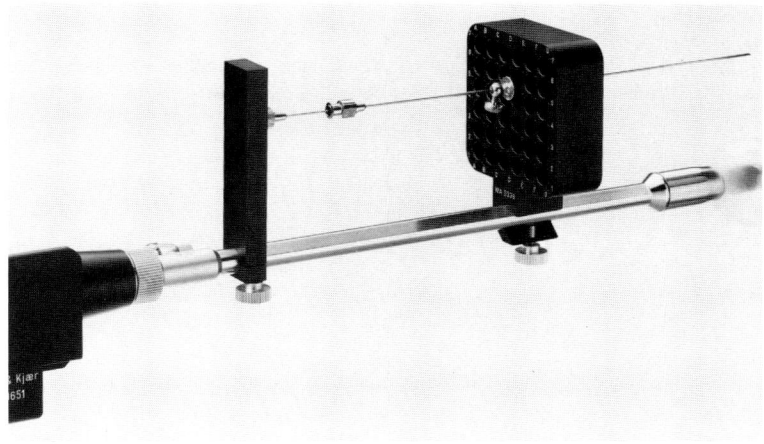

B

FIG. 11.1. Needle placement guidance device. A specially produced biopsy-type device that can place multiple needles into the prostate has been devised for use with the axially oriented scanners. This is one such device that can be used to place the needles into the prostate (**A**) and also "push" the radioactive materials from the needle into the prostate (**B**). A specially produced attachment is utilized to push the radioactive material in so that no direct hand contact to the needle is required. (Courtesy of Dr. Hans Henrik Holm.)

utilized to "push" radioactive seeds into the prostate (Fig. 11.1) The examination is performed with the axial orientation for positioning of the needles within the exact area of the prostate. The use of longitudinally oriented scanners to demonstrate the depth of seed placement is suggested. The patient is prepared in a fashion similar to that for biopsy. However, because of the length of the procedure, the scrotum must be supported more securely. The use of a stepper device simplifies accurate positioning of the needle (Fig. 11.2). A needle, without radioactive seeds, is placed through the perineum and into the prostate, stabilizing the gland and fixing the prostate to the guiding matrix so that no movement can occur.

Needles are then placed individually into the prostate for evaluation of anterior-posterior and lateral positioning using the axial orientation and for depth of insertion into the prostate using the longitudinally oriented transducer (Fig. 11.3). Once all the needles are placed,

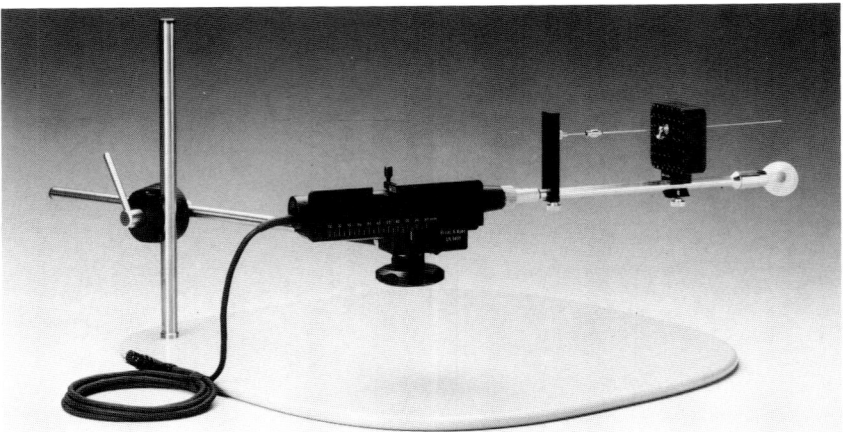

FIG. 11.2. Stepper device for radioactive seed placement. Needles with the radioactive seeds can be placed into the prostate more accurately using a "stepper" device. (Courtesy of Dr. Hans Henrik Holm.)

which requires approximately 30 min, implantation requiring an additional 30 min is begun. The ultrasound demonstrates the seeds (Fig. 11.4). A radiograph is often obtained to confirm "seeds" in the prostatic bed (Fig. 11.5) (44,203,204,497).

FOLLOW-UP STUDIES

On the first operative day, the patients are usually asked to urinate through a filter so that any possible expelled radioactive seeds are collected. Most patients are treated initially on an inpatient basis, usually requiring only 1 to 2 days of hospitalization. Outpatient procedures can also be performed.

Radiographs and/or computerized tomography can demonstrate the exact position of the seeds in relation to the prostate and periprostatic tissues.

SUCCESS OF TREATMENT

In various studies, up to 91% of patients have had clinical improvements with percutaneous placement of seeds. In all patients, tumor and prostatic size and volume have diminished. However, there has been approximately a 4% recurrence rate using this technique (44,203,497).

ANCILLARY TREATMENT

Some studies have suggested that ancillary treatment with external beam radiation be administered to the percutaneous placement of seeds.

COMPLICATIONS

Theoretical complications of percutaneous placement of radioactive seeds include intraprostatic hemorrhage and/or edema. However, preliminary studies have shown that these sequellae are rare. Follow-up studies have demonstrated the major complications to include:

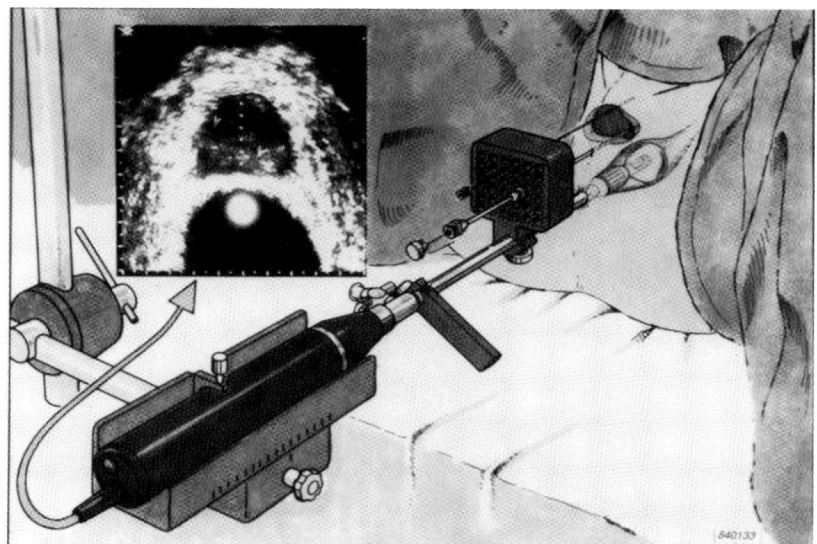

FIG. 11.3. Radioactive seed placement. The procedure is demonstrated by a schematic diagram demonstrating the study being performed and the concurrent sonogram (*upper left*). (Courtesy of Dr. Hans Henrik Holm.)

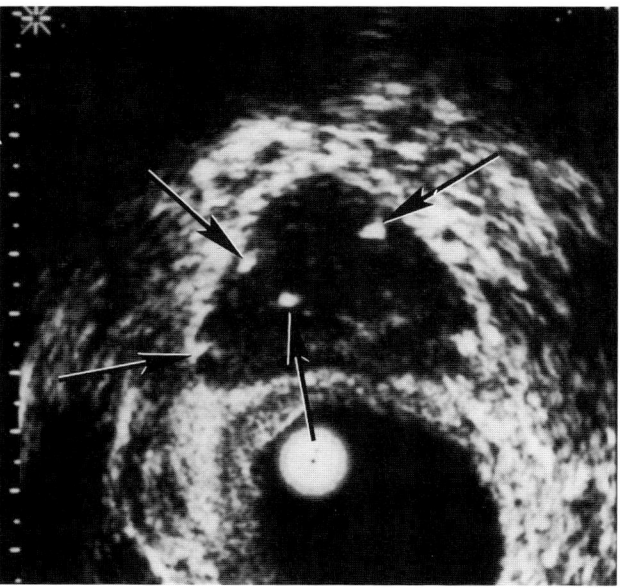

FIG. 11.4. Ultrasound during procedure. An axially oriented endorectal ultrasound demonstrates multiple acoustic reflectors (*arrows*) scattered throughout the prostate from the radioactive seed. (Courtesy of Dr. Hans Henrik Holm.)

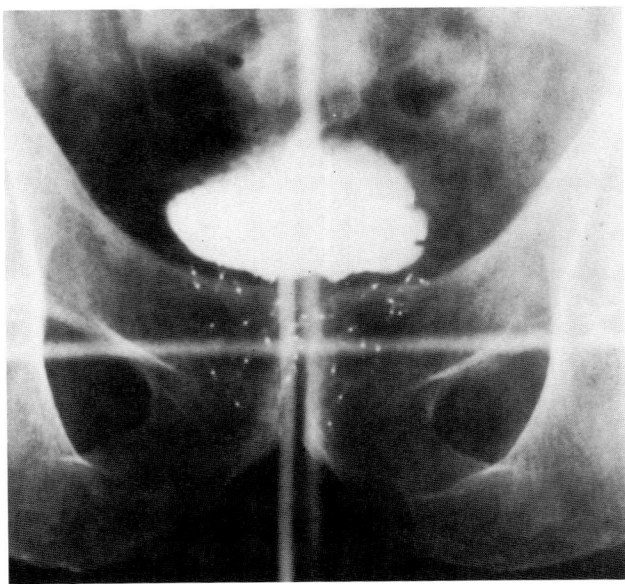

FIG. 11.5. Follow-up radiograph. This cystogram demonstrates contrast within the urinary bladder; also, in the prostatic and periprostatic area, it demonstrates multiple radioactive seeds. (Courtesy of Dr. Hans Henrik Holm.)

TABLE 11.1. Complications of percutaneous iodine-125 seed placement[a]

Complication	Minimal	Moderate	Severe
Rectal ulcer	1/31	0/31	3/31
Hematuria	3/31	1/31	0/31
Renal obstruction	4/31	0/31	2/31
Infection	4/31	1/31	1/31
Impotence	0/31	2/31	0/31
Pain	0/31	1/31	0/31

[a] Five- to 52-month follow-up in 31 patients. Data taken from ref. 497.

rectal ulcer, hematuria, renal obstruction, and infection (Table 11.1). These are generally minor, although certain severe complications may also occur.

CONCLUSION

There is still much to be learned regarding the usefulness of this technique. However, preliminary studies with both small and large numbers of patients have clearly demonstrated that radioactive seed placement appears to be an effective alternative treatment for nonoperable prostatic carcinoma. Only further studies and longer-term follow-up will demonstrate its actual benefit in the diagnostic armamentarium for prostatic disease. At the present time, seed implantation is not a completely accepted technique. Further evaluation is required to determine its exact place in the therapeutic regime for prostate cancer.

12 // *Benign Prostatic Hyperplasia*

General Considerations	191
Incidence	192
Pathogenesis	192
Clinical Manifestations	193
Imaging of Benign Prostatic Hyperplasia	193
Sonographic Characteristics	193
Conventional Ultrasound	
Transperineal Ultrasound	
The Endourethral Examination	
Endorectal Ultrasound	
Post-Transurethral Resection: Endorectal Ultrasound	200
Ultrasound Monitoring of Transurethral Resection	209
Prostatic Calculi	216
Prostatic Cysts (Cystic Changes)	219
Conclusion	220

Enlargement of the prostate gland, also known as *benign prostatic hyperplasia* (BPH), occurs in almost all older men. Its clinical implications can be both immense and debilitating.

GENERAL CONSIDERATIONS

Prostatic hyperplasia is a process that is unusual in the male patient under the age of 40 (131,191,318,376,484). However, enlargement of the gland does occur and has been estimated to affect up to 90% of the adult male population (37). Although there are a variety of possible reasons for hyperplasia of the prostate, three major etiologies (164) are suggested. These include the following:

1. Benign prostatic hyperplasia is a result of a normal prostatic cell reacting to an aberrant or abnormal endocrine environment.
2. Benign prostatic hyperplasia is a result of abnormal prostatic cells that are being stimulated to grow abnormally by the hormonal environment that is not necessarily abnormal but is probably slightly altered from the normal.
3. Benign prostatic hyperplasia is perhaps a reflection of a combination of the above two factors.

The normal prostate gland, in men between the ages of 21 and 30 years, weighs approximately 20 g. The size and weight of the prostate remains relatively constant until the development of benign prostatic hyperplasia ensues. This occurs beginning in the fourth decade (30–39 years of age). In this early age group, hyperplasia affects only a small group, or approximately 8% of all males. However, benign prostatic hyperplasia is more common as men age; 50% of men have pathologic hypertrophy by the sixth decade (37).

Studies have shown that between the ages of 31 and 50 years, the doubling time of prostatic weight is about 4.5 years. From 51 to 70 years of age, the doubling time is 10 years. Above the age of 70 years, the doubling time of prostatic weight increases dramatically, to approximately 100 years (37).

INCIDENCE

The incidence of developing benign prostatic hyperplasia is quite high (37). It is estimated that up to 80 to 90% of adult men will be affected with such pathologic processes.

PATHOGENESIS

Benign prostatic hyperplasia nodule formation occurs mostly in the preprostatic tissues, also known as the *transition zone*. Occasionally, nodules may develop in the periurethral glandular tissues. Distinct nodule development usually occurs as early as the fourth decade in life (300,302–304). Those originating in the periurethral tissues are generally smaller and purely stromal in composition, and they frequently remain small throughout life.

The hyperplastic nodules that develop in the transition zone are glandular in their origin and can enlarge to a massive size, composing the main mass of benign prostatic hyperplastic tissue. Benign prostatic hyperplastic nodules usually develop by three independent processes:

1. formation of distinct nodules;
2. enlargement of the transition zone in a diffuse manner; and
3. enlargement of the prostatic nodules (300).

Pathologically, benign prostatic hyperplasia occurs almost universally from the transition zone and the periurethral glandular tissue of the prostate. The acinar tissue is relatively immune to hyperplastic changes but can undergo other benign processes.

Microscopically, benign prostatic hypertrophy can be classified into five different entities (133). These include the following:

1. Stromal or fibroblastic nodules are the most frequent, and they are found in the sub- or periurethral epithelial tissue surrounding the prostatic urethra. These nodules have myxomatous stroma and prominent vasculature. They have also been called *fibrovascular nodules*. The lesions occur proximal to the distal portion of the verumontanum and, on the gross specimen, are clearly differentiated from the surrounding normal tissue.

2. Fibromuscular nodules (which are different from the pure muscular nodules) are associated with areas of infarction and may be infiltrated with inflammatory cells (in particular, histiocytes and plasma cells). Histologically, they may be confused with granulomatous prostatitis.

3. Smooth-muscle nodules, also known as *muscular nodules*, consist purely of smooth muscle and are uncommon. They represent true localized cellular hypertrophy of the smooth-muscle elements and usually are asymmetrical. Thus, unilateral enlargement occurs, resulting in asymmetrical benign prostatic hyperplasia.

4. Hyperadenomatous nodules are characterized by both stromal hyperplasia and epithelial hyperplasia. Histologically, these nodules usually have lower activity than do other areas of hyperplasia. The lesions are commonly associated with, or found near, areas of infarction and active healed infection. The transitional cells may undergo some squamous metaplasia.

5. Fibromyoadenomatous nodules are the lesions most commonly found in the suprapubic or retropubic specimens and are, therefore, some of the larger nodules present. Infarction and hemorrhage are common. Metaplasia is not an infrequent occurrence on histological evaluation.

CLINICAL MANIFESTATIONS

The clinical manifestations of prostatic hypertrophy are frequently related to the size and position of the hyperplastic nodules. While all hypertrophy occur from the transition zone or periurethral glandular tissue, the hypertrophic tissue may enlarge in various positions. When the middle portion of the prostate enlarges (previously known as *median* or *middle lobe hypertrophy*), there may be impingement upon the posterior portion of the urethra or impingement upon the base of the bladder and the bladder neck. With more lateral enlargment (i.e., asymmetric enlargement of the gland), there may be no clinical symptomatology. Clinically, men with benign prostatic hyperplasia may present with the following complaints:

1. decrease in the caliber and force of urine flow;
2. difficulty in initiating voiding;
3. difficulty in terminating voiding which may result in dribbling;
4. the sensation that the bladder is still filled following voiding;
5. nocturia; and
6. urinary retention.

Although clinically these manifestations may be present, an important factor in the decision for a possible interventional approach will not only be symptomatology but also postvoiding urinary bladder residual volume. A postvoid residua in the range of 100 ml or more is often considered clinically significant.

IMAGING OF BENIGN PROSTATIC HYPERPLASIA

The intravenous urogram may not necessarily be clinically useful, because of the low yield of findings (2,104,274). Benign prostatic hyperplasia may cause impingement upon the bladder base, as seen on the intravenous pyelogram. Findings of ureteral or renal pelvic dilatation may also be seen.

SONOGRAPHIC CHARACTERISTICS

Conventional Ultrasound

The conventional (suprapubic) sonographic examination can define prostatic size, shape, and position (Figs. 12.1 and 12.2). An enlarged renal collecting system or dilated ureter may be noted in these studies. Prostatic calcifications may be seen (Figs. 12.3 and 12.4).

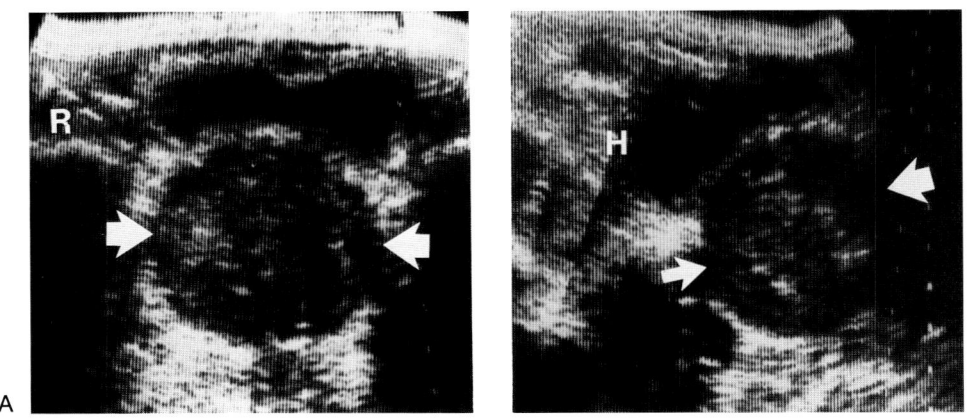

FIG. 12.1. Transabdominal scans showing benign prostatic hyperplasia. A rounded prostate (arrows) is seen in transverse (**A**) and longitudinal (**B**) orientation. Diffuse inhomogeneous echogenicity without a focal lesion is seen. (R) Patient's right side; (H) toward patient's head.

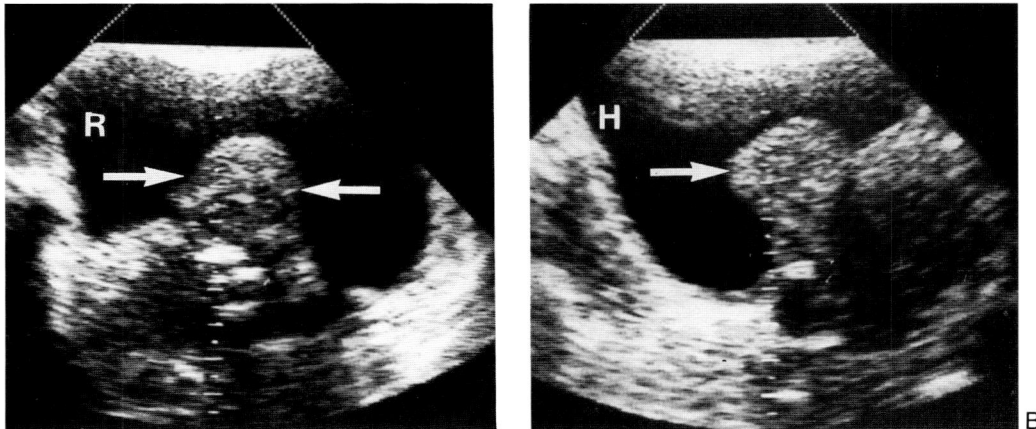

FIG. 12.2. Transabdominal approach demonstrating benign prostatic hypertrophy. The prostate in transverse (**A**) and longitudinal (**B**) orientation demonstrates a focal bulge from the periurethral glandular tissue (arrows) impinging upon the bladder base. The remainder of the prostate appears to be relatively inhomogeneous and scattered acoustic reflectors (arrowheads) consistent with calculi are seen. (R) Patient's right side; (H) toward patient's head.

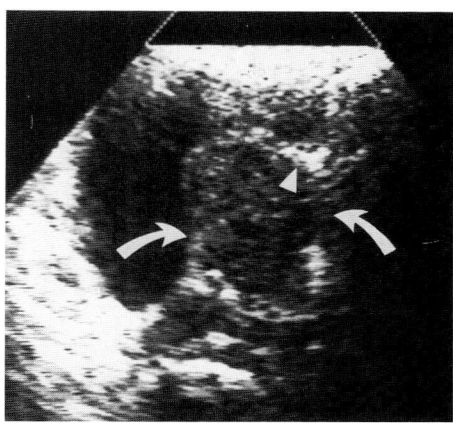

FIG. 12.3. Transabdominal scan showing benign prostatic hypertrophy. This longitudinal image, obtained using a transabdominal approach, demonstrates an enlarged prostate (*arrows*). Focal lesions (echogenic areas) are identified (*arrowhead*). Some do not cause shadowing because of the limited resolution with the transabdominal technique.

Although this is not necessarily a finding of benign prostatic hyperplasia, (it may be related to other causes) it is often seen with BPH. Distinct focal lesions may also not be identified or clearly defined. Adenomas, when present, may (Fig. 12.5) or may not be clearly defined. Conventional ultrasound is of limited value in defining focal abnormalities in the gland, particularly in a normal-sized gland with a small, but perhaps clinically significant, hyperplastic nodule.

Transperineal Ultrasound

The transperineal approach has had no better success than the suprapubic examination.

The Endourethral Examination

This technique has limited benefit in the evaluation of benign prostatic hyperplasia per se. While it can show the size and shape of the prostate (Fig. 12.6), its major use is in monitoring

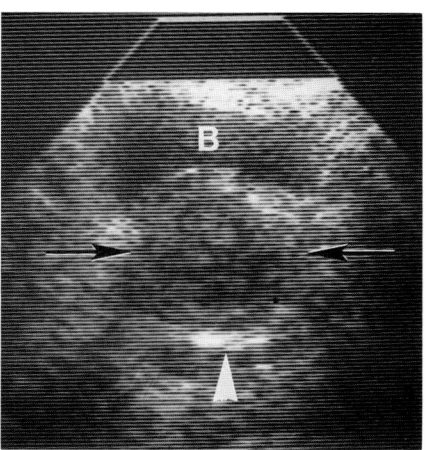

FIG. 12.4. Transabdominal sonogram showing prostatic calcification. The prostate with benign hyperplasia is seen on transverse orientation. An enlarged gland (*arrows*) is identified through the fluid-filled urinary bladder (B). A hyperechoic focus (*arrowhead*), a calculus, is seen causing acoustic shadowing.

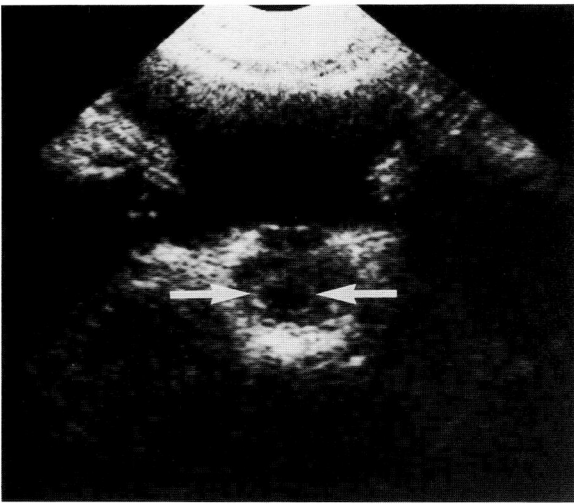

FIG. 12.5. Transabdominal approach demonstrating a cyst. A simple cyst of the prostate (*arrows*) is seen. The lesion does not appear to have the characteristics of a simple cyst because of the limited resolution of the transabdominal approach.

surgery when performed with transurethral resection of the prostate. This will be described later in this chapter.

Endorectal Ultrasound

The endorectal approach can demonstrate many areas of abnormality. Internal glandular tissue may be defined. Clearly demarcated adenomas may be seen in the periurethral areas where these originate. These lesions are frequently delineated on the ultrasound examination as well-demarcated areas (Fig. 12.7 and 12.8). When periurethrally placed and well-defined, they are classically benign-appearing on ultrasound.

Sonographic characteristics of these well-defined hyperplastic nodules can vary. They may be purely hypoechoic (Figs. 12.9 and 12.10), hyperechoic (Fig. 12.11), of mixed echogenicity (Fig. 12.12), or even isoechoic (Figs. 12.13 and 12.14), as compared to the normal tissue (403,404,409,522,530,531). The normal periurethral glandular tissue is slightly hypoechoic; thus, with hyperplastic nodule development, changes in the sonographic characteristics are frequent. The nodules may be clearly delineated and have a thin, slightly hypoechoic rim, resembling a halo surrounding the nodule (Fig. 12.15). The axial orientation can clearly define the lateral margins of the lesions better than the longitudinal orientation. The longitudinal orientation can define placement in the cephalocaudad position more accurately.

Often, multiple lesions will be seen. Lesions may be bilobed (Figs. 12.16 and 12.17), multilobed, multiple, and/or asymmetrically positioned.

Although benign hyperplastic nodules develop from the periurethral tissues and the transitional zone, they may not always be situated in the midline. Occasionally, they will be seen extending superiorly, posteriorly, or even laterally (Fig. 12.18). In these cases, bulging and distortion of the capsule may be identified. These asymmetrical areas may be of concern

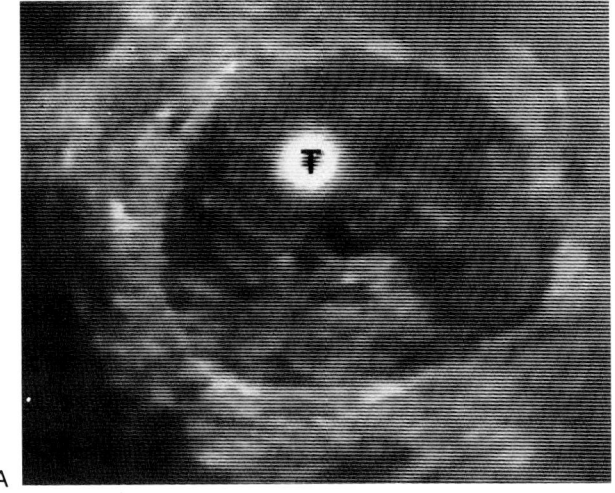

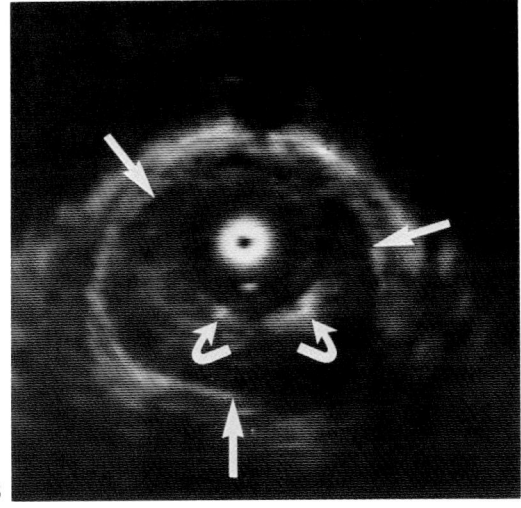

FIG. 12.6. Endourethral approach demonstrating benign prostatic hyperplasia. The transurethral approach demonstrates the tranducer (T) within the prostatic urethra. In one patient, we observe diffuse enlargement of the gland (**A**) without a focal lesion. In a second patient, benign enlargement (**B**) is identified (*arrows*) with bright echogenic reflectors (*curved arrows*), causing some acoustic shadowing (calculi surrounding the surgical capsule).

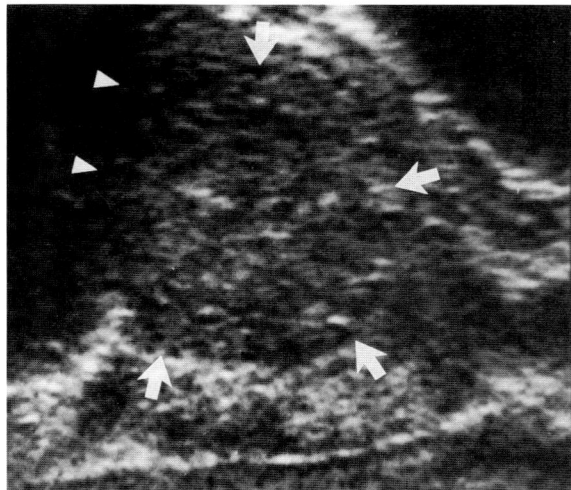

FIG. 12.7. Longitudinal endorectal sonogram showing a benign prostatic hyperplastic nodule. A well-defined, benign-appearing lesion (*arrows*) is seen involving the periurethral tissues of the prostate on longitudinal endorectal sonogram. The lesion is well-marginated and causes impingement upon the bladder base (*arrowheads*).

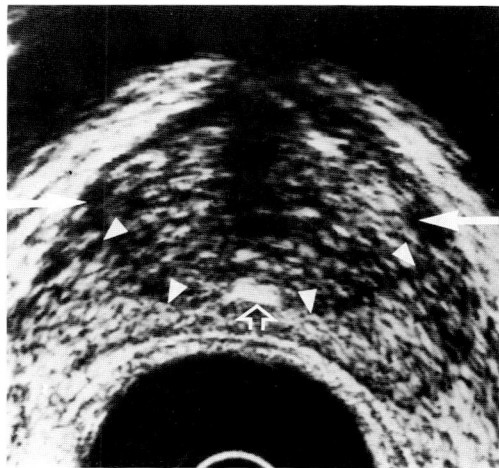

FIG. 12.8. Axial endorectal sonogram showing benign prostatic hyperplastic nodule. The endorectal sonogram in the axial orientation demonstrates a well-defined, well-marginated, mixed, but predominantly hypoechoic, lesion (*arrows*) within the prostate. A sharp demarcation between the benign hyperplastic nodule and the compressed central and peripheral zones (*arrowheads*) is identified. There is also an echogenic calculus (*open arrowhead*) with acoustic shadowing. Note that the compression of the posterior portion is more pronounced than that of the lateral margins of the peripheral zone of the gland.

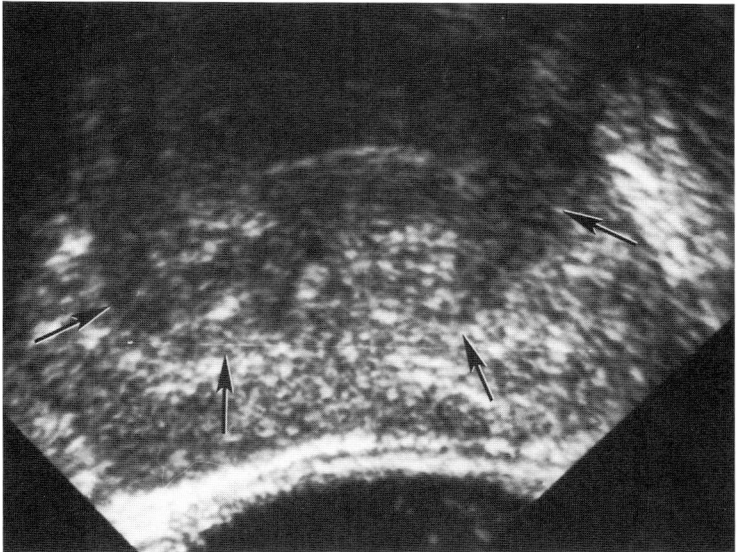

FIG. 12.9. Axial endorectal ultrasound showing benign prostatic hyperplasia. Endorectal ultrasound in the axial orientation demonstrates a relatively well-defined hypoechoic, hyperplastic nodule (*arrows*).

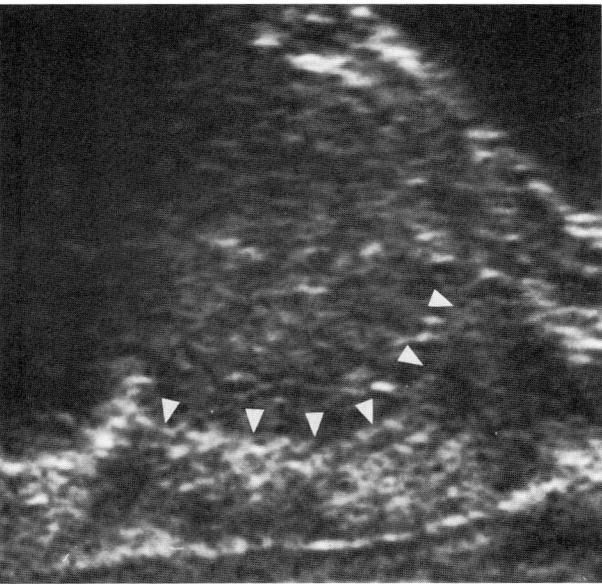

FIG. 12.10. Sagittal endorectal ultrasound showing a benign hyperplastic lesion. Endorectal ultrasound demonstrates a well-defined, well-marginated hyperplastic benign-appearing nodule, sharply demarcated from the peripheral zone (*arrowheads*). There is no impingement upon the bladder base.

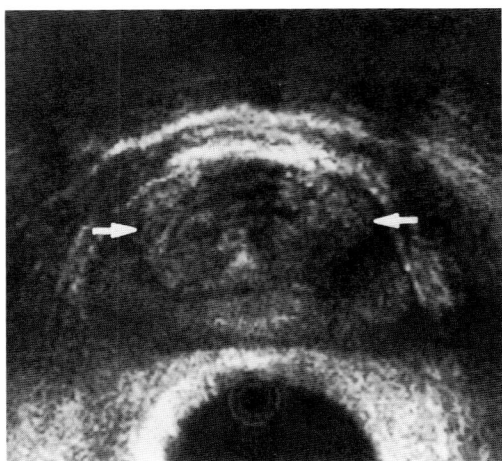

FIG. 12.11. Axial endorectal sonogram showing a hyperechoic benign-appearing nodule. This tranversely oriented endorectal sonogram demonstrates a relatively echogenic (hyperechoic) benign-appearing, well-defined nodule (*arrows*) in the periurethral tissues which is well-demarcated from the remainder of the acinar tissues.

and suggest possible malignant infiltration. However, while cancer may erode the capsule in addition to causing bulging, benign hyperplastic disease will not invade through the capsule. Distortion of the capsule without disruption can occur.

When these hyperplastic nodules become so large, they compress the normal peripheral and central zones, often extensively. The central zone appears more obviously compressed than the peripheral zone (Fig. 12.8). This compression causes an appearance of thinning and is generally more pronounced posteriorly. Histologically and clinically, benign nodules are usually well-defined. On suprapubic and retropubic resection, they can classically be peeled off from the surgical capsule. However, sonographically, all lesions may not be so clearly demarcated. In some cases of benign prostatic hyperplasia, no distinct nodule may be seen. In these cases, there may appear to be diffuse enlargement of the prostate. On the scan, the gland will appear to be rounded or globular in shape (Fig. 12.19). On the sagittal scan, the hyperplastic gland may be seen impinging upon and distorting the bladder base (Fig. 12.20). On both the axial and the sagittal orientation, there may be areas of decreased, increased, or mixed echogenicity (Fig. 12.21). In these cases, there may be no sharp delineation between normal and abnormal tissues. However, no focal lesion to suggest malignancy should be seen. Only a diffuse sonographic abnormality may be demonstrated. In these instances, while the diffuseness of the process suggests a benign disease, diffuse malignant infiltration cannot be excluded in many instances.

There are certain instances where a focal lesion that is central or peripherally oriented may be present. If these are small and relatively hypoechoic (Fig. 12.22), they may suggest the presence of cancer. Not all of the cases (also see Chapter 13, which is on inflammation) with hypoechoic lesions are malignant, and some benign processes may mimic a cancer (also see Chapter 16).

POST-TRANSURETHRAL RESECTION: ENDORECTAL ULTRASOUND

Transurethral resection of the prostate is frequently performed because patients with hyperplastic changes require relief of symptoms. Many patients will be studied by the endorectal ultrasound following surgery. This may be for recurrence of disease or for the

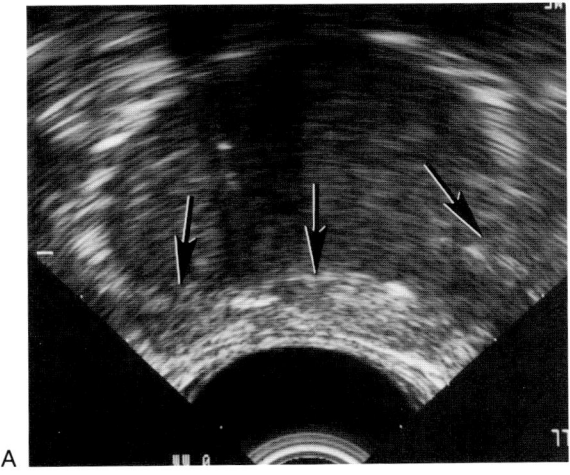

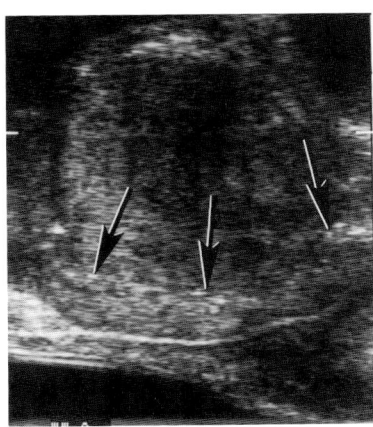

FIG. 12.12. Endorectal sonograms showing a mixed echogenic hyperplastic nodule. A hyperplastic nodule is seen on endorectal ultrasound in axial (**A**) and longitudinal (**B**) orientations. The nodule is clearly demarcated from the peripheral zone (*arrows*). Diffuse inhomogeneous echogenicity with areas of increased and decreased acoustic reflectivity are noted.

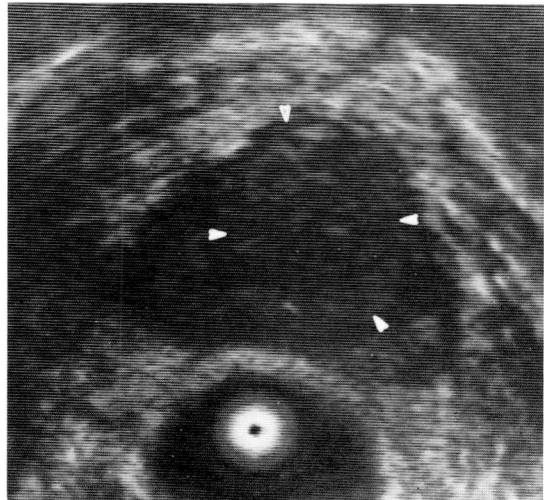

FIG. 12.13. Axial endorectal sonogram showing isoechoic lesion. This axial endorectal sonogram demonstrates an isoechoic lesion (*arrowheads*) which is poorly demarcated from the compressed normal peripheral and central zone.

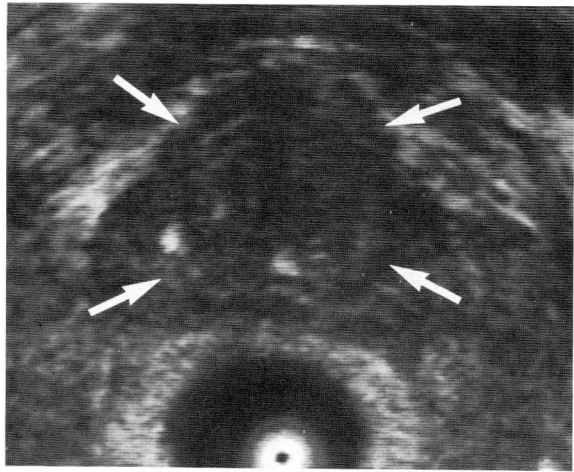

FIG. 12.14. Axial endorectal sonogram showing isoechoic lesion. This axial endorectal sonogram demonstrates an isoechoic hyperplastic (*arrows*) nodule in the periurethral tissues, causing distortion of the anterior aspect of the prostate. Subtle acoustic reflectors, calculi, and corpora amylacea are seen in the surgical capsule.

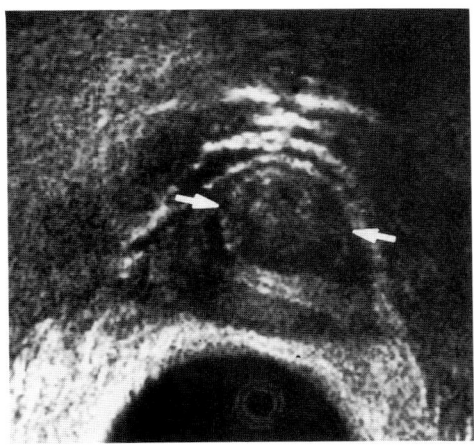

FIG. 12.15. Axial endorectal sonogram showing a halo sign. This axial endorectal ultrasound demonstrates a well-defined hyperplastic lesion of mixed echogenic reflectivity. This is seen in the periurethral tissues. The lesion is well-demarcated from the peripheral and central zones by a hypoechoic halo (*arrows*).

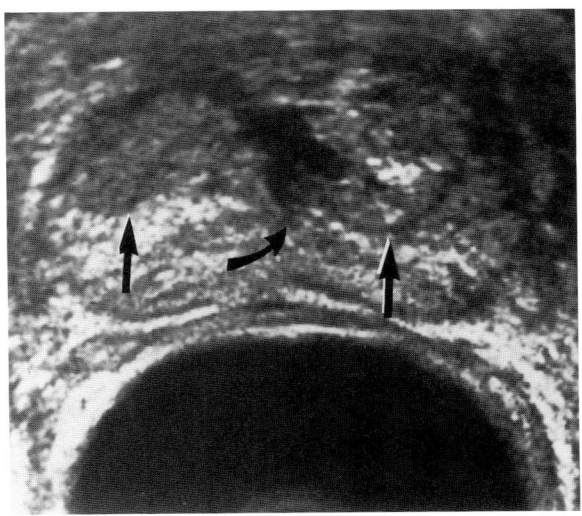

FIG. 12.16. Axial endorectal sonogram showing bilobed prostatic hyperplastic adenomas. Axially oriented endorectal sonogram demonstrates two clearly defined hyperplastic benign adenomas (*straight arrows*) with a TUR defect (*curved arrow*).

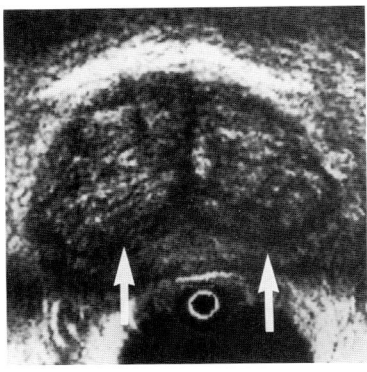

FIG. 12.17. Axial endorectal sonogram showing a bilobed adenoma. This axial image demonstrates two relatively symmetrical benign hyperplastic nodules (*arrows*).

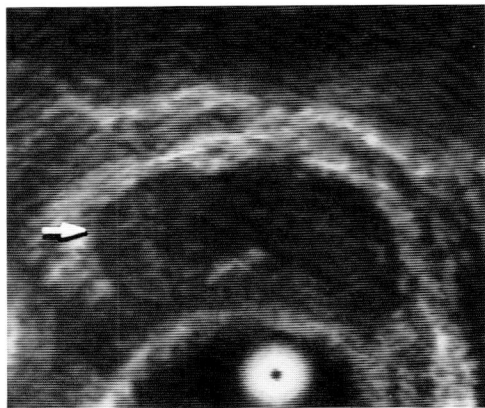

FIG. 12.18. Axial endorectal sonogram showing an asymmetric hyperplastic adenoma. This axially oriented image demonstrates a bulge (arrow) from the right lateral aspect of the prostate. This isoechoic lesion was a hyperplastic benign adenoma on biopsy.

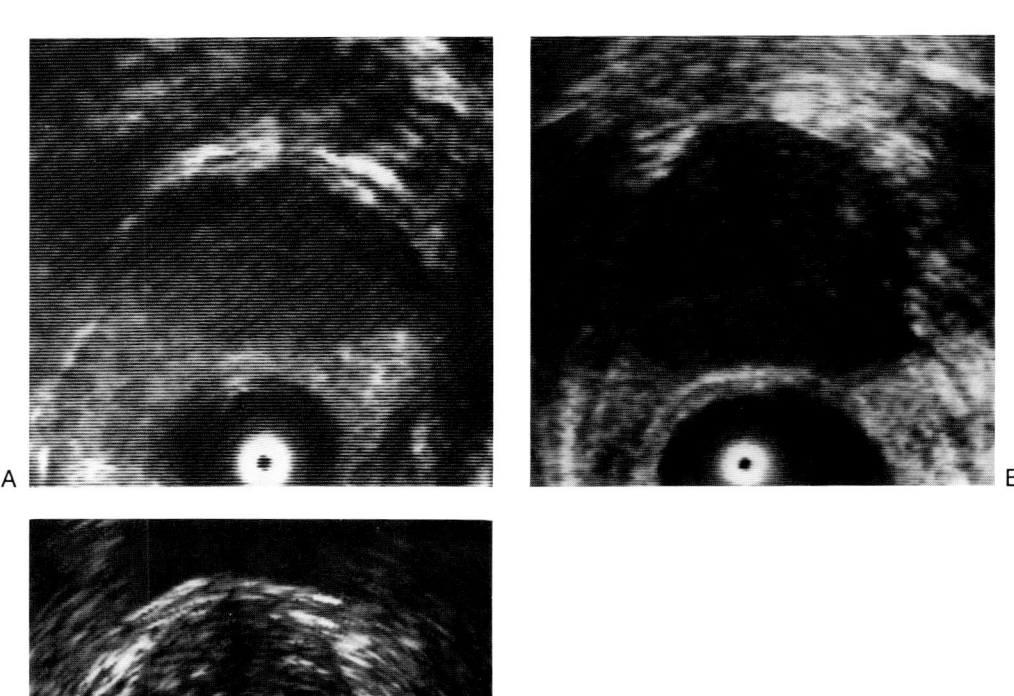

FIG. 12.19. Axial endorectal sonograms showing diffuse benign prostatic hyperplasia. Diffuse benign prostatic hyperplasia (in three different patients) shows the prostate as elongated (**A**), rounded (**B**), and globular (**C**) in shape. No focal disease is noted, yet the entire gland appears abnormal.

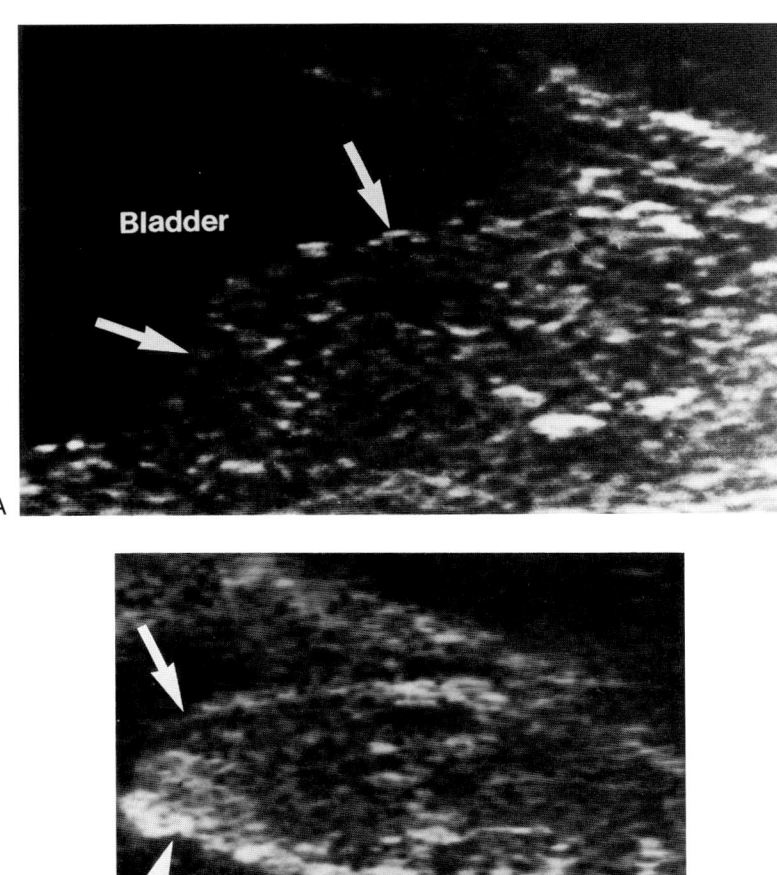

FIG. 12.20. Sagittal endorectal sonograms showing benign prostatic hyperplasia. Four different patients (**A–D**) were examined by longitudinally oriented endorectal sonograms. All have different appearances of benign prostatic hyperplastic disease causing impingement (*arrows*) upon the base of the urinary bladder.

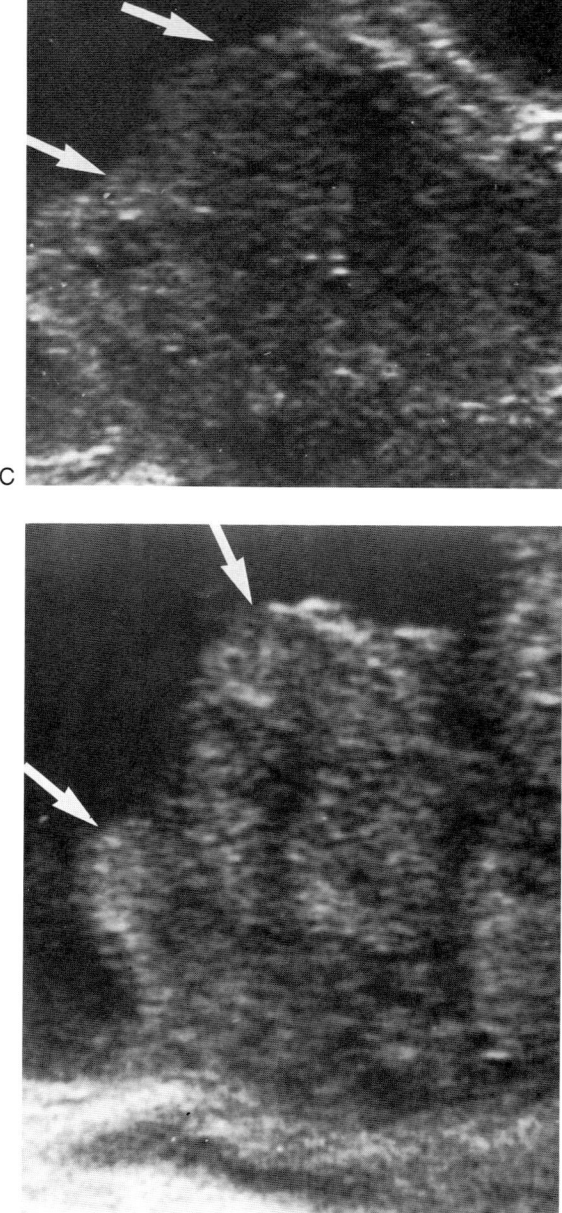

FIG. 12.20. *Continued.*

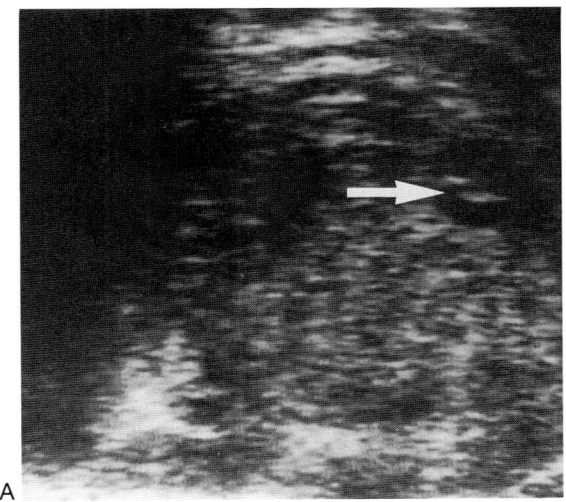

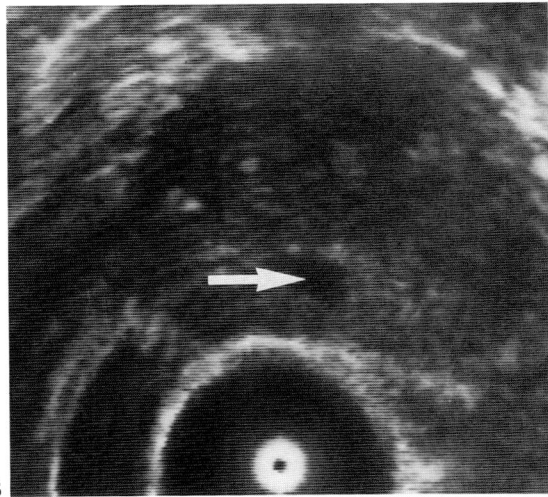

FIG. 12.21. Endorectal sonograms showing a prostatic cyst. Cystic changes of benign prostatic hyperplasia may occur. These can be seen in the longitudinally oriented (**A**) and the axially oriented (**B**) endorectal sonograms. The cystic changes (*arrows*) may be totally anechoic or may have some subtle internal echoes (debris).

208   *BENIGN PROSTATIC HYPERTROPHY*

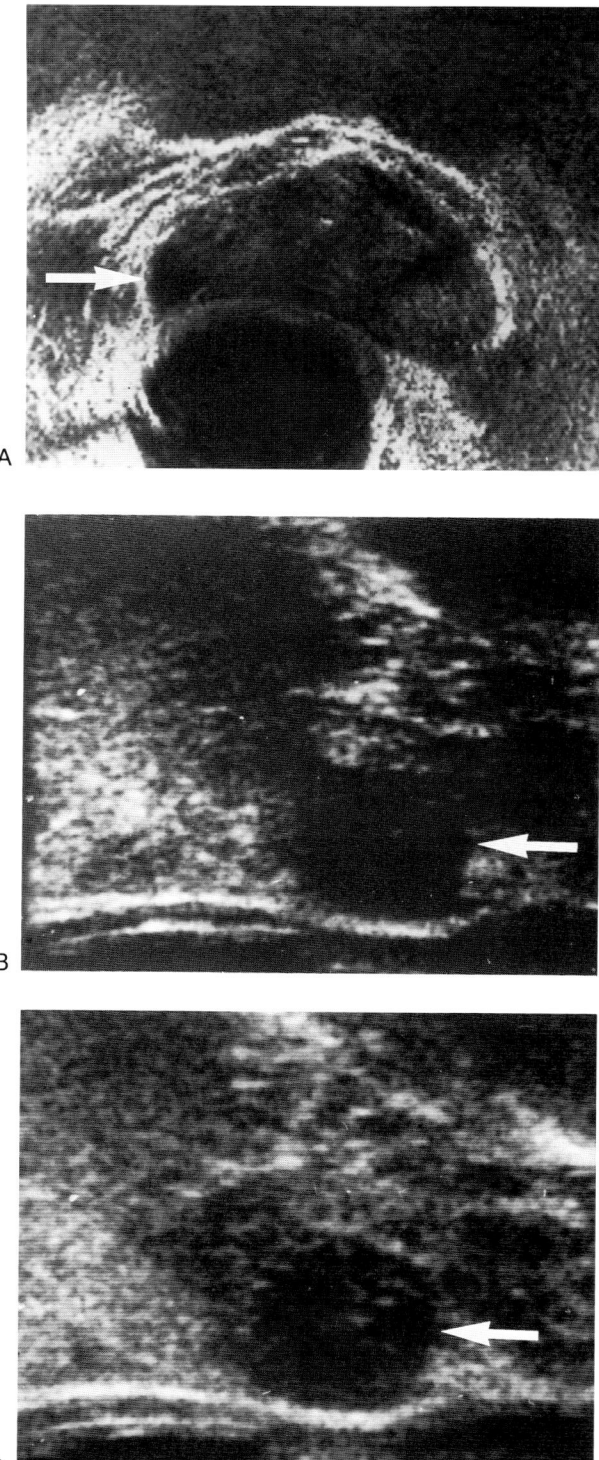

presence of a palpable abnormality suggesting the possibility of malignancy. Regardless of the clinical indication for the endorectal ultrasound, the appearance of the prostate may change following a transurethral resection. While clinically it is often felt that up to 90% of the prostatic tissue has been resected during the transurethral surgery, sonographically it appears that far less has been removed. The longitudinally oriented scan will show a defect (the area of resection) extending from the bladder base to the level of the verumontanum (Fig. 12.23). In patients who have undergone transurethral resection of the prostate, these defects are usually quite small. This is true if the ultrasound study has been performed immediately postoperatively or many years following surgery. It is not indicative of regrowth of the hyperplastic nodule, nor is it indicative of a poor surgical approach. Clinically, these patients are usually symptom-free and do quite well. This does not negate the fact that the prostate may undergo recurrent hyperplastic growth, which will be seen as impingement upon the transurethral resection defect. Occasionally, one may see larger, more elongated, or even-rounded "defects". There may be deviation or angulation of the urethra (Fig. 12.24) and the transurethral defect as the hyperplastic gland "regenerates".

The axially oriented scan will show a less obvious defect than that of the longitudinal image. Toward the periurethral area [i.e., from the base (Fig. 12.25) of the prostate to the verumontanum (Fig. 12.26)], a rounded defect in the area of the urethra will be seen. This is usually larger toward the base than toward the verumontanum and can vary in size, again depending upon the amount of resection.

TUR defects, particularly on the axial orientation, may be misinterpreted as cysts. It is therefore important that both an axially oriented scan and a longitudinally oriented one be obtained to confirm the defect.

ULTRASOUND MONITORING OF TRANSURETHRAL RESECTION

The endourethral scan can be utilized to monitor resection (182). Preoperative endourethral scanning will demonstrate the size of the gland in the axial orientation and will also demonstrate the size of the hyperplastic nodule. The gland can be defined, measurements can be obtained, and a well-defined benign hyperplastic nodule can be identified (Figs. 12.27 and 12.28). Frequently, if present around the surgical capsule, the nodule in this study will be seen with surrounding calculi. Otherwise, well-defined margins may or may not be identified. When this examination is performed at the time of resection (Figs. 12.27 and 12.28), the transducer is replaced by the resectoscope, tissue can be removed, and the transducer is then placed again into prostatic urethra following initial resection. Evaluation of the amount of remaining tissue and a demonstration of the tissue removed from the hyperplastic nodule can thus be determined. Repeat scanning following each segment of the resection is possible, to ensure adequate tissue removal and no loss of integrity of the prostate. In this way, immediate determination of the success of resection can be ascertained.

FIG. 12.22. Endorectal sonograms showing focal asymmetric benign prostatic hypertrophy. Axial (**A**) and longitudinal images of the prostate with low (**B**) and moderately high (**C**) gain controls demonstrate a 1.5-cm peripherally oriented lesion (*arrows*) in the right lateral aspect of the prostate. There are some internal echoes and some attenuation of sound. This benign lesion was diagnosed by ultrasound guided biopsy.

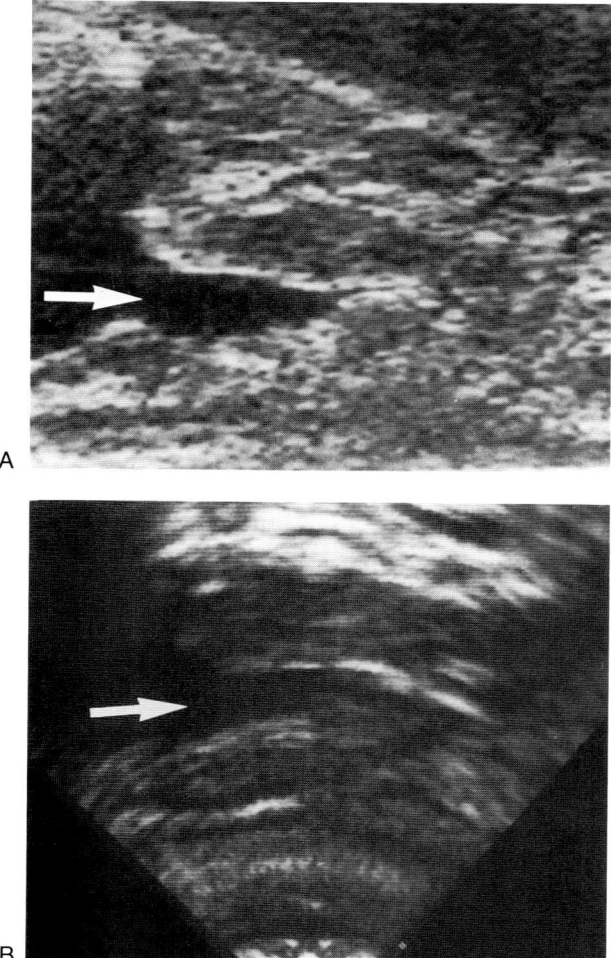

FIG. 12.23. Endorectal sonograms showing transurethral resection of the prostate defects. Four different appearances of transurethral resection defects of the prostate are visualized on longitudinally oriented endorectal sonograms. The defects (*arrows*) can be relatively thin (**A–C**) or relatively large (**D**).

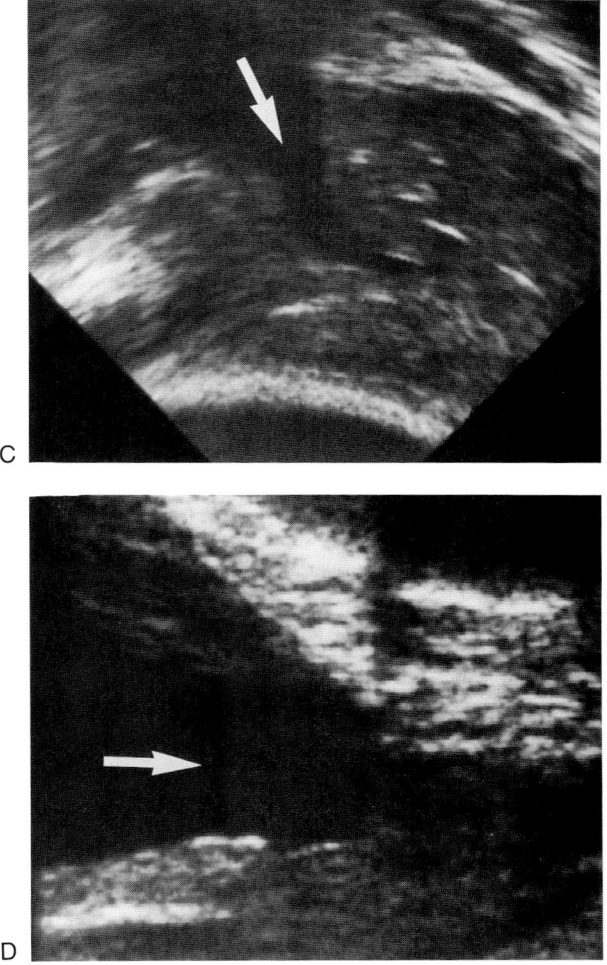

FIG. 12.23. *Continued.*

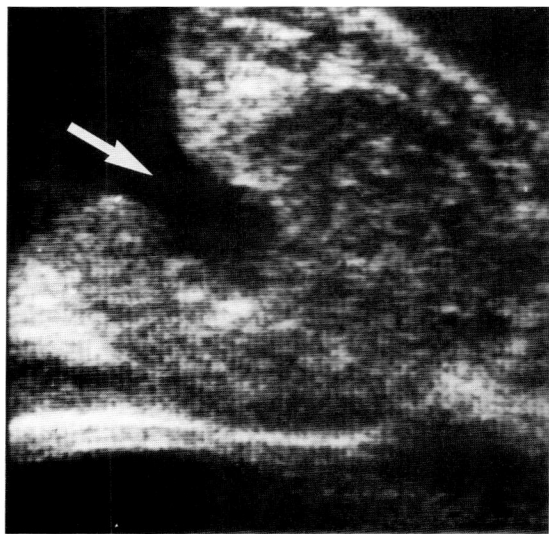

FIG. 12.24. Sagittal endorectal sonogram showing regrowth following TURP. Endorectal ultrasound of the prostate demonstrates a rounded TUR defect (*arrow*) with some anterior deviation of the prostatic urethra secondary to mild benign regrowth.

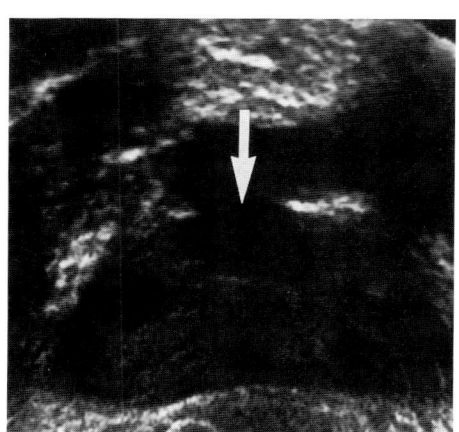

FIG. 12.25. Axial endorectal sonogram showing a TURP defect. A TURP defect (*arrow*) is seen at the bladder base.

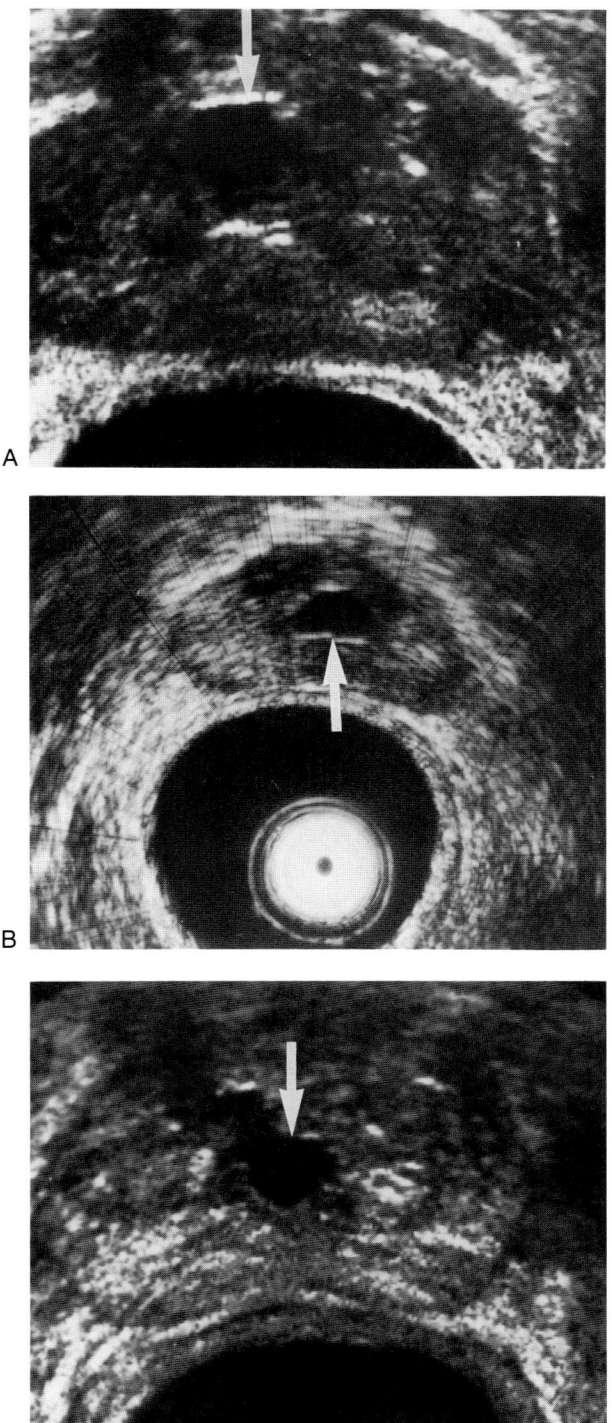

FIG. 12.26. Axial endorectal songrams showing TURP defects. Toward the body of the prostate, just proximal to the verumontanum, the axially oriented scan will show transurethral resection defects (*arrows*) in the middle of the gland. Sonograms of three different patients are shown.

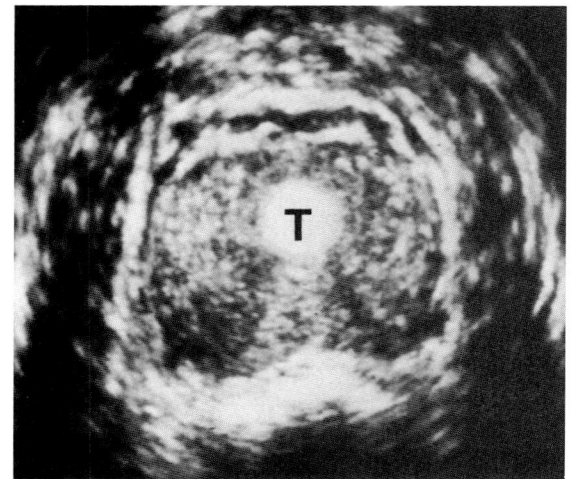

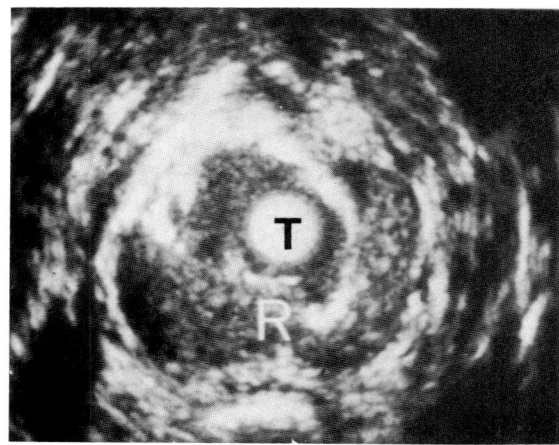

FIG. 12.27. Monitoring of transurethral resection of the prostate. Endourethral sonogram demonstrates a hyperplastic gland (**A**). Following partial resection of the gland, the probe (T) is placed back into the prostate (**B**), and the amount of residual tissue (R) is identified. Courtesy of Dr. Hans Henrik Holm.

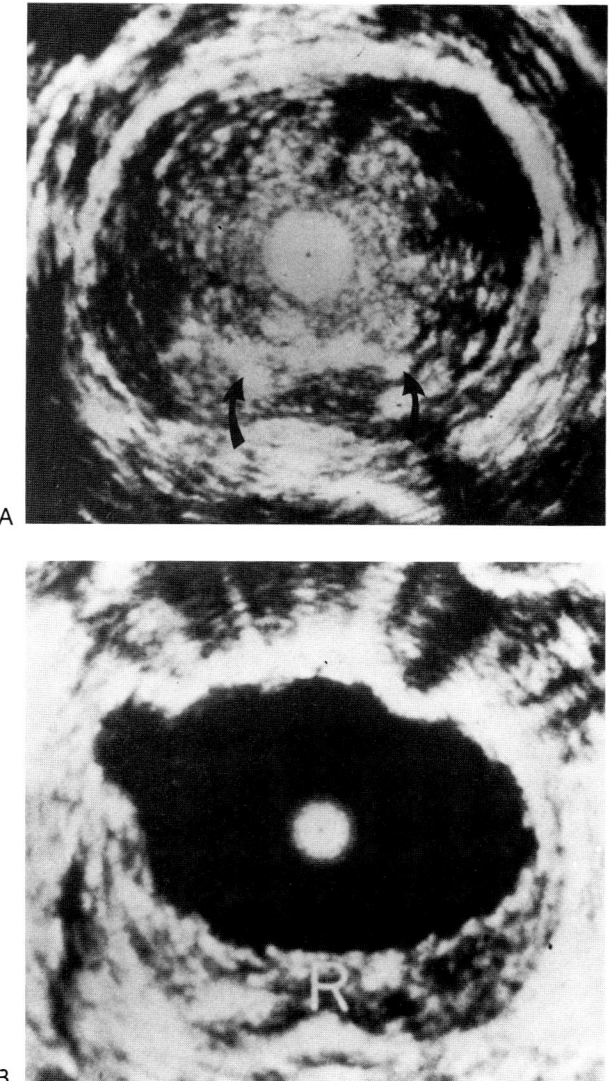

FIG. 12.28. Transurethral ultrasound for monitoring of transurethral resection of the prostate. Hyperplastic adenoma with surgical capsule calcification (*arrows*) (**A**) is identified on the endourethral ultrasound. Following a large resection (**B**), a very large defect is identified, and the amount of residual tissue (R) is minimal. Courtesy of Dr. Hans Henrik Holm.

PROSTATIC CALCULI

Prostatic calculi are a sign of benign disease. These calculi probably arise from corpora amylacea, proteinaceous material indigenous to the prostatic calculi. They may be present in a dystrophic gland secondary to prostatitis (seen in patients with no clinical symptomatology of previous inflammation) and are also frequently associated with noninflammatory benign hyperplastic changes. On the digital rectal examination, they may (on occasion) mimic malignancy. Prostatic calculi usually form in the periurethral area. When hyperplastic nodules are present, calculi may also be seen in the periphery of the nodule (i.e., the surrounding "surgical capsule") (Figs. 12.29 and 12.30).

Prostatic calculi have a typical appearance. They are brightly echogenic and may be either thin (Fig. 12.29) or thick (Fig. 12.30). All should, regardless of size, cause acoustic shadowing (acoustic attenuation), since calculi do not allow sound through-transmission. Occasionally, it may be necessary to carefully maneuver the transducer very slowly to demonstrate this acoustic attenuation. If no acoustic attenuation is present, then these bright areas (and even some of the thick echogenic areas) may not be calculi but may represent, instead, corpora amylacea (Fig. 12.31). The calcification may be focal (Fig. 12.32) or clumped (Fig. 12.33).

The shadowing secondary to calculi should always be seen regardless of the type of orientation utilized. The linear-array sector scanners, as well as the mechanical and phased-array sector scanners, should always demonstrate shadowing if the area of abnormality is placed within the focal zone of the transducer and careful maneuvering is performed. However, the rotating or radial-type image may not always demonstrate the shadowing from the bright echogenic areas (Fig. 12.34). The exact physical cause of this is not quite clear, but it may be secondary to reflection of the sound beam off multiple layers (i.e., the condom, the rectal wall, and the prostate capsule), causing some distortion of the sound beam and, thus, loss of the shadowing. In these cases, it may be difficult to define shadowing, although

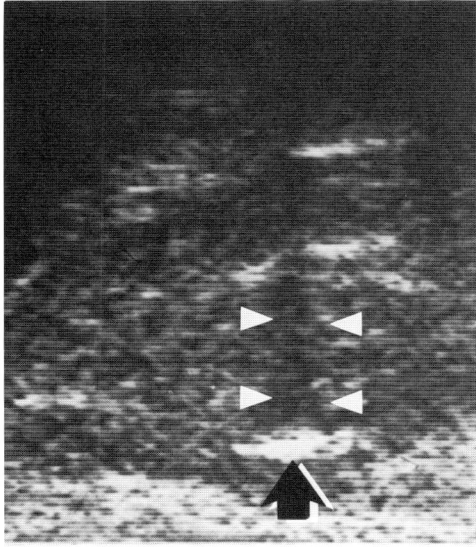

FIG. 12.29. Endorectal sonogram showing calcification. Longitudinal endorectal ultrasound with a linear-array transducer demonstrates a prostatic calculus (*arrow*) with acoustic shadowing (*arrowheads*).

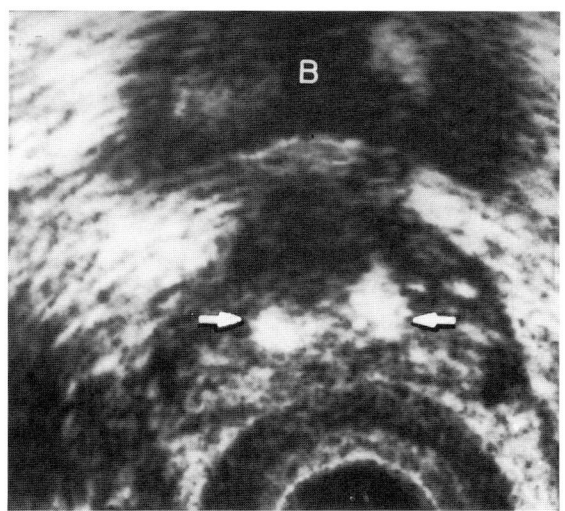

FIG. 12.30. Endorectal sonogram showing prostatic calculi. Prostatic calculi on the axially oriented radial scan are seen as a brightly echogenic foci (*arrows*). The degree of sound attenuation is less obvious than on the linear-array examinations. (B) Bladder.

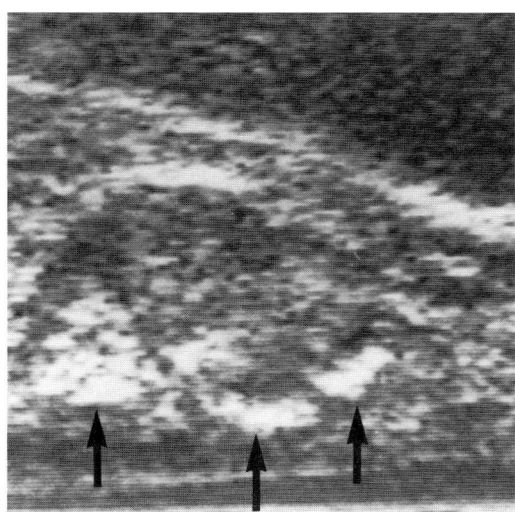

FIG. 12.31. Endorectal sonogram showing corpora amylacea. Corpora amylacea may be defined, on endorectal ultrasound, as echogenic areas without acoustic shadowing (*arrows*). Corpora amylacea is a precursor of calculi formation.

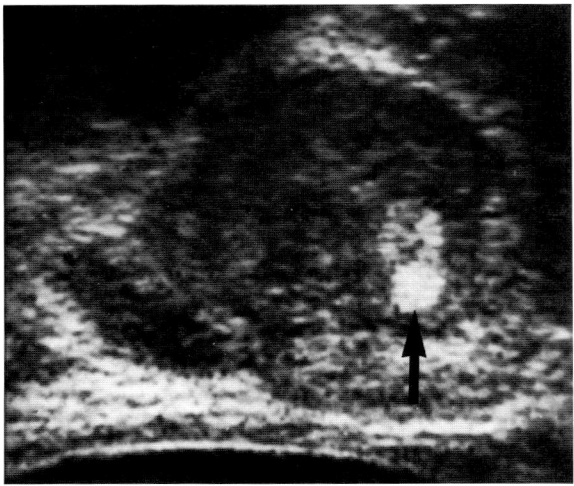

FIG. 12.32. Endorectal sonogram showing prostatic calcification. This longitudinally oriented scan demonstrates a focus of calcification (*arrow*).

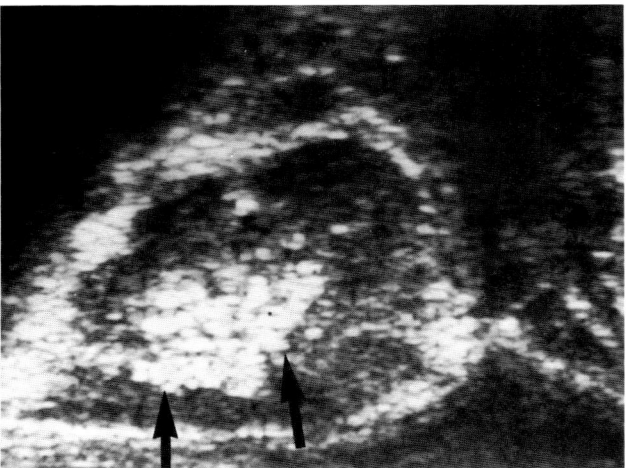

FIG. 12.33. Endorectal sonogram showing prostatic calcification. Endorectal ultrasound demonstrates a clump (*arrows*) of calcification within the prostate on longitudinal orientation.

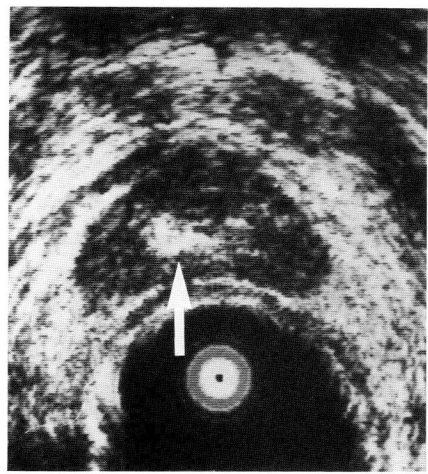

FIG. 12.34. Endorectal sonogram showing prostatic calcification. Prostatic calculi on the axial scanner (*arrow*) may not have the typical acoustic shadowing as seen with the longitudinally oriented linear array or the sector scanners.

clinically and sonographically the diagnosis of benign change versus malignancy should not be confusing.

The echogenic characteristics of calculi should not be mistaken for those carcinomas which may have subtle hyperechoic areas. With malignancy, the areas of increased echogenicity are very subtle (hyperechoic) and very thin. Calculi should always be bright, regardless of their size or the presence of shadowing.

PROSTATIC CYSTS (CYSTIC CHANGES)

Cystic changes may be present in a number of processes in the prostate. Duct dilatation, particularly that seen in the ejaculatory duct following transurethral resection, should not be confused with the cystic changes seen in necrotic hyperplastic nodules. Duct dilatation, although rounded when viewed on the axial or sagittal images, should be tubular on the other orientation. Cysts, secondary to degeneration, are usually rounded throughout.

By employing a transducer with the proper focal zone and proper scan technique, one will observe that cysts, regardless of their cause (i.e., congenital, postnecrotic, or obstructive), will have no internal echoes (as with fluid), will have sharp posterior walls, and, because of the fluid component of the cyst (Figs. 12.35 and 12.36), will cause good sound through-transmission.

These findings should always be defined on the linear-array sector scanners and on the mechanical and phased-array sector scanners. For the same reason that shadowing may not be identified with calculi by the rotating radial image, the good through-transmission seen with simple cysts may not be clearly delineated by this approach.

Many cystic changes secondary to necrotic adenomas are seen within a well-defined lesion in the prostate.

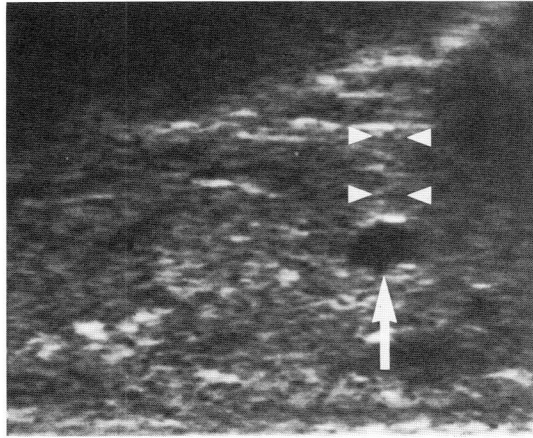

FIG. 12.35. Endorectal sonogram showing a prostatic cyst. A cyst (*arrow*) is seen on the longitudinally oriented linear-array examination. A sharp back wall and good sound through-transmission (*arrowsheads*) are identified.

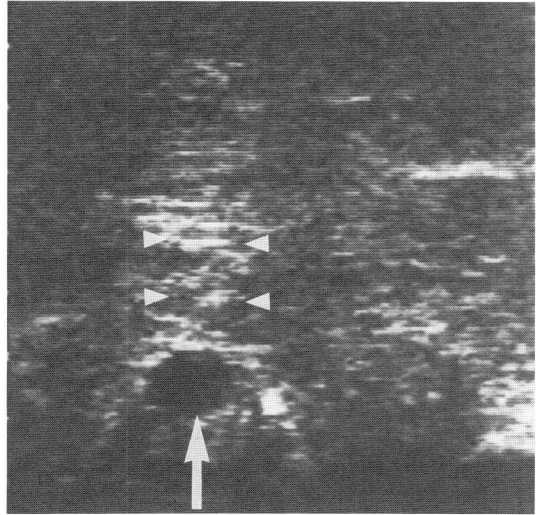

FIG. 12.36. Endorectal sonogram showing a prostatic cyst. Longitudinal image demonstrates a simple cyst (*arrow*) with sharp back wall and good sound through-transmission (*arrowheads*).

CONCLUSION

In summary, there are many cases of benign prostatic hyperplasia that are pathognomonic according to the endorectal sonogram. However, certain cases may be confusing. Most important, one should not minimize the possibility of the presence of a cancer, either palpable or nonpalpable, on the endorectal sonogram if there are changes of benign prostatic hyperplasia present. If calculi and/or cysts are seen that may, on physical examination, mimic malignancy, it is particularly important that the examination not be terminated quickly because of the presence of these lesions. There are many instances where carcinoma can develop concurrently with hyperplastic changes, cystic degeneration, and prostatic calculi. Therefore, it is essential that all types of lesions present be carefully evaluated on the ultrasound examination.

13 // Inflammation of the Prostate and Seminal Vesicles

Prostatitis: General Considerations	221
Prostatitis: Imaging Studies	222
Acute Prostatitis	
Chronic Prostatitis	
Prostatic Abscesses	224
Seminal Vesicle Inflammation	225
Seminal Vesiculitis	
Seminal Vesicle Abscesses	
Conclusion	228

Inflammatory changes of the prostate and seminal vesicles are a relatively common process that can be extremely distressing for the patient. In the acute processes, imaging is not usually needed for confirmation. However, in the subacute and chronic phases, confirmation and/or diagnostic needs may require an ultrasound or occasionally may require other types of imaging studies.

PROSTATITIS: GENERAL CONSIDERATIONS

There are a variety of causes of inflammation of the prostate (prostatitis), the most common being nonbacterial (362). Some of these processes are difficult to diagnose and to treat. Classification of prostatitis is currently divided into three categories that are based on the digital rectal examination and characteristics of the expressed prostatic secretion from this examination (362). The three types include: (a) bacterial prostatitis in both the acute and chronic form; nonbacterial prostatitis; and prostadynia (where there is a negative prostatic secretion and a negative digital rectal examination).

Bacterial prostatitis is usually caused by the same gram-negative organisms that affect and cause infection in the remaining urinary tract. More than 80% of bacterial prostatitis can be attributed to *Escherichia coli*, whereas 10% to 15% are due to other organisms such as klebsiella, seratia, proteus, pseudomonas, and enterobacter. The remaining 5% of cases are due to gram-positive organisms, which include enterococcus, staphylococcus, and streptococcus. Following transrectal or transperineal biopsy, anaerobic bacteria are usually the cause and are due to *Bacteroides fragilis* or *Clostridium perfringens*. Both of these frequently cause a fulminant prostatitis (309,362).

The granulomatous prostatitides include tuberculosis, blastomycosis, coccydioidmycosis, and cryptococcus, although other granulomatous-type prostatitides are frequently diagnosed as resolving acute bacterial prostatitis.

Histologically, prostatitis was initially thought to affect the entire gland. Recent studies, however, have shown that instead of diffuse involvement, there is more often a focal inflammatory process of the peripheral zone's acinar glandular tissue (297). In the acute process, the gland may become symmetrically edematous. In chronic prostatitis, diffuse or asymmetric involvement may occur. Enlargement of the gland may also result, but the latter process is often secondary to concurrent inflammatory benign prostatic hypertrophy, since both processes can occur in a single individual. Neither of these processes predispose to the occurrence of the other.

Prostatic calculi are a suspected sequellae of prostatitis, although they may occur in men with no history of glandular inflammation. In these cases, calcification is due to other causes. The exact role of the prostatic calculi in accentuating and perpetuating inflammation of the gland is controversial.

PROSTATITIS: IMAGING STUDIES

Acute Prostatitis

The use of imaging studies to diagnose acute or chronic prostatitis is limited. In the acute process, the plain radiograph can demonstrate irregularity of the bladder, particularly at the base. In the chronic stage, prostatic calculi may be identified. However, neither of these findings are pathognomonic of prostate inflammation.

There are no radionuclide studies that delineate inflammation of the prostate with accuracy; similar limitations are noted with computed tomography.

The transabdominal suprapubic sonogram may delineate and identify the prostate. Non-radio-opaque prostate calculi may also be identified as acoustically bright foci and shadowing. These findings are certainly not pathognomonic.

Endorectal sonography of the prostate delineates the gland more clearly. Studies have reported that in acute prostatitis, three main characteristics may be identified: (i) a hypoechoic rim surrounding the entire prostate gland (Fig. 13.1); (ii) a low-level or echo-free halo surrounding the periurethral zone (Fig. 13.2); or (iii) low-level echo areas scattered irregularly within the prostate (172).

Chronic Prostatitis

In chronic prostatitis, the endorectal sonogram may demonstrate diffuse inhomogeneous echogenicity of the prostate, with areas of fluid and/or decreased acoustic reflectivity. Similar sonographic characteristics may also be seen in noninflammatory, nonmalignant conditions of the prostate (i.e., prostate hypertrophy) (397).

In subacute and more indolent cases of inflammation, sonographic appearances on the endorectal ultrasound may mimic more ominous processes. Small peripherally oriented hypoechoic lesions that could represent carcinomas have been biopsied using sonographic guidance (259,262,407–411). On occasion, in up to 20% of cases, these areas have represented indolent inflammation or even infarction, one of the sequellae of infection.

The diagnosis of chronic prostatitis is not pathognomonic on ultrasound. There may be examples of inflammation and other types of pathology (including BPH) that have similar sonographic appearances.

INFLAMMATION OF THE PROSTATE AND SEMINAL VESICLES 223

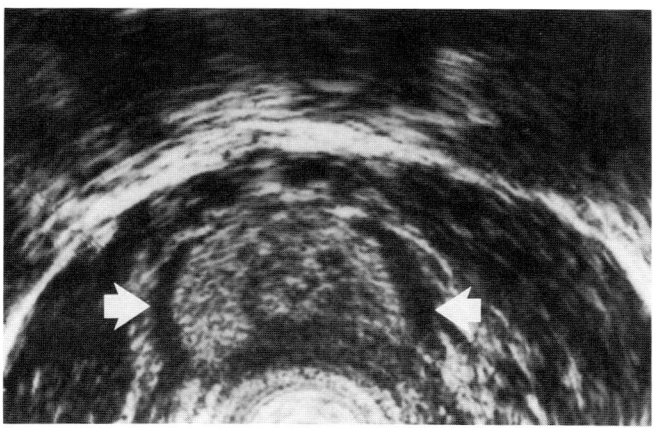

FIG. 13.1. Axial endorectal sonogram showing acute prostatitis. A hypoechoic rim is seen (*arrows*) surrounding the lateral aspects of the prostate. This abnormal area is secondary to acute prostatitis. (Courtesy of Dr. G. J. Griffiths.)

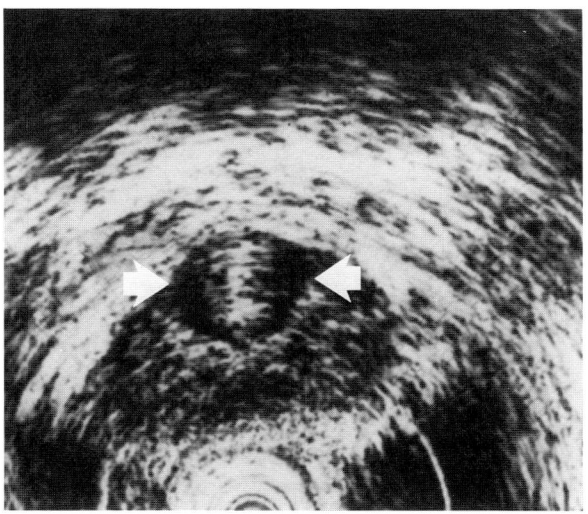

FIG. 13.2. Axial endorectal sonogram showing acute prostatitis. An endorectal ultrasound demonstrates a hypoechoic rim (*arrows*) surrounding the periurethral area of the prostate. (Courtesy of Dr. G.J. Griffiths.)

PROSTATIC ABSCESSES

Prostatic abscesses usually develop as processes secondary to prostatitis but can also develop from hematogenous spread from another source (34). Most of the imaging techniques are nonspecific. Whereas conventional imaging has had limited benefit in the diagnosis of abscesses, computerized tomography (CT) and magnetic resonance imaging (MRI) may delineate abnormal areas. However, experience with these imaging techniques has been limited. Endorectal sonography can show areas of irregularity and abnormal echogenicity as well as size differences (Figs. 13.3 and 13.4). The abnormal focus is usually slightly hypoechoic, suggesting the liquefied components of the abscess. Although the ultrasound characteristics may be nonspecific, the diagnosis can be suggested (262) in conjunction with clinical presentation. Additionally, the transrectal ultrasound permits accurate ultrasound guided transperineal aspiration for diagnosis.

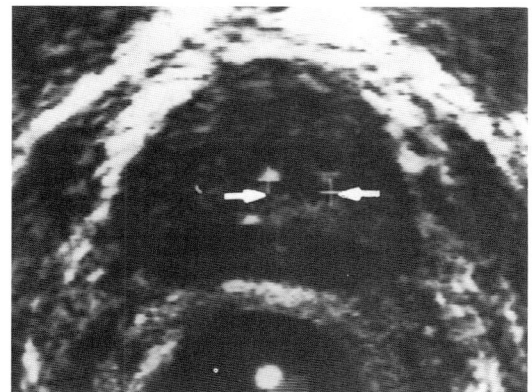

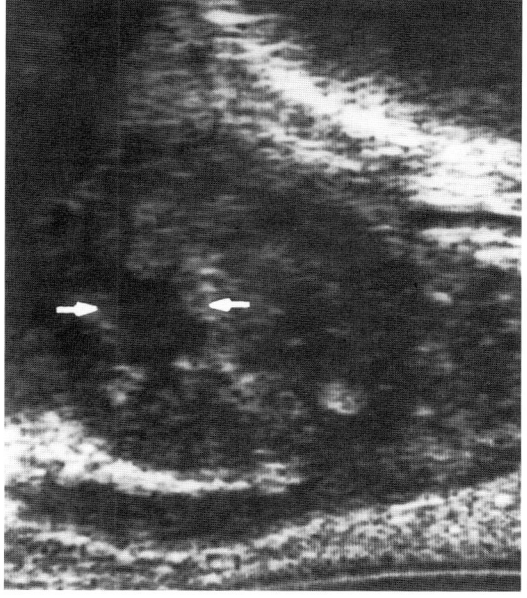

FIG. 13.3. Endorectal sonogram showing a prostatic abscess. A prostatic abscess (*arrows*) is seen in the axial (**A**) and the longitudinal (**B**) endorectal sonograms. Sonographically guided biopsy diagnosed the abscess. Although the sonographic findings are not pathognomonic for prostatic abscess, it can be suggested with clinical correlation. (Courtesy of Dr. Fred Lee.)

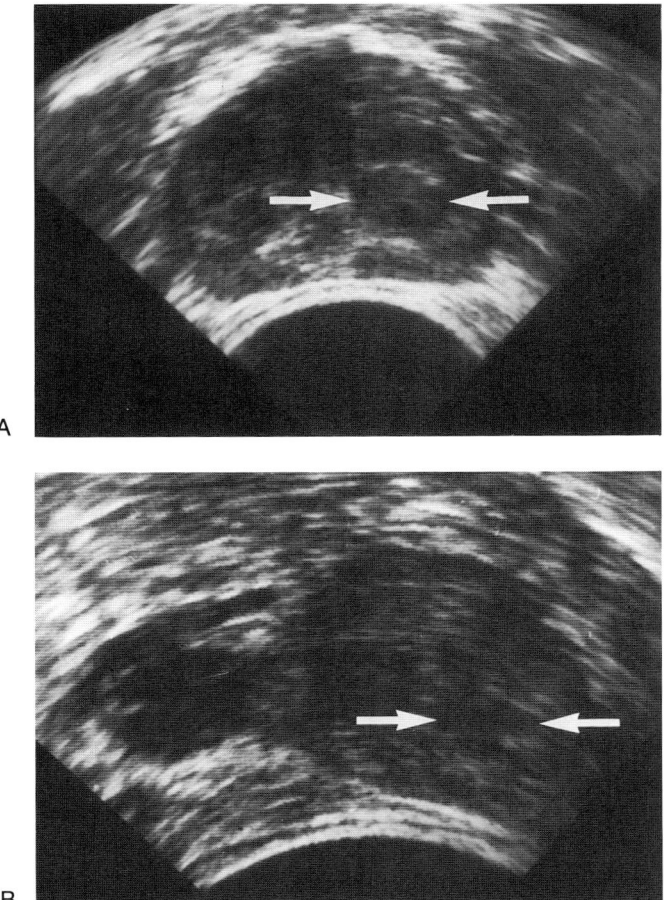

FIG. 13.4. Endorectal sonogram showing a prostatic abscess. Sonogram in the axial (**A**) and the longitudinal (**B**) view demonstrates a poorly defined, slightly hypoechoic area (*arrows*), an abscess, on the patient's left side. This patient had undergone a transurethral resection of the prostate 1 month earlier.

SEMINAL VESICLE INFLAMMATION

Seminal Vesiculitis

Seminal vesiculitis or seminal vesicle inflammation is usually a secondary inflammatory process due to prostatitis. It is unusual to have inflammation of the seminal vesicle without inflammation of the prostate, although it can occur.

Imaging studies are presently of limited diagnostic benefit. The plain film and excretory urogram are usually not useful. Ultrasound may show enlargement and decreased echogenicity of the seminal vesicles, and is best appreciated by endorectal sonography (Fig. 13.5) (397). However, there has been only limited use of this technique for evaluation of possible inflammation.

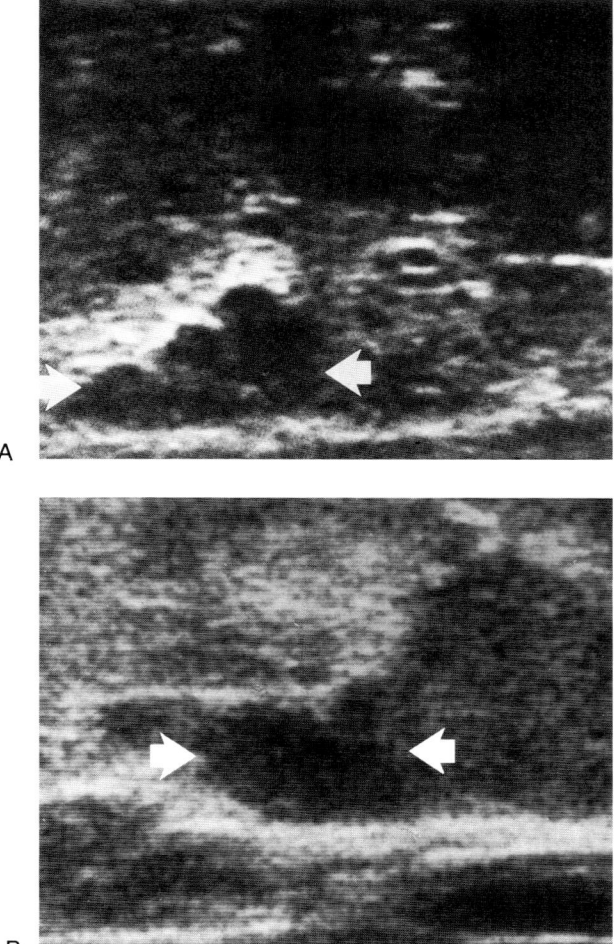

FIG. 13.5. Endorectal sonograms showing seminal vesiculitis. Longitudinally oriented sonograms in two different patients demonstrate an enlarged, slightly hypoechoic seminal vesicle (*arrows*) in both individuals. This was compared to the contralateral side (not shown), which was normal.

Seminal Vesicle Abscesses

Seminal vesiculitis may lead to seminal vesicle abscess (264). In these cases, asymmetric enlargement of one seminal vesicle—confirmed by CT, ultrasound, or MRI—can be observed (Fig. 13.6). The ultrasound (probably defined only by the endorectal approach) may show an anechoic or hypoechoic partially fluid-filled lesion.

Seminal vesicle abscesses may also be due to congenital anomalies, the most common being ectopic ureteral insertion into the seminal vesicles. In these cases, as the seminal vesicle enlarges, a mass causing impression upon the fluid-filled bladder may be seen on the urogram, sonogram (Fig. 13.7), or other imaging study.

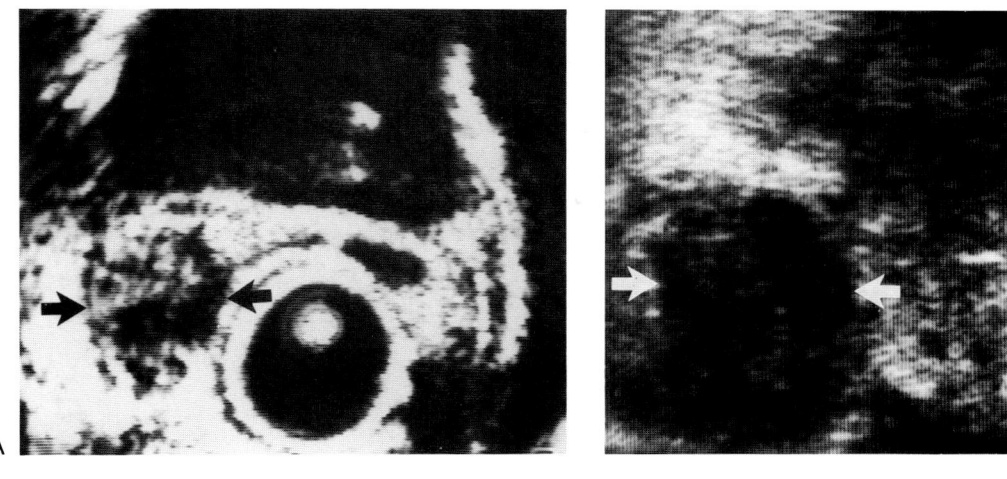
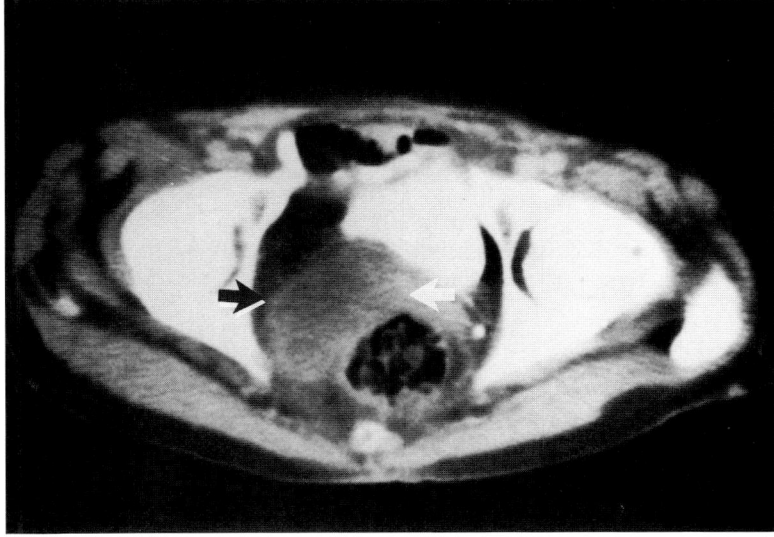

FIG. 13.6. Endorectal sonograms showing a seminal vesicle abscess. Transverse (**A**) and longitudinal (**B**) endorectal sonograms demonstrate an abnormal right (*arrows*), as compared to the normal left, seminal vesicle. There is good through-transmission, but there is also the presence of internal echoes, suggesting a complicated fluid collection—in this case, a seminal vesicle abscess. The findings were confirmed on a computed tomogram (**C**). (Courtesy of Dr. Fred Lee.)

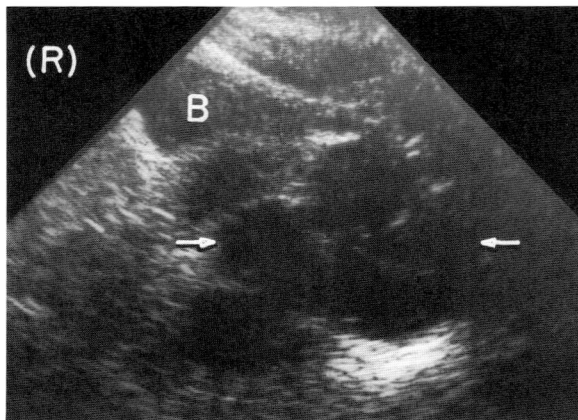

FIG. 13.7. Transabdominal sonogram showing a seminal vesicle abscess. A patient with recurrent epididymitis presented with a mass (*arrows*) posterior to a compressed, partially fluid-filled urinary bladder (B) on this transversely oriented transabdominal sonogram. The mass has a septate appearance with some fluid components and is suggestive of seminal vesicle abscess, which was confirmed at surgery. (R) Patient's right side.

CONCLUSION

In general, inflammatory conditions of the prostate and seminal vesicles are usually diagnosed by clinical symptomatology and the physical examination. The imaging studies are often used as complementary, but not necessarily diagnostic, studies.

14 // *Infertility and Seminal Vesicle Disease*

Infertility	229
Seminal Vesicle Disease	232
Congenital Abnormalities	
Absence of the Seminal Vesicle	
Cysts	
Postsurgical Aquired Disease	
Primary Neoplasms	
Conclusion	239

INFERTILITY

There are many causes of male infertility. Almost all of them are beyond the scope of this text. Thus, the evaluation of most cases of male infertility is not aided by sonographic evaluation.

However, there are certain (unusual) entities that may be diagnosed or identified by the sonogram. In general, most of these require the endorectal approach, which can define the internal structures of the prostate and the periprostatic tissues more clearly than the other imaging techniques.

These include the following:

1. *Absence of the seminal vesicles.* An unusual cause of male infertility is absence of the seminal vesicles, which can be determined by the endorectal ultrasound. Absence of the vas deferens may also be seen.

2. *Ejaculatory duct dilatation.* This is most commonly seen in patients with transurethral resection defects in the older male population. In these cases, the longitudinally oriented scan is best to determine ejaculatory duct dilatation with perhaps secondary seminal vesicle dilatation.

Ejaculatory duct obstruction and dilatation may also be a cause of male infertility. In these cases, bilateral obstruction is usually present. These are often due to congenital ejaculatory duct obstruction and dilatation.

On occasion, men have presented with unilateral obstruction of the ejaculatory duct. In many instances, the exact cause is unclear, but the sonogram findings are obvious (Fig. 14.1). This may not be cause of infertility.

For evaluation of all cases of possible ejaculatory duct dilatation, the longitudinally oriented scanner is necessary (Fig. 14.2).

Ultrasound has also been utilized in the operating room in an attempt to dislodge the cause of obstruction. Studies have been undertaken using the longitudinally oriented en-

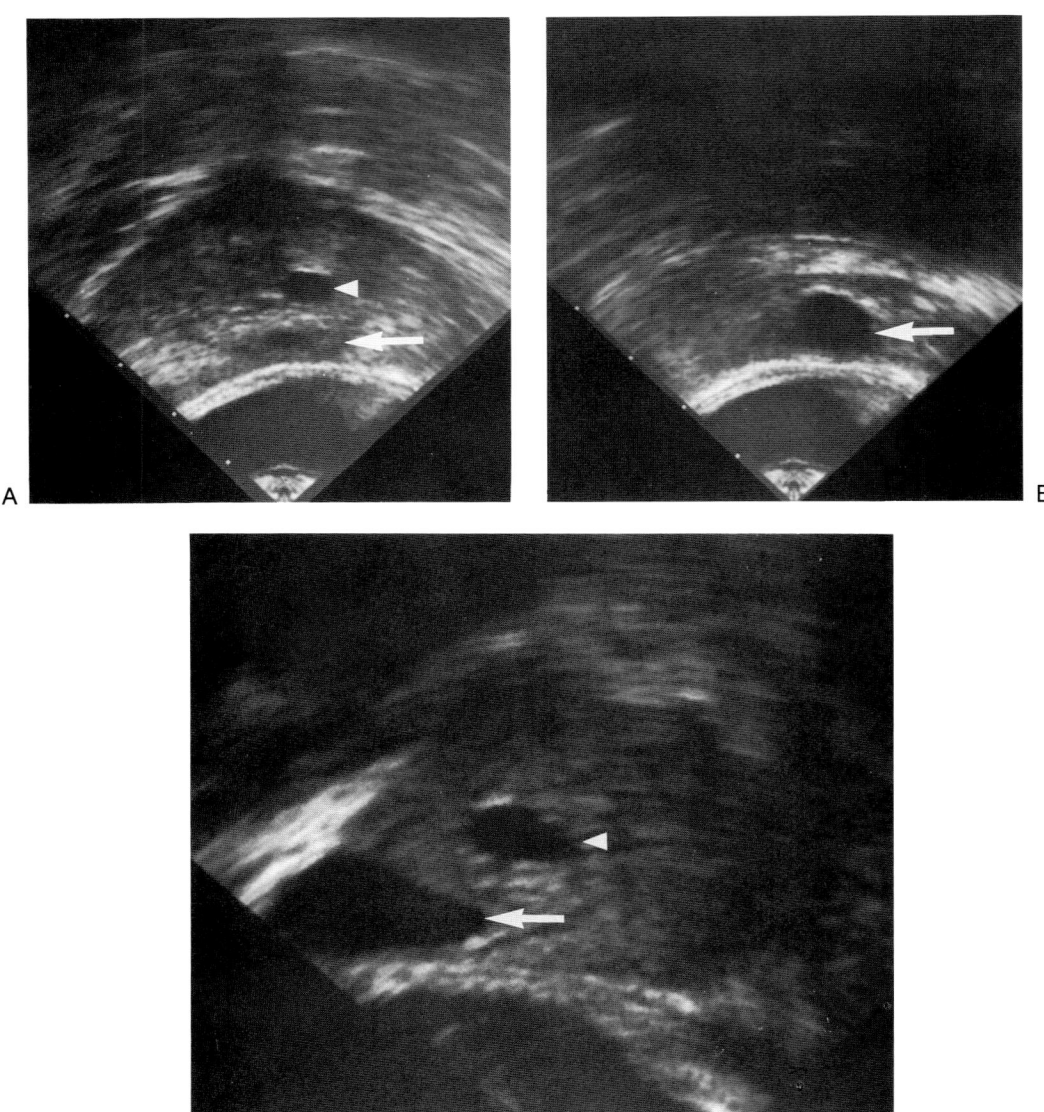

FIG. 14.1. Ejaculatory duct and seminal vesicle dilatation secondary to obstruction. The axially oriented endorectal sonogram (**A**) at the level of the base of the prostate demonstrates dilatation of a portion of the left seminal vesicle (*arrow*) and the left ejaculatory duct (*arrowhead*). An axial section slightly more cephalad at the level of the seminal vesicle (**B**) demonstrates marked dilatation of the left seminal vesicle (*arrow*) at the level of the origin of the left ejaculatory duct. The longitudinal endorectal sonogram (**C**) demonstrates dilatation of the ejaculatory duct (*arrow*) at the level of insertion into the verumontanum and more proximally (*arrowhead*) as it exits from the seminal vesicle.

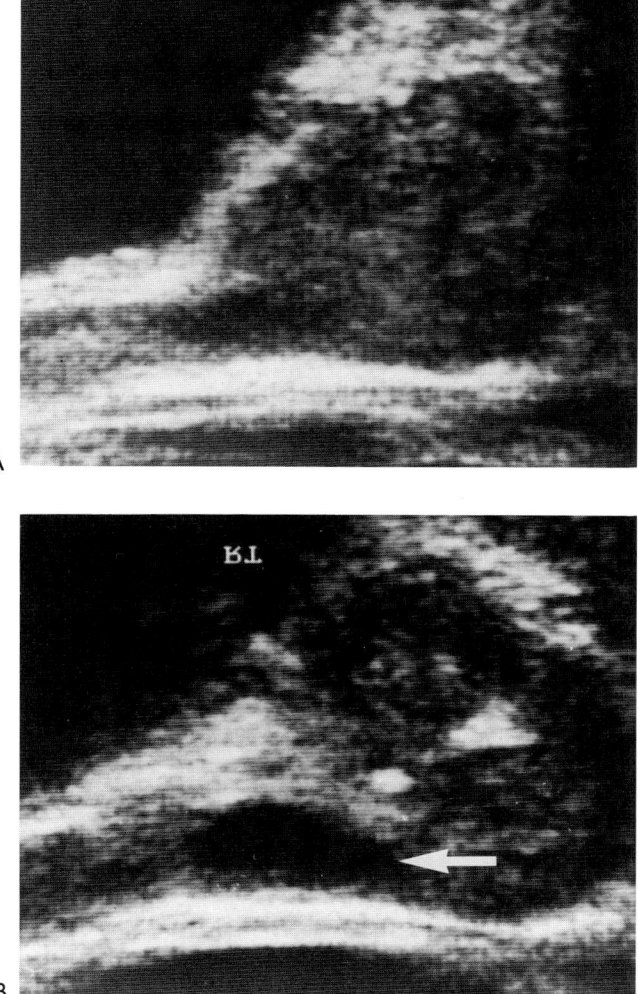

FIG. 14.2. Right-sided ejaculatory duct dilatation. Longitudinal endorectal ultrasound on the left (**A**) and right (**B**) sides demonstrates a normal left, but an obstructed right, ejaculatory duct (*arrow*).

dorectal scanner used concurrently with a cystoscopic study in an attempt to unroof the blocked insertion of the ejaculatory duct into the seminal vesicle. Only minimal experience has been obtained with this technique, and further work is required to define its true benefit.

SEMINAL VESICLE DISEASE

There are certain indications for evaluation of the seminal vesicles by endorectal ultrasound. The most frequent is determining prostatic cancer extension. These ultrasound findings have already been covered in Chapter 10. Other pathologic entities may also be present, and thus identified, during ultrasound scanning. A review of these is included below.

Congenital Abnormalities

There are certain congenital abnormalities that may involve the seminal vesicles. One is ectopic insertion of the ureter (a ureterocele) into the seminal vesicle. This is frequently associated with ipsilateral renal agenesis or dysgenesis and contralateral renal hypertrophy. The ipsilateral hemitrigone may be absent in these cases. A mass may be palpable on the digital rectal examination; also, there may be retrograde flow of sperm into the epididymis, causing recurrent epididymitis. There may also be perineal or testicular pain, which is often related to sexual intercourse. However, urinary symptoms may be absent, and surgical treatment may be necessary.

The sonographic appearance may include the following:

1. a mass that is either cystic-, semicystic-, semisolid-, or solid-appearing in nature, either involving the implicated seminal vesicle or in the area of the seminal vesicle;
2. dysgenesis or agenesis of the ipsilateral kidney; and
3. inflammation of the epididymis (due to retrograde flow of material into the epididymis).

When a mass is palpated on the digital rectal examination or present on the sonogram, either in an abdominal or endorectal study, it is essential that evaluation of the kidney be undertaken. Additionally, examination of the epididymis may be helpful to demonstrate clinical (or even subclinical) cases of epididymitis. These findings will show enlargement and will usually demonstrate inhomogeneous (frequently decreased) echogenicity of the involved epididymis.

Absence of the Seminal Vesicle

Absence of the seminal vesicle is an unusual finding and may be bilateral or unilateral. It has been associated with mucoviscidosis but may also occur in men without this disorder. Assuming the technique of the examination is optimized, the axial endorectal sonogram will demonstrate the absence of one or both structures. Unilateral absences is a more obvious finding and is easier to diagnose (Fig. 14.3). The longitudinal orientation can also be used, but closer attention to anatomical detail may be required (Fig. 14.4).

When there is bilateral absence, there is no asymmetry. Particular care is essential in performing the sonogram. This will ensure that high quality and complete study are achieved so that the lack of visualization of the seminal vesicles is real, as opposed to being caused by technical difficulties.

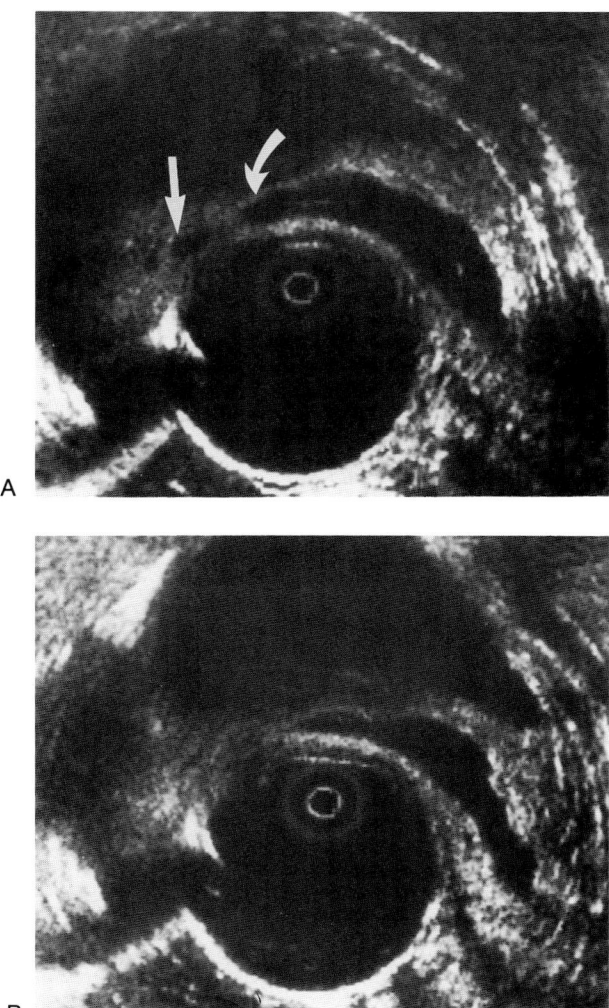

FIG. 14.3. Absence of the seminal vesicles—axial orientation. Axially oriented endorectal ultrasound demonstrates the presence of the right (*straight arrow*) and the left (*curved arrow*) vas deferens (**A**). A section slightly more caudad (**B**) demonstrates complete absence of the right seminal vesicle.

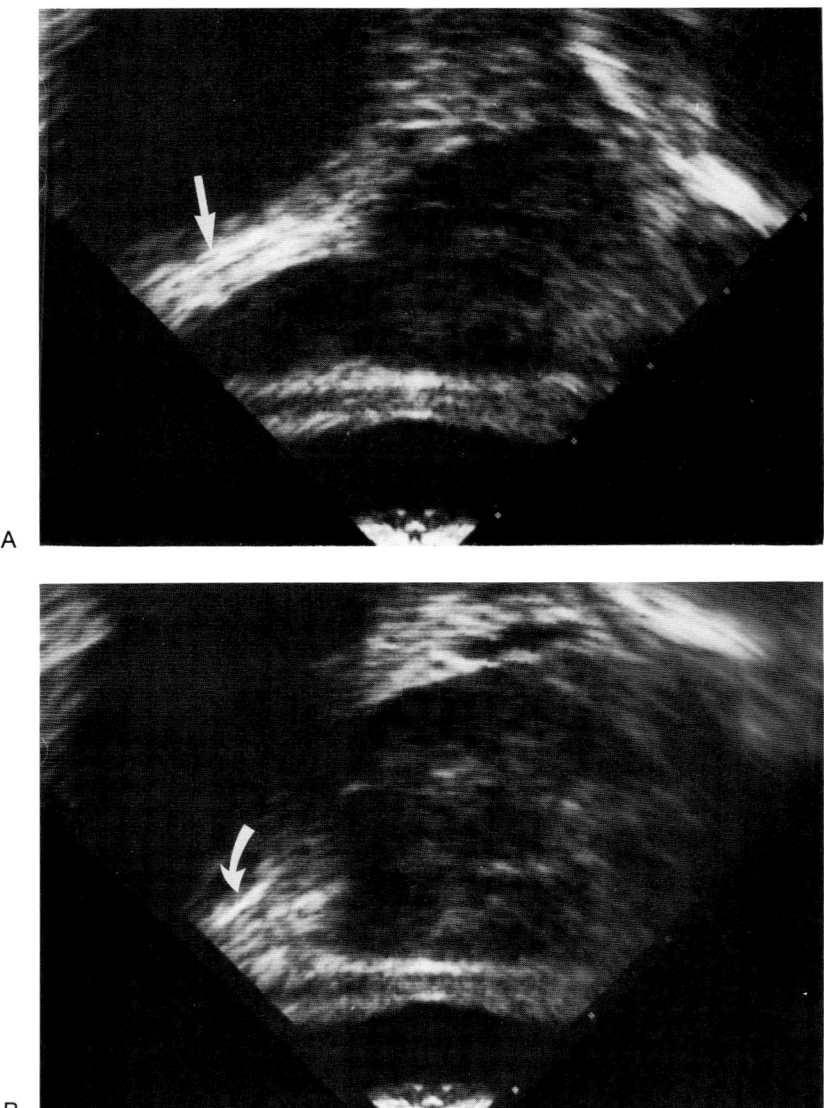

FIG. 14.4. Absence of the right seminal vesicle—longitudinal orientation. These longitudinally oriented endorectal sonograms demonstrate a normal (*straight arrow*) left seminal vesicle (**A**) and absence (*curved arrow*) of the right seminal vesicle (**B**).

Cysts

The cysts are unusual lesions. They are frequently congenital and may be secondary to a congenital obstruction of the seminal vesicle and the ejaculatory duct. Sonographically, they will appear as simple cysts in the seminal vesicle. On occasion, they may be difficult to distinguish from tubular dilatation. They may, on occasion, be seen on the conventional sonogram (Figs. 14.5 and 14.6), but small cysts will only be identified on the endorectal sonogram (Fig. 14.7).

The differential diagnosis includes Wolffian duct cysts, müllerian duct remnant cysts, prostatic cysts, diverticula of the ejaculatory duct, and, as stated, seminal vesicle dilatation (i.e., cystic changes) due to obstruction.

Postsurgical Acquired Disease

Many patients will develop bilateral or unilateral dilatation of the seminal vesicles following a transurethral resection. In these cases, the ejaculatory duct is usually dilated as well. They can be seen on the endorectal ultrasound as tubular dilatation of the ejaculatory ducts from the verumontanum to the seminal vesicle. The onset of dilatation is quite variable. The sonographic findings are identical to those seen in congenital ejaculatory duct dilatation.

Primary Neoplasms

Neoplasia can be divided into benign and malignant lesions. The most common growth of the epididymis is adenocarcinoma, although sarcoma has occasionally been reported (328). Benign lesions can include fibromas, myomas, and cystic adenomas. Sonographically, it is difficult (if not impossible) to differentiate these lesions from each other, although the lesion can be identified (328). Some lesions may be seen on the conventional sonogram (Fig. 14.8). To delineate a small tumor, the findings on the endorectal ultrasound study may be more obvious (Fig. 14.9). Diagnostic criteria include the following:

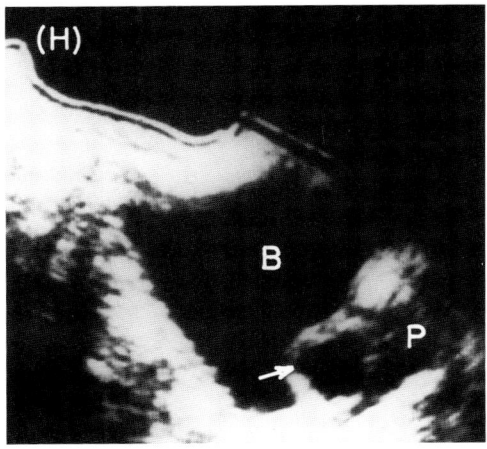

FIG. 14.5. Transabdominal sonogram showing a seminal vesicle cyst. Transabdominal ultrasound through a fluid-filled urinary bladder (B) demonstrates a simple-appearing cyst (*arrow*) superior to the prostate (P). This cyst has sonographic characteristics of a simple cyst and extends off the seminal vesicle. (H) Toward patient's head.

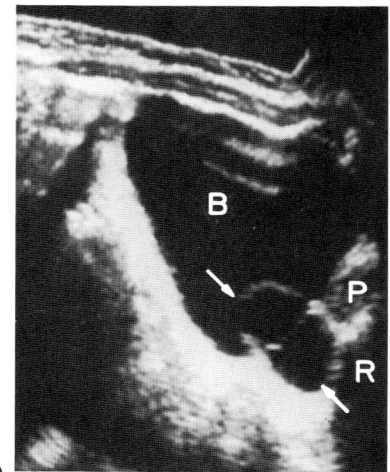
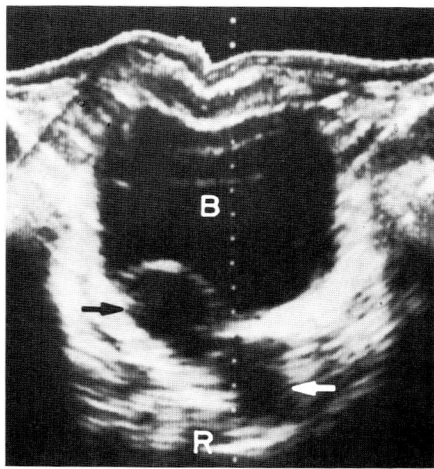

FIG. 14.6. Transabdominal sonograms showing a bilobed seminal vesicle cyst. Longitudinally oriented (**A**) and transversely oriented (**B**) sonograms using the transabdominal approach demonstrate a bilobed (*arrows*) seminal vesicle cyst superior to the prostate (P). (B) Bladder; (R) rectum.

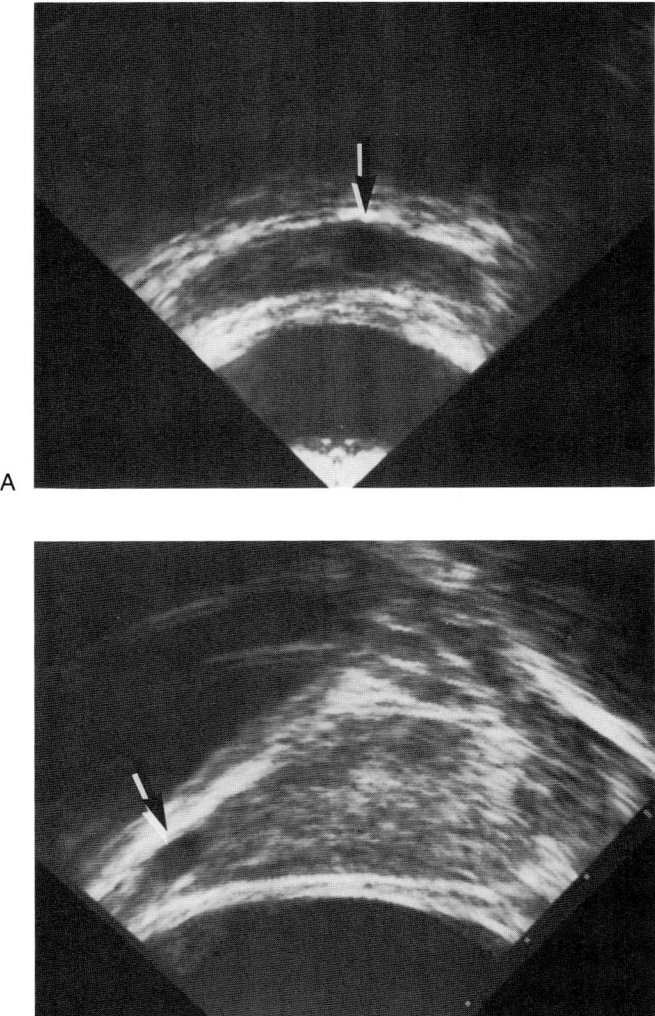

FIG. 14.7. Endorectal sonograms showing a seminal vesicle cyst. Axially oriented (**A**) and longitudinally oriented (**B**) sonograms demonstrate a simple-appearing cyst (*arrows*) involving the medial aspect of the left seminal vesicle.

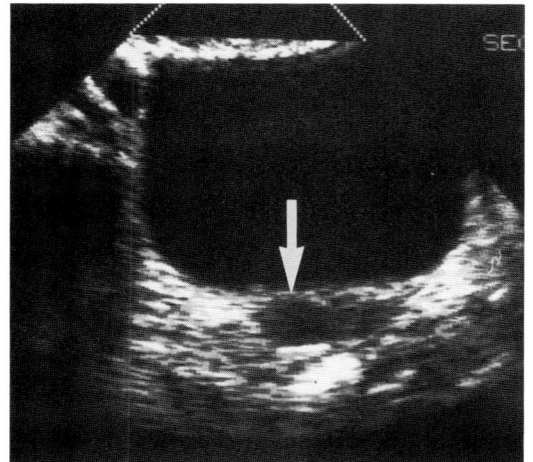

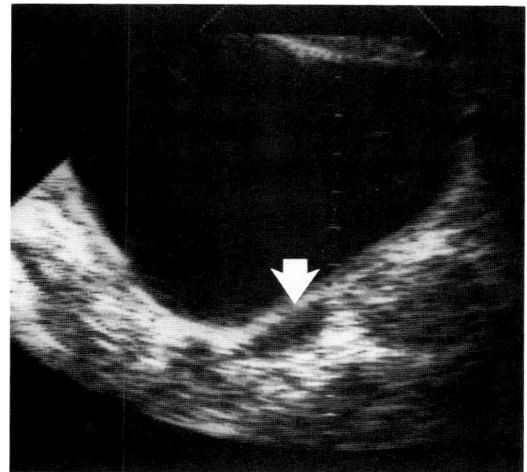

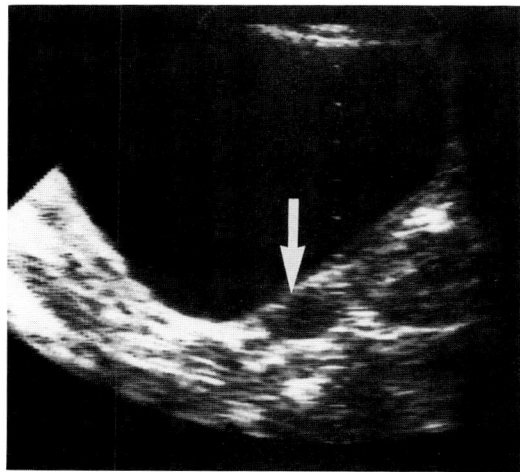

FIG. 14.8. Fibroma of the seminal vesicle. Transabdominal ultrasounds in transverse view (**A**) and longitudinal orientations of the left (**B**) and right (**C**) seminal vesicles demonstrate a solid, asymmetric mass on the right (*arrows*) as compared to the normal (*arrowhead*) left seminal vesicle. This mass, on histologic evaluation, was a fibroma.

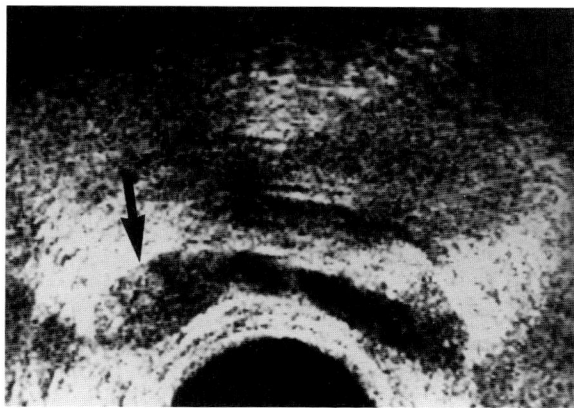

FIG. 14.9. Epididymal carcinoma. Endorectal ultrasound in an axial orientation demonstrates asymmetry of the seminal vesicles, with the right side (*arrow*) being larger and more echogenic than the left side. On histologic evaluation, this was an epididymal carcinoma.

1. Asymmetry in size.
2. Asymmetry in shape.
3. An obvious mass in one seminal vesicle.
4. Asymmetry in echogenicity. The abnormal side should appear more echogenic than the normal side.

Thus, the presence of a unilateral solid mass involving the seminal vesicles should be sufficient enough to suggest the need for surgery and histologic diagnosis (328). The sonogram is not adequate to make a tissue diagnosis.

CONCLUSION

In summary, regardless of the pathology present, the following are suggested for evaluation of the seminal vesicles:

1. An axially oriented scanner using endorectal technique will demonstrate the presence of both right and left seminal vesicles.
2. An axially oriented scanner is best used to demonstrate the presence of symmetry of both vas deferens as they join with seminal vesicles.
3. Symmetry in size, shape, and echogenicity should be present.
4. Solid lesion of the seminal vesicle suggests tumor.
5. Cystic changes in the seminal vesicle suggest the possibility of ureterocele, cystic change, or obstruction.
6. The longitudinally oriented scanner is best used to define the prostatic–seminal-vesicle angle and asymmetry in this area.

15 // The Prostatic Urethra

Neuromuscular Disorders	241
Autonomic Nervous System Abnormalities	241
Spinal Cord Injury	243
Drug-Induced Disorders	243
Urodynamic Studies	243
Electromyogram	244
Cystometrogram	244
Urethrometrogram	244
Bladder Neck Obstruction	245
Imaging Techniques	245
Imaging of Bladder-Neck Obstruction	250
Imaging of Bladder Hyperreflexia	255
Imaging of the Prostatic Nodules	255
Conclusion	258

Voiding is the final step in the elimination of urine. This intermittent (but ongoing) process, known as *micturition*, is dependent on vesical filling until tension within the bladder rises above a certain threshold. When this level is reached, bladder pressure stimulates the micturition reflex and causes a conscious need to urinate. The micturition reflex then acts to stimulate signals from the nervous system that facilitate the complex process of voiding.

Since the majority of urethral abnormalities occur in the male, the emphasis of this chapter will be on the proximal, or prostatic (posterior), urethra and on the various imaging techniques that can be utilized to evaluate this area.

NEUROMUSCULAR DISORDERS

Voiding abnormalities due to neuromuscular dysfunction affect more than 25 million Americans. Neuromuscular disorders of voiding can be grouped into those associated with either a contracted (Table 15.1) or a noncontracted (Table 15.2) bladder. Diabetes mellitus is the most common cause of a hypotonic areflexic bladder, affecting more than 50% of all diabetics over age 50 (361). Other neuromuscular disorders include detrusor-muscle–bladder-neck dyssynergia, detrusor-muscle–sphincter dyssnergia, or detrusor-muscle hyperreflexic abnormalities (135A,360).

AUTONOMIC NERVOUS SYSTEM ABNORMALITIES

Subjects with detrusor-muscle–bladder-neck and detrusor-muscle–sphincter dyssynergia usually manifest autonomic dysreflexia. Clinically, they may present with headache, high

Table 15.1. Causes of contractile bladder[a]

Type	Dysfunction	Common causes

Uninhibited	Incontinent because voiding reflex triggers before bladder is full	Suprapontine
		  Cerebral atherosclerosis
		  Early multiple

	Also voluntary voiding	Neoplasm of brain Pernicious anemia

Reflex	Voiding via spinal cord reflex
	No voluntary control
		Subpontine
		Cord injury
		Neoplasm
		  Extradural abscess
		  Disc lesion
		  Degenerative arthritis
		  Vertebral collapse
		  Syringomyelia

		Suprapontine
		  Extensive brain injury
		  Advanced multiple sclerosis

Hyperreflexic	Bladder contrast involuntarily (volume under 100 ml)	Suprapontine lesion
		  Cervical cord lesion
		  Irritated reflex bladder (by infection or catheter)

[a]From reference 393.

Table 15.2. Cause of a poorly contractile (hypoereflexic) or noncontractile (areflexic) bladder[a]

Lower motor neuron lesions: sensory and motor
  Cauda equina lesions
  Herniated disc
  Acute transverse myelitis
  Guillain-Barré syndrome
  Extensive rectal carcinoma
  Abdominoperineal resection
  Perivesical fibrosis (pelvic surgery or injury)

Motor paralysis, sensory intact (motor nerves to bladder)
  Injury, neoplasm, or herniated disc
  Poliomyelitis

Cord infarction (anterior cord syndrome)

Overdistension areflexia

Sensory loss
  Diabetes mellitus
  Tabes
  Alcoholic neuropathy
  Untreated chronic overdistension from upper motor lesion

[a]From reference 393.

blood pressure, bradycardia, and sweating. Patients with spinal cord lesions at the T5 level and above may show similar symptoms. The mechanism of autonomic dysreflexia is as follows (136,361):

1. As the detrusor muscle contracts (detrusor-muscle–bladder-neck dyssynergia), the bladder neck fails to relax and is forced open against resistance.
2. The adrenergic fibers are overstimulated.
3. Excessive noradrenalin is secreted, resulting in peripheral vasoconstriction and sweating.
4. Lesions below T5 cause the splanchnic veins to dilate, and blood pressure does not rise; lesions above T5 do not cause the splanchnic veins to dilate, and blood pressure does rise.
5. Baroreceptors in the carotid sinus are stimulated, resulting in bradycardia; decreased cardiac output is then insufficient, and blood pressure rises (sometimes substantially).

SPINAL CORD INJURY

Spinal cord injury, which affects up to one million people in the United States alone, is a common cause of voiding abnormalities (136,361). Twenty thousand subjects are afflicted yearly (361). Because these individuals frequently encounter difficulties with micturition and subsequent development of complications, they are often required to undergo reexamination and reevaluation in order to determine the extent of disease and/or disability. An understanding of these studies and their findings can further patient care.

DRUG-INDUCED DISORDERS

There are various drugs (Table 15.3) that, because of their effects on the peripheral autonomic nervous system, cause contraction of the detrusor muscle, bladder neck, or the urethra. There are also pharmacological agents that cause relaxation of these structures (Table 15.4) (136,361).

URODYNAMIC STUDIES

A complete set of urodynamic studies should be obtained in order to evaluate voiding difficulties appropriately. These studies should include: measurement of bladder pressure

Table 15.3. Drugs that contract the detrusor, bladder neck, or urethra[a]

Group of drugs	Area affected	Drug
Cholinergic drugs	Detrusor contracts	Acetylcholine Bethanecol Methacholine Nicotine
α-Adrenergic drugs	Increased bladder neck and urethral pressure	Phenylephrine Ephedrine Imipramine
β-Blockers	Increased urethral pressure	Propranalol

[a]From reference 393.

Table 15.4. Drugs that relax the detrusor, bladder neck, or urethra[a]

Group of drugs	Area affected	Drugs
Anticholinergics	Decreased bladder contractility	Propantheline α-Tubocarine Reserpine Guanethedine Phenothiazine Antihistamines
α-Blockers	Decreased bladder neck and urethral pressure	Phentolamine Phenoxybenzamine Prozacin HCl
β-Stimulants	Decreased urethral pressure	Isoproterinol Progesterone

[a]From reference 393.

during filling and voiding; urine flow and urethral pressures during voiding; and electromyography of the periurethral striated sphincter.

ELECTROMYOGRAM

The electromyogram can be performed by inserting a small needle through the perineum into the surrounding striated muscle of the lower section of the urethra. Electrical activity from striated muscle can then be measured. When muscles contract, electrical activity will be present; when the muscle is relaxed, the absence of electrical activity will be noted. There is always some muscle contraction present, even when the muscle is at rest. In the normal individual, this is to prevent incontinence. Normal subjects can contract the perineal muscles at will, which increases electromyographic electrical activity. The initial phase of normal voiding encompasses relaxation of striated muscle. Electrical activity in the EMG will cease at this level (445).

CYSTOMETROGRAM

The cystometrogram records bladder pressure. In theory, it can determine the exact area of vesical or urethral narrowing or stricturing. However, this measure requires catheterization. Because of the insertion of the catheter, which is a foreign body, the resulting information may be slightly altered from the true state. In the normal adult, the normal bladder pressure during voiding does not rise above 70 cm water. It is slightly less, in the range of 40 cm, in normal children. Elevation above these normal pressures suggests obstruction at the bladder neck or in the urethra (445).

URETHROMETROGRAM

The cystometrogram can also be used to measure urethral pressures. The catheter is withdrawn from the bladder slowly. As this is done, pressures are taken from within the bladder neck and prostatic urethra. If the urethral pressures are elevated above those in the bladder, voiding cannot occur.

BLADDER NECK OBSTRUCTION

The most common etiology of bladder neck obstruction involves neuromuscular dysfunction. This can include: (a) detrusor-muscle–bladder-neck dyssynergia; (b) a bladder neck flap of mucosa which forms in the posterior aspect of the bladder neck as a result of repeated traumatic insults (i.e., frequent catheterizations); and (c) benign prostatic hyperplasia in which either diffuse enlargement or smaller focal nodules cause an impression on the bladder neck and cause subsequent voiding difficulties.

In patients with destrusor-muscle–bladder-neck dyssynergia, the bladder neck opens either minimally or not at all. When treated with intravenous phentolamine, which is an α-adrenergic blocking agent, the dyssynergia will respond; that is, the bladder neck will open. Drug inducement, however, has no effect on patients with a posterior-placed mucosal bladder flap or adenomatous nodules (136,361,445).

IMAGING TECHNIQUES

Until recently, imaging studies to evaluate voiding were performed with iodinated contrast [i.e., the X-ray voiding cystourethrogram (VCU)]. Following an intravenous pyelogram, or in a retrograde fashion via a Foley catheter, the urinary bladder is distended with contrast, and the voiding images are obtained. Both the posterior and anterior urethra can be clearly defined by this technique. The internal and external sphincter may be demonstrated as subtle concentric rings around the contrast-distended posterior urethra. These rings can be seen at the levels of the base and apex of the prostate.

The suprapubic sonogram may define the posterior urethra when dilated or following transurethral resection of the prostate, but this is usually an incidental finding (see Chapter 12). Conventional sonography has little benefit for diagnosis in the adult. In the child, however, the abdominal sonogram can demonstrate the dilated trigone canal, proximal posterior urethra, and wall thickness of the bladder. The posterior urethral valve, which can be delineated by the VCU, is generally not seen by ultrasound.

Magnetic resonance imaging rarely defines the nondilated urethra; however, it can demonstrate the dilated urethra, particularly when secondary to previous transurethral prostatic resection. Signal intensity will be similar to that of urine.

Recently, voiding sonourethrography has been utilized for evaluation of patients with neuromuscular dysfunction (136,361,445) and anatomic irregularities of the prostatic and periprostatic urethral area (398). The sonourethrogram can be performed either as a primary examination or following a transrectal sonoendoscopic study of the prostate. The technique is similar to the routine transrectal ultrasound examination. A linear-array probe with longitudinally oriented images is essential. The condom covered sonoendoscope, is inserted into the patient's rectum following lubrication with gel. The area from the bladder neck to the membranous urethra can be evaluated with this technique.

Although many patients can urinate in the lithotomy position, positioning the patient in the decubitus position is preferable (398). The normal sonourethrogram will demonstrate early distension of both the bladder neck and the proximal posterior urethra. The normal bladder base is initially flat. The urethral angle is rounded. As voiding proceeds, the prostatic urethra straightens (Fig. 15.1). The normal prostatic urethra courses parallel to the rectum. Rounding of the posterior tip of the bladder base may be seen with mild hyperplasia (Fig.

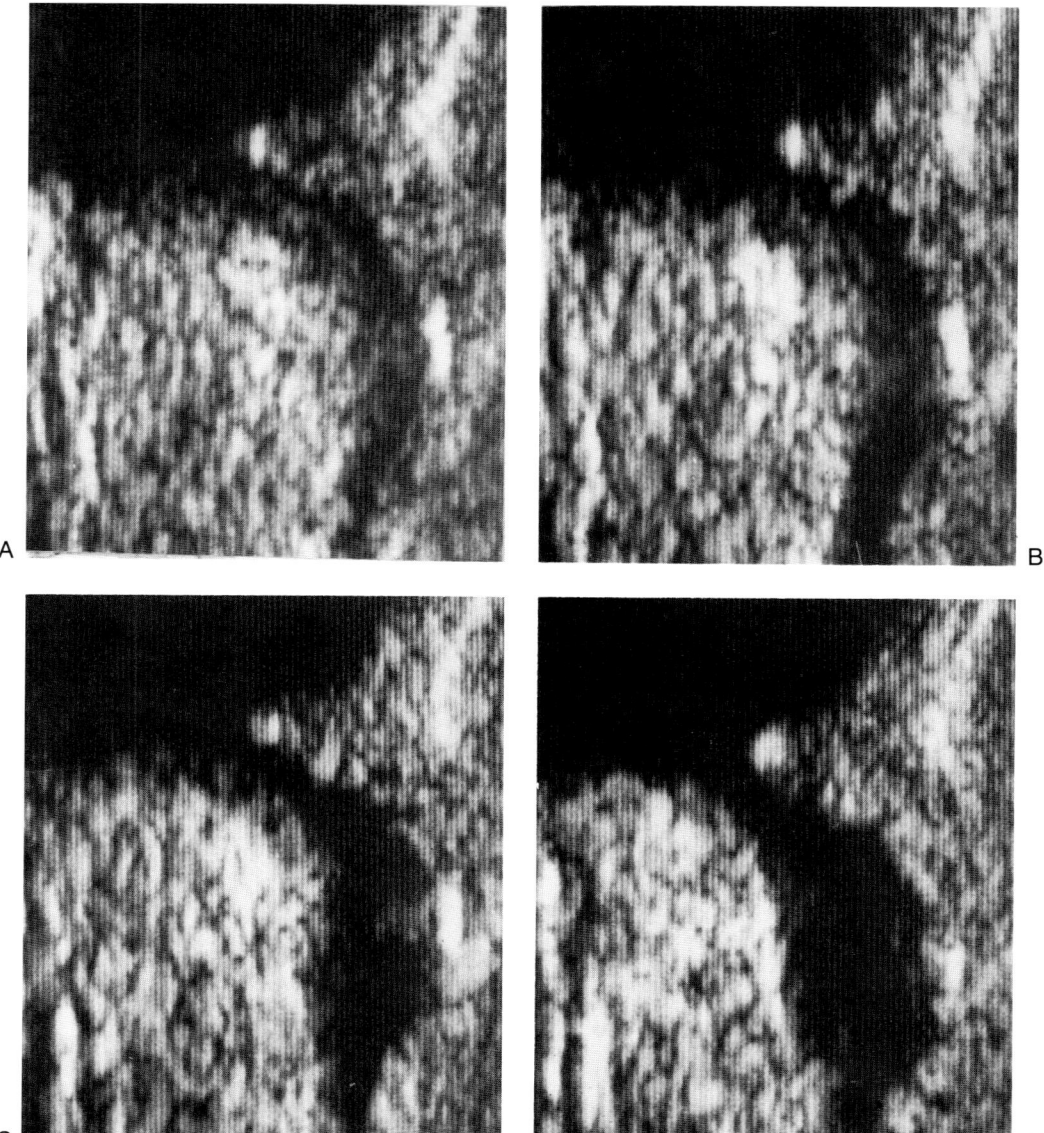

FIG. 15.1. Normal sonographic voiding cystourethrogram. Sequential images (**A–D**) and a line diagram of the same images (**E**) demonstrate normal voiding. The urethra angle flattens as voiding progresses. The internal sphincter is seen as it opens during normal voiding. The anterior wall of the urethra straightens as it moves forward during micturition. (From reference 393.)

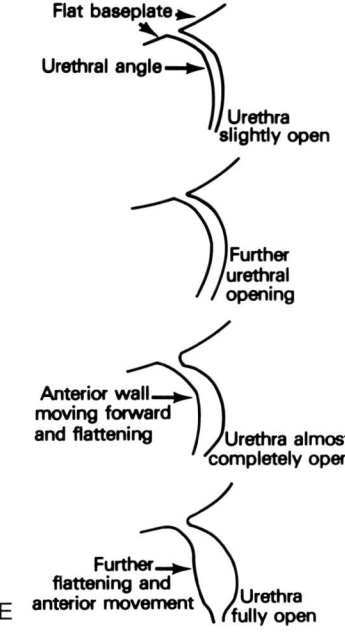

FIG 15.1 *Continued.*

15.2). The proximal prostatic urethra may appear very prounounced and large (although normal) below the bladder neck (Fig. 15.3).

The sensation or pressure of the probe within the rectum does not inhibit voiding in men without normal neurosensory function (i.e., patients with spinal cord injuries). If necessary, the Credé maneuver can be used to induce voiding in subjects with neurosensory deficiencies. Gentle pressure upon the bladder with fingers placed just above the symphysis pubis and application of gentle continuous increasing pressure on the fluid-filled bladder in a posterior-caudad projection will usually initiate urination (Fig. 15.4). Gentle tapping at, or just superior to, the pubic bone is another maneuver that can also result in opening of the bladder neck and the posterior prostatic urethra (Fig. 15.5). These techniques are generally ineffective in patients without neurosensory dysfunction. However, having the bladder overdistended prior to the transrectal study does improve the success rate of the examination.

Although Polaroid or X-ray film can be used as the sole modality for preserving a voiding study, the use of a videotape for a permanent dynamic recording and later review is useful, particularly when a follow-up study is planned to evaluate for possible changes. If possible, when examining patients for evaluation of neurogenically induced (or other) abnormalities of micturition, the voiding X-ray cystourethrogram and/or sonourethrogram should be performed simultaneously with neurodynamic studies (136,361,445). However, if only the imaging techniques are available, extensive information can be obtained (136,361,445).

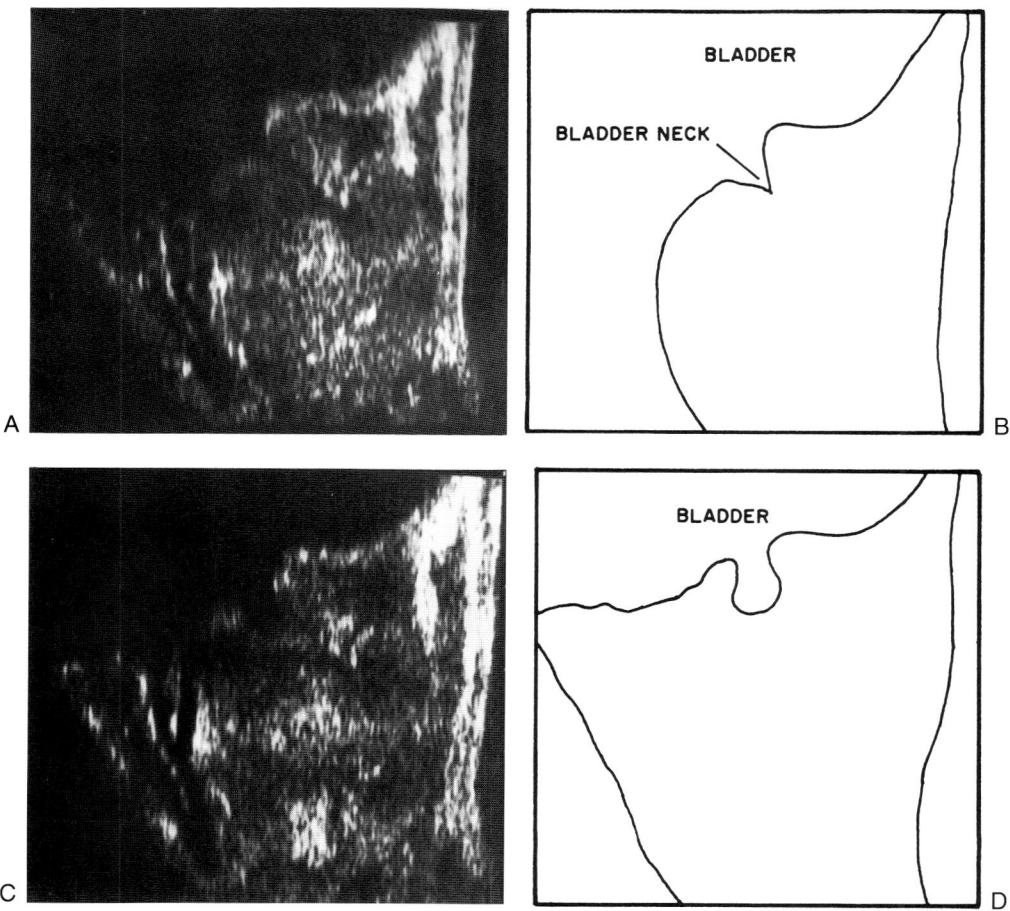

FIG. 15.2. Rounding of the posterior lip with mild benign prostatic hyperplasia. When mild benign prostatic hyperplasia occurs, mild rounding of the posterior portion (lip) of the base of the bladder may be seen. This finding may also be demonstrated during early voiding (**A** and **B**). (From reference 393.)

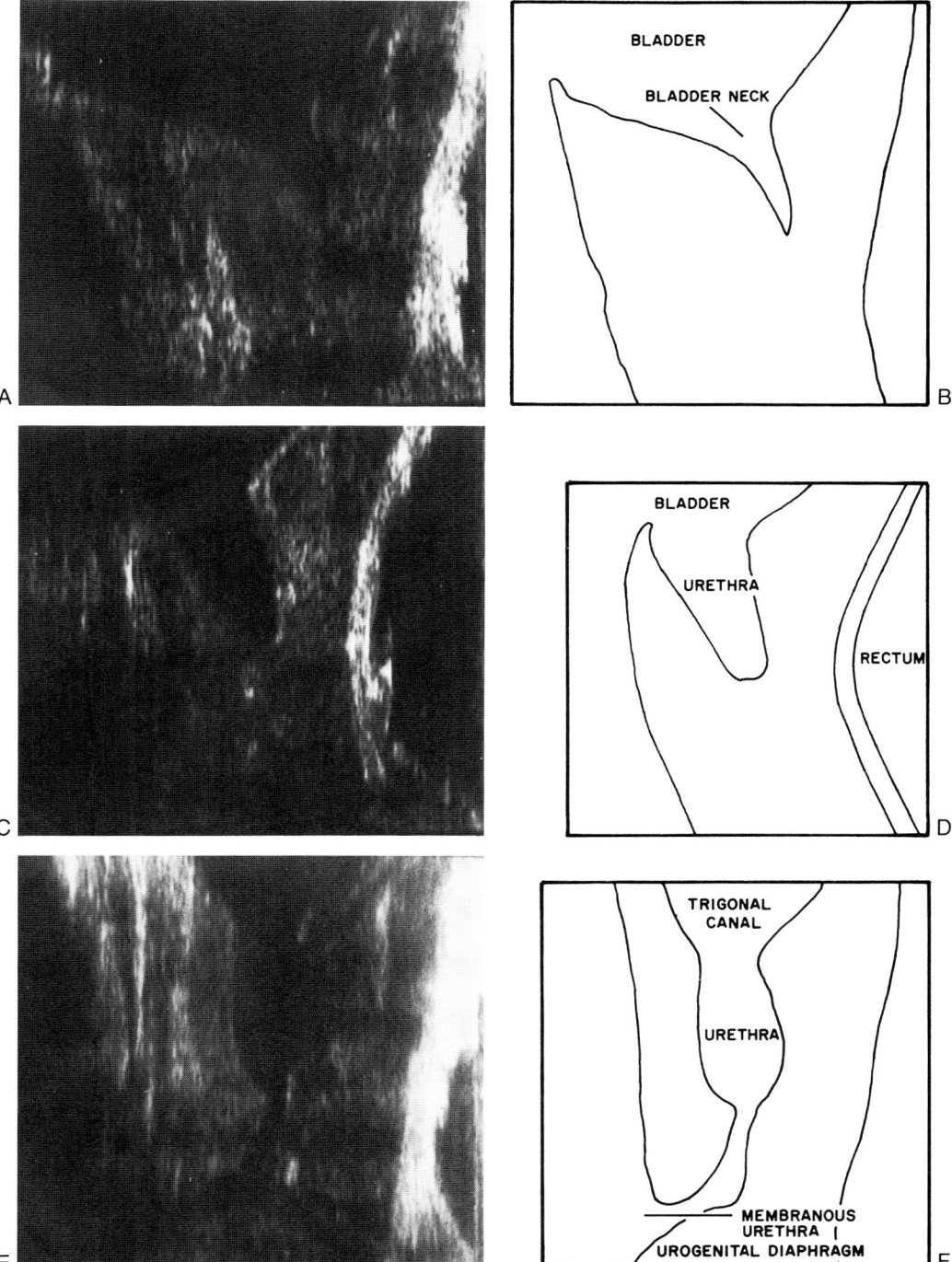

FIG. 15.3. Pronounced proximal urethra demonstrated during voiding sonourethrogram. An endosonourethrogram during early voiding demonstrates the bladder neck (**A** and **B**) as it begins to distend. As micturition continues (**C** and **D**), the proximal urethra begins to dilate; during mid-stream flow (**E** and **F**) seen in this male patient, the trigonal canal and urethra proximal to the dilated verumontanum begin to dilate. The distal prostatic urethra and the membranous urethra may also be demonstrated by the voiding sonourethrogram at the level of the urogenital diaphragm (**E** and **F**). (From reference 393.)

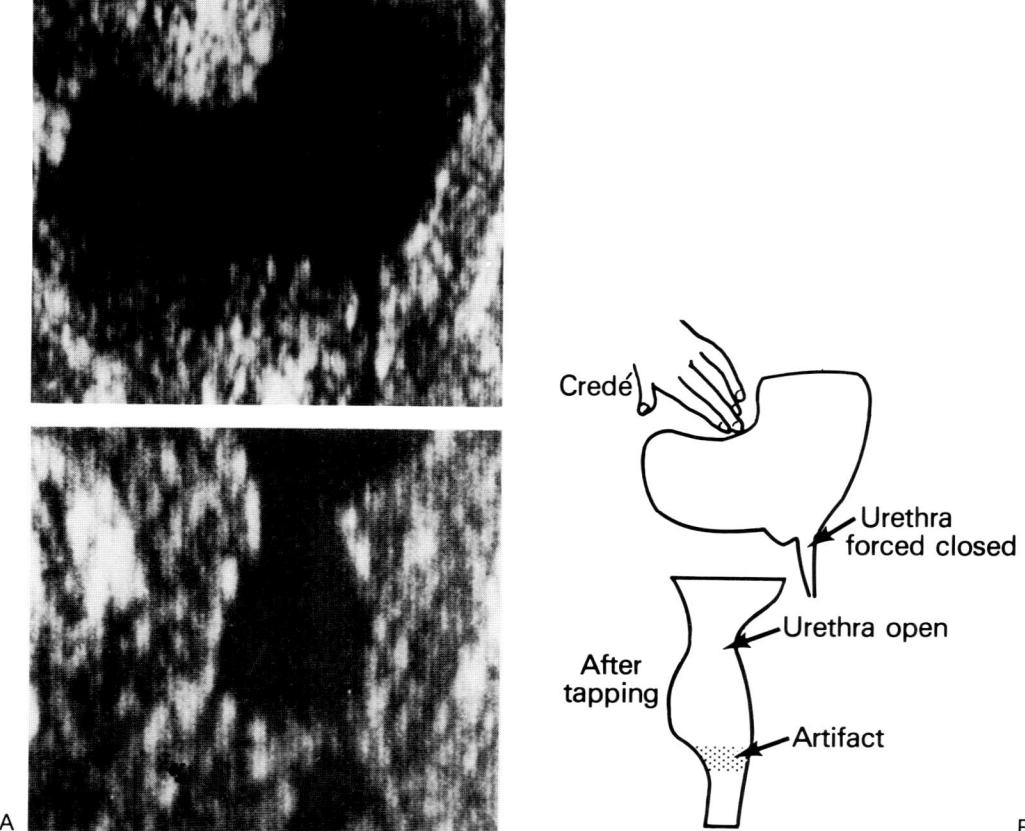

FIG. 15.4. Voiding with the Credé maneuver. The Credé manuever (pressure applied to the urinary bladder just superior to the symphysis pubis) is seen during a voiding sonourethrogram. This technique may be used successfully to initiate voiding in some patients with hyperreflexic bladders. (From reference 393.)

IMAGING OF BLADDER-NECK OBSTRUCTION

Urodynamic imaging studies, particularly with the transrectal sonographic approach, have demonstrated that in patients with detrusor-muscle–bladder-neck dyssynergia, the bladder either does not open at all or opens only minimally. Intravenous administration of a test dose of phentolamine can produce normal voiding. This functional test can be monitored by the sonographic examination (Fig. 15.6). Although the intravenous test dose is higher than the normally prescribed oral dose, repeat sonourethrograms can be performed following a 10-day trial dose. The results can determine the need to continue or alter the administered amount of medication. Adequate clinical response is ascertained by continued opening of the bladder neck. If bladder-neck opening remains deficient, the amount of oral phentolamine must be increased. Because no radiation is used for these sonographic voiding cystourethrograms, multiple examinations can be performed without hazard to the patient (136,361,445).

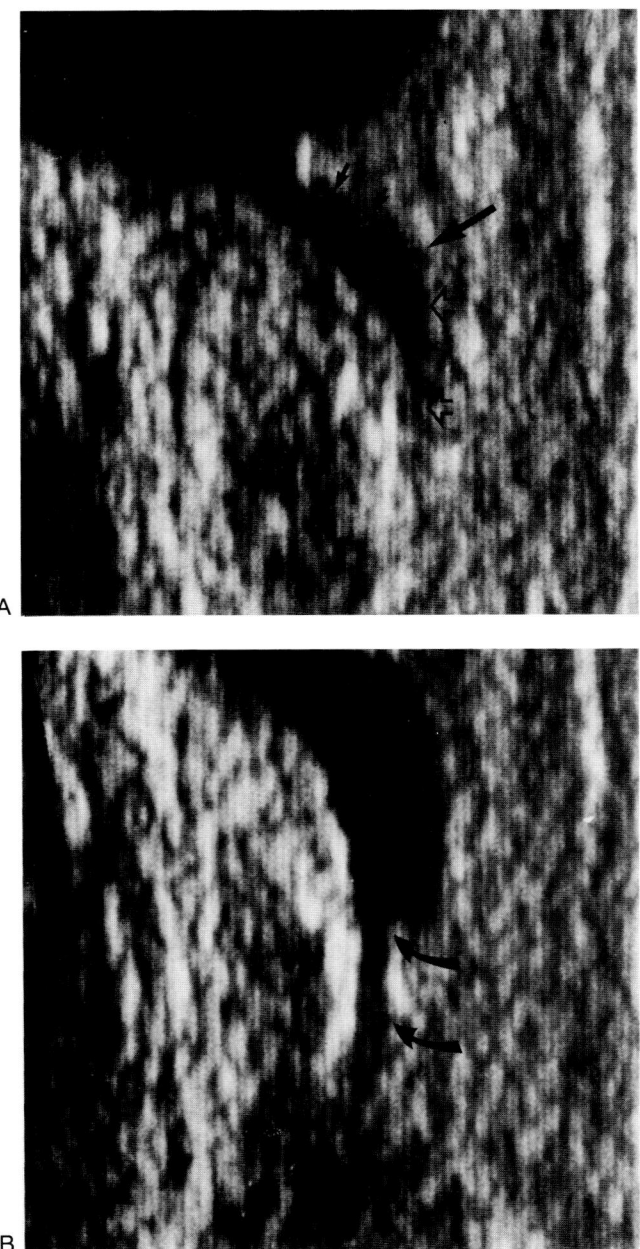

FIG. 15.5. Voiding by tapping maneuver. Voiding may occur in patients with neurosensory deficits by a tapping maneuver. An endorectal sonourethrogram prior to tapping (**A**) demonstrates the urethral angle (*large arrow*) and the level of the urethra at the bladder neck (*small arrows*) and just proximal to the verumontanum (*open arrowheads*). Note the difference in the angle between the proximal portion and the mid-portion of the proximal prostatic urethra. Following tapping, the urethra dilates (**B**). The verumontanum (*curved arrows*) is noted. (Courtesy of Dr. Gerald W. Friedland.)

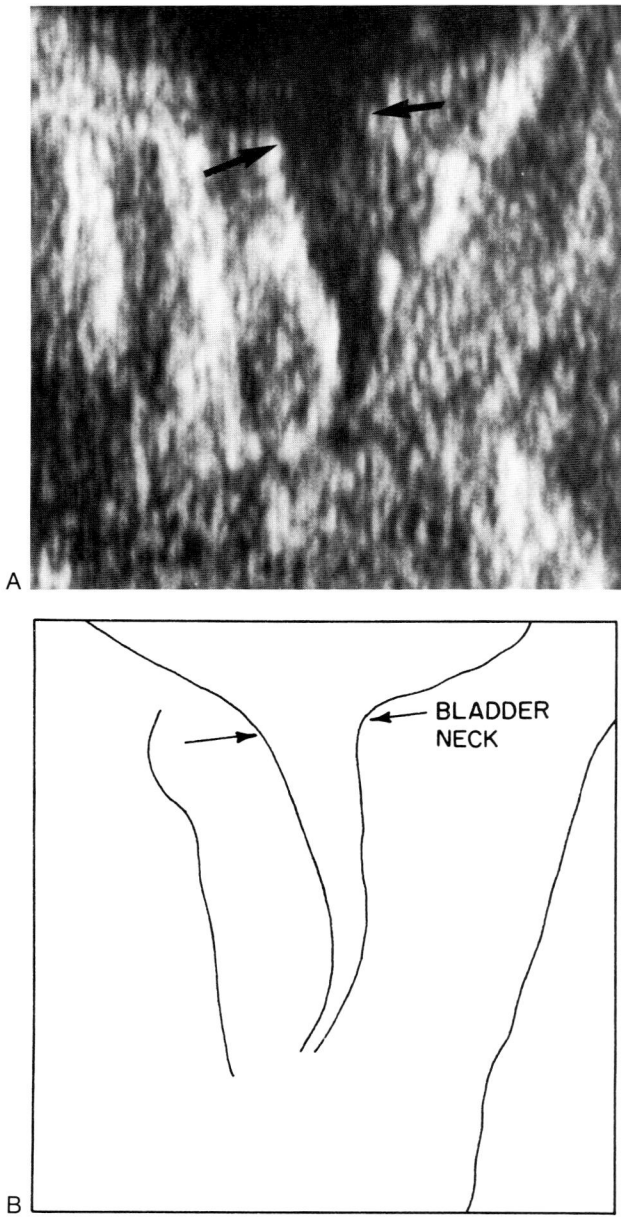

FIG. 15.6. Detrusor-muscle–bladder-neck dyssynergia. Voiding endorectal sonourethrogram demonstrates a bladder neck that is only slightly dilated (**A** and **B**). Following a test dose of phentolamine administered intravenously (**C** and **D**), the bladder neck distends following a successful test of treatment. (Courtesy of Dr. Gerald W. Friedland.)

THE PROSTATIC URETHRA

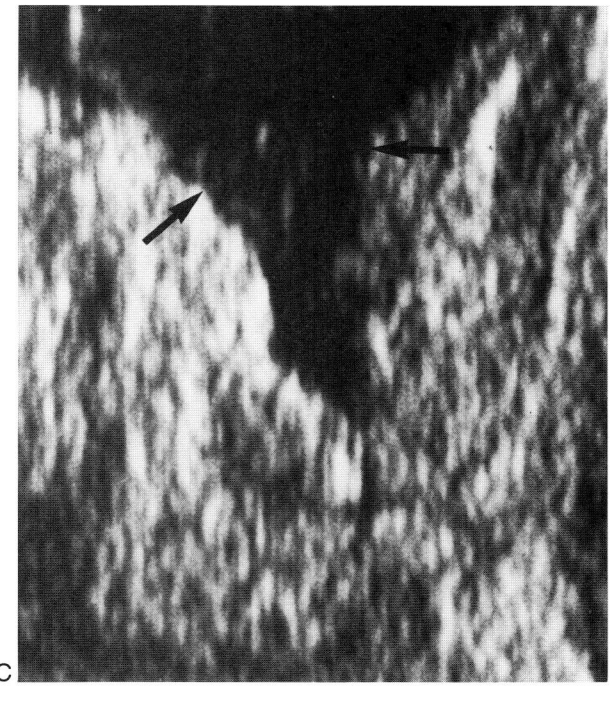

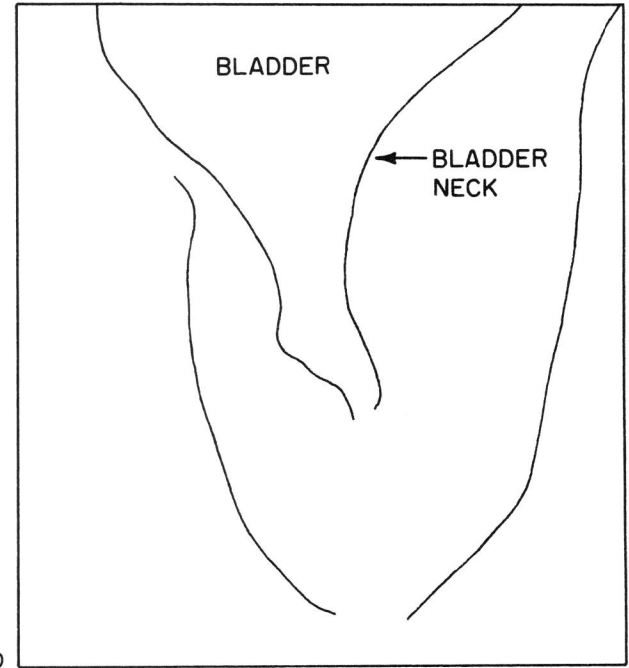

FIG. 15.6 *Continued.*

A prominent-sized proximal urethra may be a normal finding (Fig. 15.3). This should be differentiated from a markedly dilated proximal posterior urethra, which is secondary to chronic bladder outlet obstruction (Fig. 15.7).

It was once thought that adequate treatment of voiding abnormalities due to neurosensory deficits could be done by chronic intermittent catheterization. Recent evidence now indicates that a posterior bladder flap composed of mucosa and granulation tissue can form at the region of the bladder neck (Fig. 15.7). The development of this flap not only inhibits voiding but, in itself, is a contraindication for continuous bladder catheterization. Frequently it is not seen at all on the normal radiographic cystogram and cystourethrogram and is only demonstrated by the transrectal sonographic voiding study.

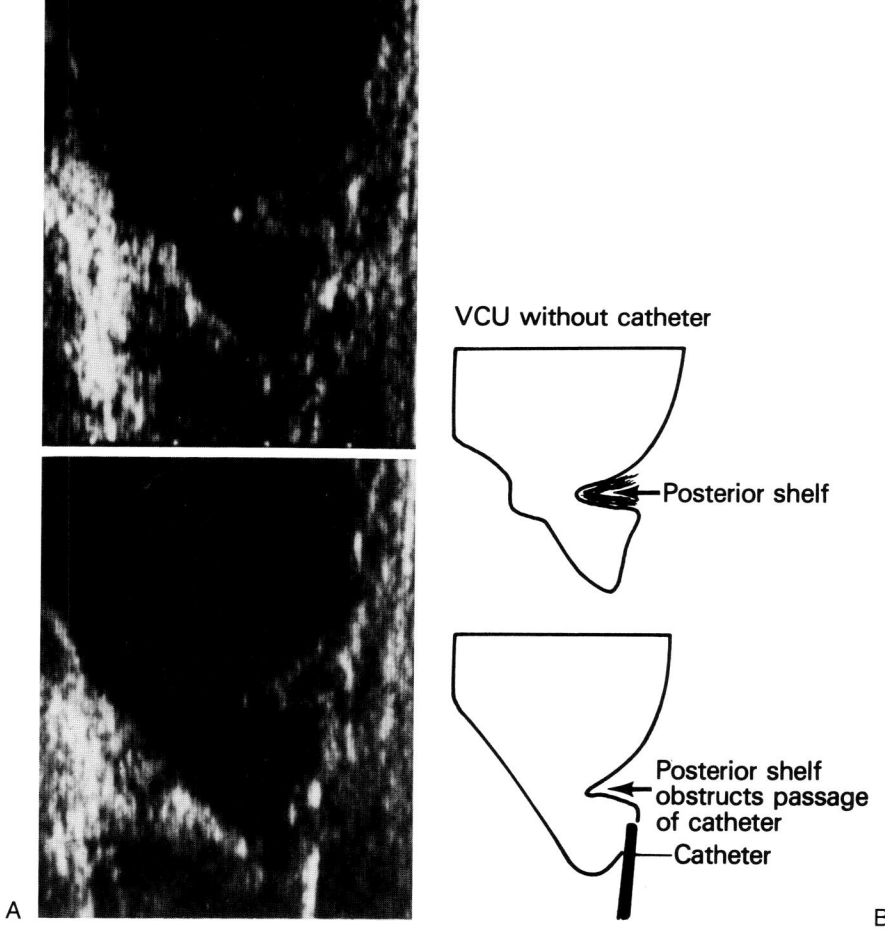

FIG. 15.7. Granulation tissue of the posterior shelf with a markedly dilated proximal urethra. Mucosa and granulation tissue of the posterior shelf may be a complication of constant, chronic intermittent catheterization. The endorectal sonourethrogram demonstrates a posterior shelf and a catheter which may be obstructed by entering the urinary bladder. The proximal ureter is markedly dilated. (From reference 393.)

IMAGING OF BLADDER HYPERREFLEXIA

Patients with bladder hyperreflexia feel an urge to micturate with a small, partially filled bladder. This often occurs when a catheter is inserted into a minimally distended urinary bladder. It has been seen with only 30 ml of urine present. Drastic and immediate contraction of the urinary bladder occurs. Before the use of the transrectal sonourethrogram, this hyperreflexic syndrome was not known. Immediate withdrawal of the urethrally placed catheter eliminates the bladder's hyperactive response to the foreign object (136,361,445).

IMAGING OF THE PROSTATIC NODULES

Benign prostatic hypertrophy may cause diffuse compression or, more commonly, may cause a clearly demarcated nodule impinging upon the urethra or bladder neck.

These nodules, which originate in the periurethral tissues, can occupy any area of the prostate. When they extend toward the peripheral tissues of the gland, voiding may be unaffected. However, when impinging upon the urethra or bladder neck, compression on the prostatic urethra may occur (5). Although the radiographic cystourethrogram may demonstrate subtle or marked impingement upon the prostatic urethra, direct visualization of the causative mass is not possible. The transrectal sonographic study can, in great detail, define the bladder, bladder neck, bladder neck nodules (Fig. 15.8), and the prostatic urethra (Fig. 15.9). It can delineate the exact size, shape, and echogenic texture of the impinging lesions. Other lesions (i.e., unsuspected carcinoma) may also be detected during the sonographic cystourethrogram (398,445).

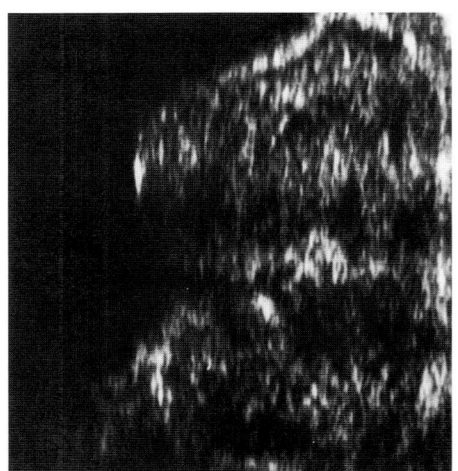
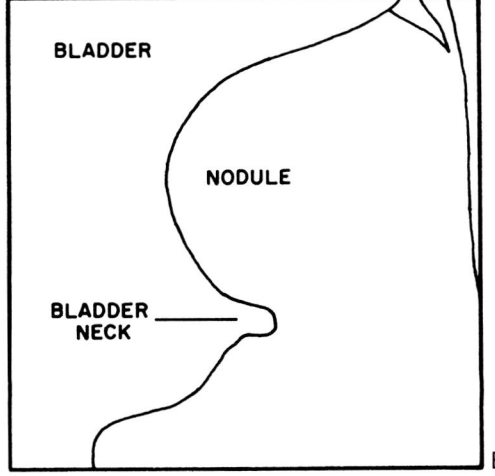

FIG. 15.8. Bladder neck nodules. Endorectal ultrasound of the prostate and urethra during voiding demonstrates homogeneous echogenicity to the prostate. There is enlargement to the posterior lip of the urinary bladder **(A–B)**; during sequential voiding **(C–J)**, this area of abnormality is noted to impinge upon the proximal urethra. The urethra is abnormally deviated. Despite the large size of these hyperplastic nodules, normal voiding occurs. (From reference 393.)

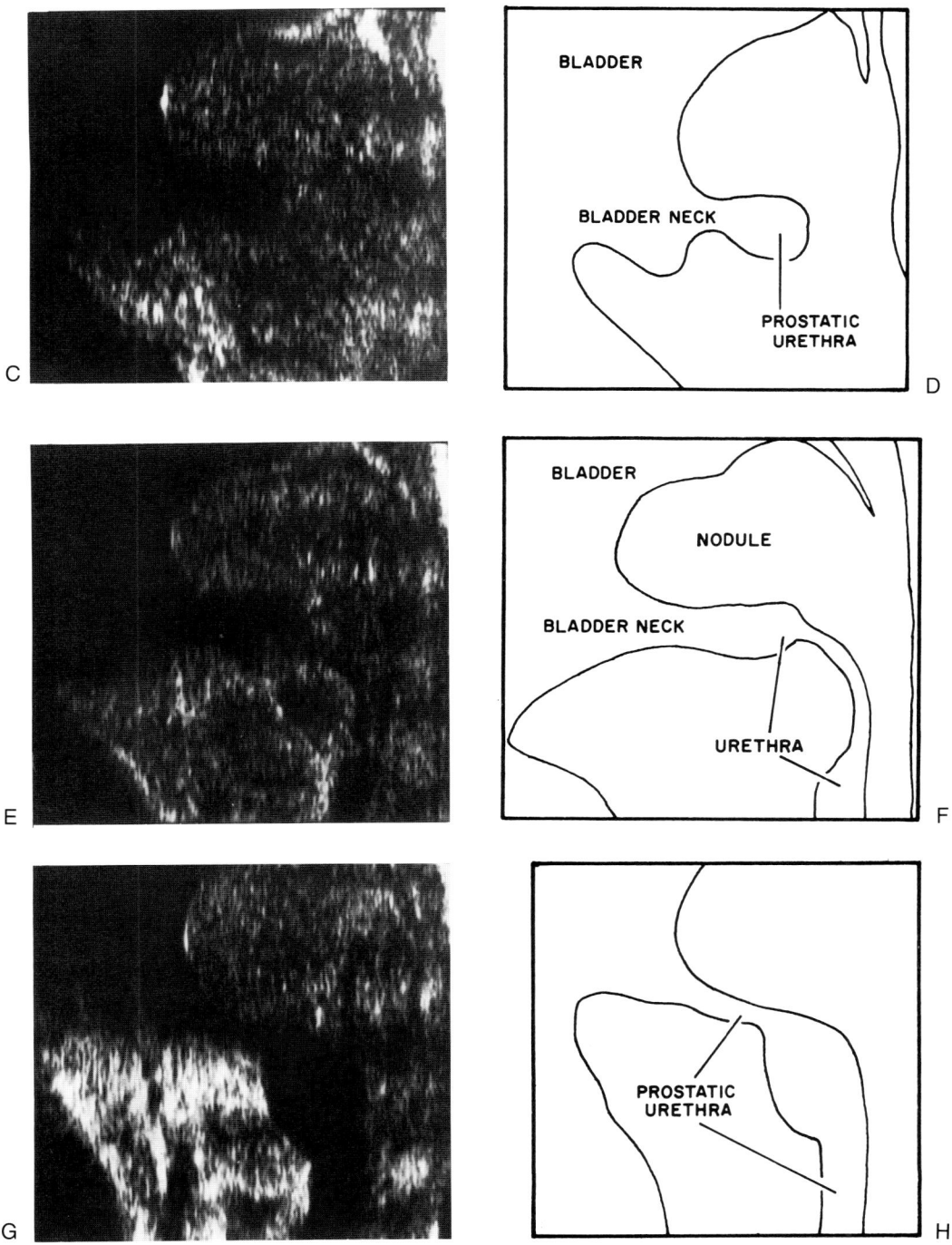

FIG. 15.8. Continued.

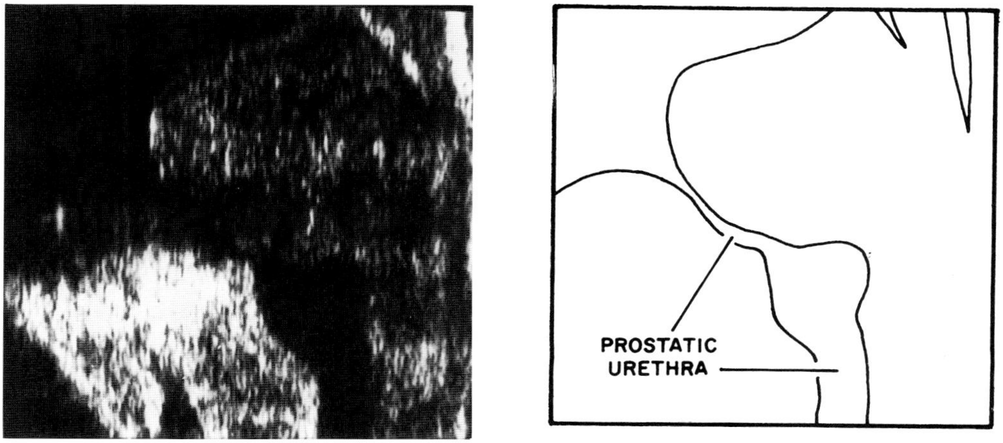

FIG. 15.8. *Continued.*

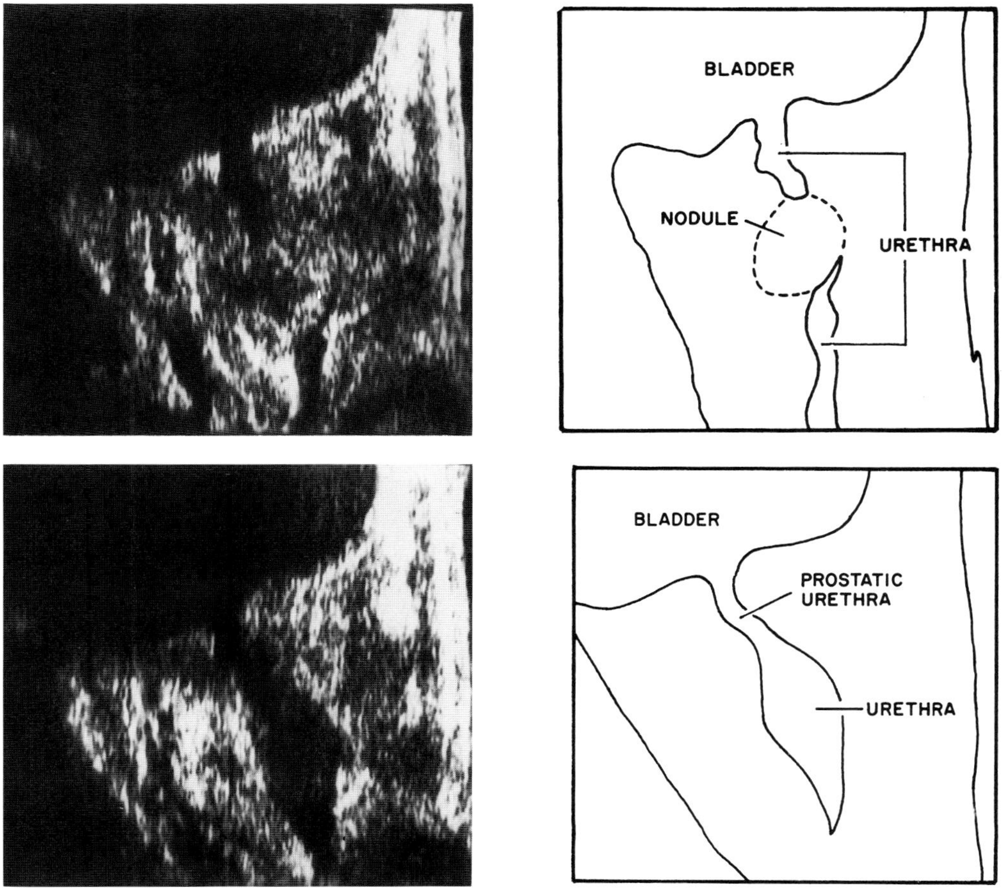

FIG. 15.9. Small benign prostatic nodule causing urethral impingement. An endorectal sonourethrogram demonstrates a benign prostatic hyperplastic nodule just anterior to the prostatic urethra causing impingement upon the flow or urine during voiding, just proximal to the level of the verumontanum. The nodule is seen best in the midline (**A** and **B**). As the probe is rotated slightly (**C** and **D**), the nodule is less clearly defined.

CONCLUSION

The endorectal voiding sonourethrogram is a relatively new technique whose potential has not yet been realized. As the technique is used more frequently, its benefit for diagnosis and evaluation of other disorders will certainly become evident.

16 // Endorectal Prostatic Ultrasound: Clinical Indications and Clinical Implications

Differential Diagnoses in Endorectal Ultrasound	259
Prostate Cancer	
Sonographic Characteristics of Benign Disease	
The Peripherally Oriented Hypoechoic Lesion	
Screening	260
Present Clinical Indications	264
Evaluation of a Palpable Mass	
The Clinically Normal Prostate	
Biopsy Guidance	
Evaluation of Inflammatory Disease	
Sonourethrography	
Screening	
Future Indications for Endorectal Prostatic Ultrasound	266
Conclusion	266

DIFFERENTIAL DIAGNOSES IN ENDORECTAL ULTRASOUND

The previous chapters have dealt with the sonographic characteristics of various disease processes that may affect the prostate, the seminal vesicles, and the surrounding structures. While certain sonographic findings may suggest a specific disease process, there is still great overlap between the many entities which involve the gland. Because of this, certain criteria have been developed to suggest or differentiate one disease process from another. These are summarized below. (Reference to each specific chapter is recommended for further elaboration.)

Prostate Cancer

Prostate cancer can have a variety of appearances, but the most characteristic appearance, particularly for the smaller lesion, is the peripherally oriented, hypoechoic lesion. These lesions are usually irregularly marginated, although portions of the mass may actually appear well delineated. Extension along the capsule of the prostate into the inner prostatic tissues or outside of the gland may occur. The hypoechoic mass, however, is not pathognomonic for malignancy. (This is discussed later in this chapter.)

Capsular bulge is an indication, but not an absolute diagnostic characteristic, of prostate cancer. Some benign prostatic hyperplastic lesions may also bulge the capsule.

Capsular infiltration is a sign of malignancy. The most important characteristic to suggest prostate cancer is sonographic asymmetry of the peripheral zone. This is true regardless of echogenicity. Disruption of portions of the peripheral zone, be they hypo-, iso-, or hyperechoic, or have sonographically mixed areas, are highly suspicious for possible malignancy.

Seminal vesicle extension is a sign of malignant infiltration as opposed to benign disease. This can be delineated by the loss of the "nipple," or a change in the normal seminal vesicle-prostatic "angle."

Regardless of these "signs" of cancer, tissue diagnosis is essential and thus, biopsy is necessary. An algorithm (Fig. 16.1) is suggested to determine those masses that may require biopsy.

Sonographic Characteristics of Benign Disease

The classic benign prostatic hyperplastic lesion is a well-defined mass in the periurethral areas. These lesions can be single or multiple, and, although they may cause a bulge in the capsule, they will not cause capsular disruption. The echogenic characteristics are varied. Occasionally, a "halo" sign may be delineated.

There are peripherally oriented hypoechoic lesions that may also be benign. These have been seen in a variety of studies and can include normal prostatic tissue, musculature surrounding the ejaculatory ducts, inflammatory or necrotic tissue, fibrotic material, or even benign prostatic hyperplastic tissue.

The Peripherally Oriented Hypoechoic Lesion

A hypoechoic lesion oriented in the peripheral zone of the prostate, which is asymmetrically situated, is highly suspicious for malignancy. However, the peripherally oriented hypoechoic lesion is not pathognomonic for malignant tumor. The exact significance of the peripherally oriented lesion in relation to the diagnosis of cancer is not definite. The positive predictive value for cancer of this lesion is far less than 100%. Various studies have shown that the chance of malignancy in a hypoechoic peripherally oriented lesion in the prostate ranges from approximately 0–52% (Table 16.1) (73,253,257,286,291,407–411,418). However, several of these studies may have included biopsy of smaller lesions and would, therefore, because a small cancer may be misdiagnosed, be less predictive of malignancy than biopsy of large lesions. There may be a slightly higher false-negative biopsy rate for the smaller lesion than for the larger lesion. In any event, there are benign lesions (normal tissue, benign prostatic hypertrophy, inflammation, fibrosis, infarction, normal muscle, etc.) that may mimic a hypoechoic cancer on the endorectal sonogram. Additional work is needed to further elucidate these findings. Even a positive predictive value of less than 100% may be acceptable if endorectal ultrasound is to be used as a screening tool. But the question remains— is screening a possibility or even a reality?

SCREENING

Is endorectal ultrasound of the prostate an appropriate screening modality? Much has been written with regard to prostatic screening, both in the medical and the nonprofessional journals. Before attempting to determine the benefits or possible uses of prostate ultrasound for screening, certain parameters should be reviewed.

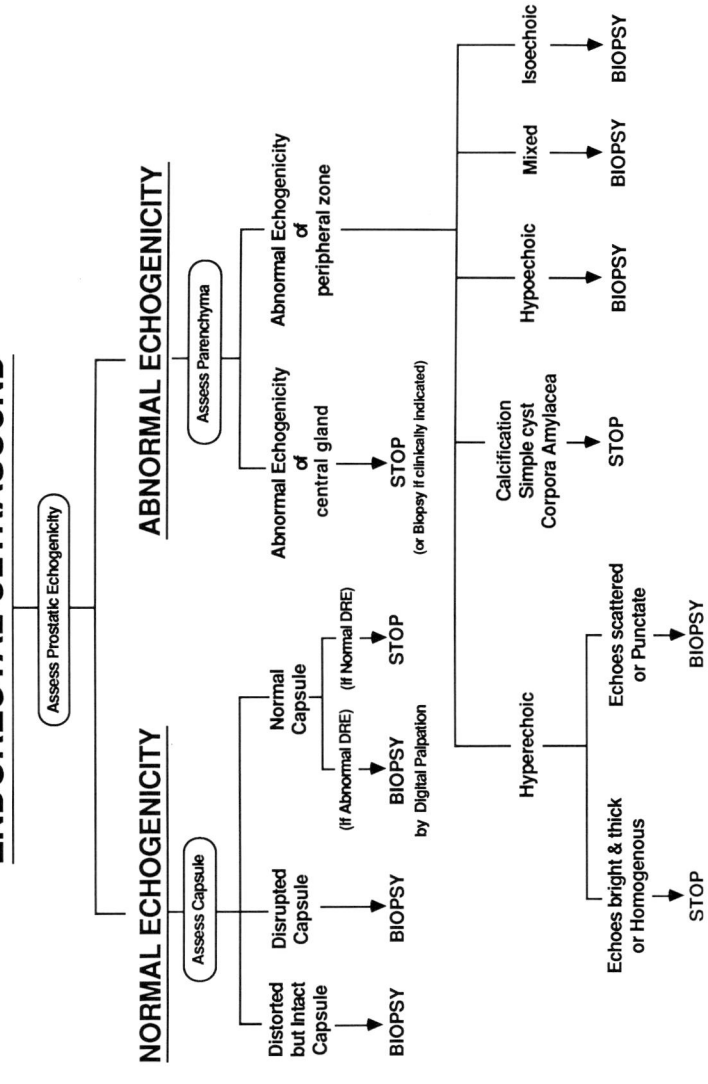

FIG. 16.1. Algorithm for sonographic diagnosis of prostatic disease.

Table 16.1. The positive predictive value of the peripherally oriented hypoechoic prostatic lesion

Number of lesions	Number of cancers	PPV(%)	Study
80	17	21.3	Rifkin (410)
43	0	0	McHugh (291)
14	0	0	Chancellor (73)
109	20	18	MacIntyre (287)
149	77	52	Lee (257)

What is sensitivity, specificity, positive predictive value, and negative predictive value? These are terms that are used frequently, but too often, inappropriately or inaccurately. A consistent and proper use of this terminology is essential for comparisons between studies and for possible determination of a specific technique and its ability for use in the diagnostic armamentarium.

The following are the statistical definitions of these parameters:

- Sensitivity is the ability of a test to accurately predict the presence of disease;
- Specificity is the ability of a test to accurately predict the absence of disease;
- Positive predictive value is the percentage of subjects with a positive examination who actually have the abnormality;
- Negative predictive value is the percentage of subjects with a negative examination who do not have the abnormality.

For example, the positive predictive value of an examination to determine cancer would equal the percentage of actual cancer patients in a group of all patients with a positive study.

The formulas used to calculate these parameters are as follows:

$$\text{Sensitivity} = \frac{\text{True positive}}{\text{True positive} + \text{False negative}}$$

$$\text{Specificity} = \frac{\text{True negative}}{\text{True negative} + \text{False positive}}$$

$$\text{Positive predictive value} = \frac{\text{True positive}}{\text{True positive} + \text{False positive}}$$

$$\text{Negative predictive value} = \frac{\text{True negative}}{\text{True negative} + \text{False negative}}$$

Several preliminary studies have suggested that ultrasound can be used as an effective and appropriate screening tool. Others have shown the reverse. Examples of a few screening studies are presented below.

A study by Watanabe included an examination of 10,000 consecutive men (520). Only 137 cancers were detected, and of those, 129 were palpable. The limitations of this study include the following: (a) the use of older equipment, (b) a lack of digital rectal examination of all subjects, and (c) sonographic criteria that are not necessarily in use today or applicable to identification of very small lesions.

Another early study by Rosenberg et al. examined 2,214 men (417). Of these 766 (80%) of the men had a negative ultrasound, and a normal digital rectal examination. Twenty-four men (1% of the total population) had a negative ultrasound, but a positive digital rectal examination. Two of these had cancer on biopsy. Four-hundred and twenty-four men (19%

of the population) had a positive ultrasound. Of these, 352 (16%) had a negative digital rectal examination and 72 (3%) had a positive rectal examination. Not all men in the latter two groups underwent biopsy. Of those who had a positive ultrasound and a negative rectal examination, there was one positive biopsy out of 90 men. Three of 24 men with a positive ultrasound and a positive digital rectal examination had cancer—a 12% positive predictive value. Deficiencies in this study include the following:

1. Not all patients with abnormal rectal exams or ultrasounds had biopsy;
2. The diagnostic criteria for the determination of abnormal ultrasound studies were not delineated; and
3. Older equipment was utilized in this study.

A more recent study undertaken by Lee et al. examined 784 men (257). There were 20 subjects with cancer detected. Eighteen of the 20 had malignancy determined by ultrasound, and ten of the 20 (there was overlap) had cancer detected by the digital rectal examination. The detection rate was 2.3% by ultrasound and 1.3% by digital rectal examination.

In a fourth study, combining the early results reported by Chancellor (73) and the later results by McHugh (291), individuals who were undergoing a transurethral resection of the prostate for benign prostatic hyperplasia were examined. None of the men had an abnormal digital rectal examination, with the exception of prostatic hypertrophy. Endorectal ultrasound was performed prior to the transurethral prostatic resection and, if an abnormality was detected in the peripheral zone, biopsies were undertaken. These biopsies were performed using endorectal sonographic guidance. There were 43 peripherally oriented hypoechoic lesions detected by ultrasound (nonpalpable) that were biopsied and none had cancer on the pathologic specimen (291). This was not a true "screening" population.

A study by Ragde (the fifth "screening" study) evaluated 1,051 men who were examined because of self-referral (379). The breakdown of subjects by age is as follows:

$$<50 \text{ years of age} = 16\%$$
$$50-59 \text{ years of age} = 28\%$$
$$60-69 \text{ years of age} = 37\%$$
$$70-79 \text{ years of age} = 15\%$$
$$\geq 80 \text{ years of age} = 4\%$$

In the Ragde study, 138 men had a sonographically abnormal area (defined as a hypoechoic, peripherally oriented lesion) and sonographically guided biopsies. There were 50 cancers detected (a detection rate of 4.8%). None of the subjects had a digital rectal examination during the study.

In a sixth study by Rifkin, 112 men had endorectal ultrasound because of self-referral (405). There were 3 cancers (3%) that were detected by endorectal ultrasound and none of these men had a suspicious digital rectal examination. These studies, although varied in method and technique, do suggest some indication or future possibility of using endorectal prostatic ultrasound to detect clinically unsuspected malignancy. However, the data appear, at present, to be inconclusive in evaluating the ability to use this technique as a screening tool. A few questions must be answered before we can successfully determine if prostate ultrasound is a viable screening modality.

1. Do we really understand the pathogenesis and the biological life of all prostatic cancers?
2. Will the patient benefit by treatment of these nonpalpable cancers which will be detected by the endorectal sonogram?

3. Will we be offering the patient more help than harm from the possible complications incurred in treating the newly discovered cancer?
4. Will we be inflicting greater damage to the patient by treating the malignancy than if we had left the cancer untreated?
5. Is the technique cost effective?

Some people have alluded to prostate ultrasound as a screening tool equivalent to the mammogram for detection of breast cancer. Unfortunately, while this may appear initially to be a valid comparison, there are many differences between prostate cancer and breast cancer. For example, the autopsy rate for undetected malignancy of the prostate appears to be far higher than that for breast cancer. However, breast cancer may affect a younger population and it is still considered a more "lethal" disease than prostate cancer.

Thus, while it would be beneficial and useful to equate screening for breast and prostate cancers, it is not always possible. The effectiveness of the mammogram as a screening for evaluation of breast cancer and breast disease has taken a number of years to develop. Additionally, there are many lesions seen on the mammogram that do not necessarily require biopsy or excision. This is not always true for the endorectal prostate sonogram. It may be necessary to biopsy all prostate lesions. Thus, the biopsy rate may be far higher for the prostate than it is for the breast.

While most of the questions regarding prostate screening cannot be answered fully at this time, there is great hope for the future. There is no doubt that endorectal ultrasound can detect clinically unsuspected and nonpalpable lesions. Many of these will be cancers. There is also no question that endorectal ultrasound will have great benefit in the evaluation of prostatic disease. However, while endorectal ultrasound may become a screening tool at this point there are no long-term studies with results to substantiate this claim. Further work and long-term, large scale studies must be undertaken to confirm that endorectal prostate ultrasound is a viable, cost-effective, and useful technique as a screening tool. Additionally, early work has suggested that by using serum prostatic specific antigen (PSA) as a biological marker for the presence (and perhaps size) of cancer, ultrasound may become even more specific for the detection of cancer (9,24,68,150,177,227,247,248,330,371,433, 473,519).

PRESENT CLINICAL INDICATIONS

There are a number of clinical indications for the use of prostate ultrasound today. These include the following:

- Evaluation of a palpable mass;
- Evaluation for prostatic disease in a man without a palpable mass;
- Biopsy guidance;
- Evaluation of inflammatory diseases of the prostate and seminal vesicles;
- Sonourethrography;
- Treatment procedures.

These are discussed below in more detail.

Evaluation of a Palpable Mass

On physical examination, many men present to their physicians with a distinctly abnormal prostate, or with a prostatic mass on the digital rectal examination. While many of these may be malignant (and others, benign), the need for further evaluation can definitively exclude certain entities. These include calculi, corpora amylacea, clearly defined prostatic cysts, and in certain instances, benign prostatic hyperplastic change. Additionally, many men present clinically with a subtle but not necessarily a definitively abnormal area in the prostate on the digital rectal examination. In these patients, the endorectal sonogram is of great benefit.

The Clinically Normal Prostate

Men may present to their physicians with a normal rectal examination. However, other abnormalities may be found, i.e., bone lesions, metastatic adenocarcinoma without a known primary or abnormal blood studies. The serum studies include elevated prostatic specific antigen and/or elevated prostatic acid phosphatase. The endorectal prostatic ultrasound may define areas of abnormality which are not palpable and which can be biopsied using endorectal sonographic guidance to help make diagnoses and thus, expedite treatment. The exact ability to definitively exclude malignancy in a "normal" feeling gland is still yet to be determined.

Biopsy Guidance

As mentioned in detail in Chapter 8, sonography is an accurate technique for biopsy guidance. This is obviously more important for the subtle lesion than for the palpable lesion. There is also some benefit of sonographic guidance for patients with a distinctly abnormal palpable mass who have an abnormal digital rectal examination but a negative digitally guided biopsy. A biopsy may be avoided if the sonogram detects benign disease, i.e., a calculus, as the cause of a palpable abnormality. There is an important subgroup of individuals who may not benefit by the endorectal sonographically guided biopsy. This includes those patients with the "isoechoic" cancer who have a palpable abnormality. In these cases, the sonographically guided biopsy is more a blind procedure than the digital rectal guided biopsy, where a mass is detected (Fig. 16.1).

Evaluation of Inflammatory Disease

Clinically, when inflammation of the prostate and/or the seminal vesicles is suggested, endorectal ultrasound or other sonographic techniques are not necessarily indicated. However, if treatment is incomplete or ineffective, abscesses may form and endorectal ultrasound may delineate these purulent pockets within the prostate and/or the seminal vesicles.

Sonourethrography

There are subgroups of men, as described in Chapter 15, who may benefit by the sonographic voiding studies (sonourethrography).

Screening

As previously stated, there is tremendous hope for the future that prostate ultrasound may become a screening tool. However, further work is necessary to actually ellucidate the true impact of this technique.

FUTURE INDICATIONS FOR ENDORECTAL PROSTATIC ULTRASOUND

While there are many indications (as mentioned throughout this text) for the use of prostate ultrasound, the future holds even greater promise. Techniques are being developed daily that will define, refine, and re-define the uses of this promising, innovative and exciting new technology. Only as further work is undertaken and the results made known, will even greater implications of this technology be appreciated.

CONCLUSION

Sonography of the prostate during the past 20 years has evolved into a highly sophisticated technological advancement. With the advent of the high resolution endorectal ultrasound, disease processes, diagnostic applications and even therapeutic innovations have developed that have made this a clinically important tool. There are many present indications for the use of prostate ultrasound. The future appears to hold even more promise for its development and use.

References and Selected Bibliography

1. Abe M, Hashimoto T, Matsuda T, Saitoh M, Watanabe H: Prostatic biopsy guided by transrectal ultrasonography using real-time linear scanner. *Urology* 1987; 29:567–569.
2. Abrams PH, Roylance J, Feneley RCL: Excretion urography in the investigation of prostatism. *Br J Urol* 1976; 48:681–684.
3. Abu-Yousef MM: Benign prostatic hyperplasia: Tissue characterization using suprapubic ultrasound. *Radiology* 1985; 156:169–173.
4. Abu-Yousef MM, Narayana AS: Prostatic carcinoma: Detection and staging using suprapubic US. *Radiology* 1985; 156:175–180.
5. Abu-Yousef MM, Narayana AS: Transabdominal ultrasound in the evaluation of prostate size. *J Clin Ultrasound* 1982; 10:275–278.
6. Ackermann R, Frohmuller HGW: Complications and morbidity following radical prostatectomy. *World J Urol* 1983; 1:62–67.
7. Ackermann RJ: Problematic prostatic prediction [Letter to the Editor]. *JAMA* 1985; 254:1171–1172.
8. Aguilar M, Gaffney EF, Finnerty DP: Prostatic melanosis with involvement of benign and malignant epithelium. *J Urol* 1982; 128:825–827.
9. Ahmann FR, Schifman RB: Prospective comparison between serum monoclonal prostate specific antigen and acid phosphatase measurements in metastatic prostatic cancer. *J Urol* 1987; 137:431–434.
10. Aito H, Kataja ja Matti Saarialho M: Eturauhasen koon maarittaminen kaikukuvauksella vatsanpeitteiden lapi. *Duodecim* 1980; 101:54–58.
11. Akiyama T: Bladder Tumors. Transrectal scanning. In: *Diagnostic Ultrasound in Urology and Nephrology* (H Watanabe, JH Holmes, HH Holm, BB Goldberg, Editors). Igaku-Shoin, New York, 1981, pp. 90–95.
12. Ando K, Sawamura Y, Tajima M: Real-time image. In: *Diagnostic Ultrasound in Urology and Nephrology* (H Watanabe, JH Holmes, HH Holm, BB Goldberg, Editors). Igaku-Shoin, New York, 1981, pp. 111–117.
13. Ando K, Sawamura Y, Tajima M: Ultrasound of the scrotal contents. In: *Diagnostic Ultrasound in Urology and Nephrology* (H Watanabe, JH Holmes, HH Holm, BB Goldberg, Editors). Igaku-Shoin, New York, 1981, pp. 191–203.
14. Apple JS, Paulson DF, Baber C, Putman CE: Advanced prostatic carcinoma: Pulmonary manifestations. *Radiology* 1985; 154:601–604.
15. Aragona F, Serretta V, Marconi A, Spinelli C, Arganini M, Fiorentini L: Leiomyosarcoma of the prostate in adults. *Ann Chir Gynaecol* 1985; 74:191–194.
16. Arger PH: Computed tomography of the lower urinary tract. *Urol Clin North Am* 1985; 12:677–686.
17. Arima M: Renal blood flow measurement by Doppler technique. In: *Diagnostic Ultrasound in Urology and Nephrology* (H Watanabe, JH Holmes, HH Holm, BB Goldberg, Editors). Igaku-Shoin, New York, 1981, pp. 211–221.
18. Armenian HK, Lilienfeld AM, Diamond EL, Brossi DJ: Relation between benign prostatic hyperplasia and cancer of the prostate: A prospective and retrospective study. *Lancet* 1974; 2:115–117.
19. Ayiomamitis A: Epidemiology of cancer of the prostate in Canada: 1950–1984. *Br J Urol* 1987; 60:157–161.
20. Babaian RJ, Lowry WL, Finan BF: Intraluminal antibiotic regimen for patients undergoing transrectal needle biopsy of prostate. *Urology* 1982; 20:253–255.
21. Bagshaw MA: Radiotherapeutic treatment of prostatic carcinoma with pelvic node involvement. *Urol Clin North Am* 1984; 11:297–304.
22. Baker ME, Silverman PM, Korobkin M: Computed tomography of prostatic and bladder rhabdomyosarcomas. *J Comput Assist Tomogr* 1985; 9:780–783.
23. Baker WJ: Carcinoma of the prostate: Analysis of 200 cases. *J Urol* 1959; 81:197–202.
24. Ban Y, Wang MC, Chu TM: Immunologic markers and the diagnosis of prostatic cancer. *Urol Clin North Am* 1984; 11:269–276.
25. Banner MP, Hassler R: The normal seminal vesiculogram. *Radiology* 1978; 128:339–344.
26. Baran GW, Golin AL, Bergsma CJ, Stone TE, Wilson PR, Reichardt BA, Lobert PF, Carlson JC: Standardized endosonography of prostate carcinoma. *J Urol* 1987, 137(4 Part 2):357A.

27. Baran GW, Golin A, Bergsma C, Stone T, Wilson P, Reichardt B, Lobert P, Locke CS, Calson JC, Holly LE: Standardized endosonographic evaluation of prostate cancer: Receiver-operator-characteristic analysis. *AJR* 1987; 149:975–980.
28. Barnes RW, Ninan CA: Carcinoma of the prostate: Biopsy and conservative therapy. *J Urol* 1972; 108:897–900.
29. Bartsch G, Egender G, Hubscher H, Rohr H: Sonometrics of the prostate. *J Urol* 1982; 127:1119–1121.
30. Bartsch G, Dietze O, Hohlbrugger G, Marberger H, Mikuz G: Incidental carcinoma of the prostate—Grading and tumor volume in relation to survival rate. *World J Urol* 1983; 1:24–28.
31. Bartsch G, Hohlbrugger G, Mikuz G, Marberger H: Transurethral resection in prostatic carcinoma. A cause of accelerated metastatic growth. *World J Urol* 1983; 1:36–39.
32. Bauer DL, Garrison RW, McRoberts JW: The health and cost implications of routine excretory urography before transurethral prostatectomy. *J Urol* 1980; 123:386–389.
33. Beck PH, McAninch JW, Lewinsky B, Whitlock NW, Stutzman RE, Goebel JL: Vasoseminal vesiculography in staging adenocarcinoma of the prostate. *Urology* 1978; 11:239–242.
34. Becker LE, Harrin WR: Prostatic abscess: A diagnostic and therapeutic approach. *J Urol* 1964; 91:582–585.
35. Beisland HO, Laerum F: Transrectal ultrasonography before and after neodymium-YAG laser irradiation of localized prostatic carcinoma. *Eur Urol* 1986; 12:39–42.
36. Benoit G, Boccon-Gibod L, Steg A: Anatomical study of total cystoprostatectomy. *Eur Urol* 1985; 11:228–232.
37. Berry SJ, Coffey DS, Walsh PC, Ewing LL: The development of human benign prostatic hyperplasia with age. *J Urol* 1984; 132:474–479.
38. Bertermann H: The European experience: Use of transrectal ultrasound in the diagnosis and management of prostate cancer. In: *The Use of Transrectal Ultrasound in the Diagnosis and Mangement of Prostate Cancer* (F Lee, RD McLeary, Editors). Alan R. Liss, New York, 1987, pp. 177–194.
39. Billis A: Latent carcinoma and atypical lesions of prostate. An autopsy study. *Urology* 1986; 28:324–329.
40. Bissada NK, Finkbeiner AE, Redman JF: Accuracy of preoperative estimation of resection weight in transurethral prostatectomy. *J Urol* 1976; 116:201–202.
41. Blackard CE, Soucheray JA, Gleason DF: Prostatic needle biopsy with perineal extension of adenocarcinoma. *J Urol* 1971; 106:401–403.
42. Blacklock NJ: Anatomical factors in prostatitis. *Br J Urol* 1974; 46:47–54.
43. Blair A, Fraumeni JF Jr: Geographic patterns of prostate cancer in the United States. *J Natl Cancer Inst* 1978; 61:1379–1384.
44. Blasko J, Ragde H: Seattle experience with transperineal percutaneous radioisotope implantation for prostatic carcinoma utilizing transrectal ultrasound and template guidance. Presented at the Second International Symposium on Transrectal Ultrasound in the Diagnosis and Management of Prostate Cancer, Detroit, Michigan, September 21–22, 1987.
45. Blennerhassett JB, Vickery AL Jr: Carcinoma of the prostate gland. An anatomical study of tumor location. *Cancer* 1966; 19:980–984.
46. Blum MD, Bahnson RR, Lee C, Deschler TW, Grayhack JT: Estimation of canine prostatic size by *in vivo* ultrasound and volumetric measurement. *J Urol* 1985; 133:1082–1086.
47. Blute ML, Zincke H, Farrow GM: Long-term followup of young patients with Stage A adenocarcinoma of the prostate. *J Urol* 1986; 136:840–843.
48. Bocking A, Kiehn J, Heinzel-Wach M: Combined histologic grading of prostatic carcinoma. *Cancer* 1982; 50:288–294.
49. Boyce WH, Yeaman L: Ultrasonography in urologic practice; Benign diseases of the prostate gland. *J Urol* 1987; 137(4 Part 2):241A.
50. Brawer M, Chodak G: Prostate cancer detectable by ultrasound. *Diagn Imag Clin Med* 1987; 9:154–157.
51. Brawn PN, Ayala AG, von Eschenbach AC, Hussey DH, Johnson DE: Histologic grading study of prostate adenocarcinoma: The development of a new system and comparison with other methods—A preliminary study. *Cancer* 1982; 49:525–532.
52. Breslow N, Chan CW, Dhom G, Drury RAB, Franks LM, Gellei B, Lee YS, Lundberg S, Sparke B, Sternby NH, Tulinius H: Latent carcinoma of prostate at autopsy in seven areas. *Int J Cancer* 1977; 20:680–688.
53. Brooman PJC, Griffiths GJ, Roberts E, Peeling WB, Evans K: Per rectal ultrasound in the investigation of prostatic disease. *Clin Radiol* 1981; 32:669–676.
54. Buonocore E, Hesemann C, Pavlicek W, Montie JE: Clinical and *in vitro* magnetic resonance imaging of prostatic carcinoma. *AJR* 1984; 143:1267–1272.
55. Burkholder GV, Kaufman JJ: Local implantation of carcinoma of the prostate with percutaneous needle biopsy. *J Urol* 1966; 95:801–804.
56. Burks DD, Fleischer AC, Kulkarni MV, Lidell HT, Karl EM: Transrectal prostate sonography: Evaluation of sonographic features in benign and malignant lesions. *AJR* 1986; 146:1187–1191.
57. Buttyan R, Olsson CA: Androgen receptor assays in advanced prostatic cancer. *Urol Clin North Am* 1984; 11:311–317.
58. Byar DP: Survival of patients with incidentally found microscopic cancer of the prostate: Results of a clinical trial of conservative treatment. *J Urol* 1972; 108:908–913.

59. Cantrell BB, DeKlerk DP, Eggleston JC, Boitnott JK, Walsh PC: Pathological factors that influence prognosis in stage A prostatic cancer: The influence of extent versus grade. *J Urol* 1981; 125:516–520.
60. Carpentier PJ, Schroeder FH, Blom JHM: Transrectal ultrasonography in the followup of prostatic carcinoma patients. *J Urol* 1982; 128:742–746.
61. Carpentier PJ, Schroeder FH: Transrectal ultrasonography in the followup of prostatic carcinoma patients: A new prognostic parameter? *J Urol* 1984; 131:903–905.
62. Carpentier PJ, Schroeder FH, Schmitz PIM: Transrectal ultrasonometry of the prostate: The prognostic relevance of volume changes under endocrine management. *World J Urol* 1986; 4:159–162.
63. Cariou G, Vuong-Ngog P, Merran S, Le Duc A, Plainfosse MC: Correlations between radiography, ultrasonography, computed tomography and pathologic findings in prostatic disease. *Urology* 1985; 26:599–602.
64. Carroll PR, Leitner TC, Yen TSB, Watson RA, Williams RD: Incidental carcinoma of the prostate: Significance of staging transurethral resection. *J Urol* 1985; 133:811–814.
65. Carter SSC, Thin RN, Pryor JP, O'Donoghue EN: The use of transrectal ultrasound in the investigation of benign diseases of the prostate and seminal vesicles. *J Urol* 1987; 137(4 Part 2):367A.
66. Cascione CJ, Bartone FF, Hussain MB: Transabdominal ultrasound versus excretory urography in preoperative evaluation of patients with prostatism. *J Urol* 1987; 137:883–885.
67. Catalona WJ, Scott WW: Carcinoma of the prostate: A review. *J Urol* 1978; 119:1–8.
68. Catalona WJ, Menon M: New screening and diagnostic tests for prostate cancer and immunologic assessment. *Urology* (Suppl) 1981; 17:61–65.
69. Catalona WJ, Stein AJ: Staging errors in clinically localized prostatic cancer. *J Urol* 1982; 127:452–456.
70. Catalona WJ: Grading and staging of prostate cancer. *J Urol* 1982; 128:747–748.
71. Catalona WJ, Dresner SM: Nerve-sparing radical prostatectomy: Extraprostatic tumor extension and preservation of erectile function. *J Urol* 1985; 134:1149–1151.
72. Catalona WJ, Scott WW: Carcinoma of the prostate. In: *Campbell's Urology* 5th edition (PC Walsh, RF Gittes, AD Perlmutter, TA Stamey, Editors). W.B. Saunders, Philadelphia, 1986, pp. 1463–1534.
73. Chancellor MB, McHugh TA, Dorr RP, VanAppledorn CA: Transrectal prostate ultrasonography before transurethral prostatectomy, its value in screening for stage A cancer. *J Urol* 1987; 137(4 Part 2):241A.
74. Chodak GW, Schoenberg HW: Early detection of prostate cancer by routine screening. *JAMA* 1984; 252:3261–3264.
75. Chodak GW, Schoenberg HW: Problematic prostatic prediction. *JAMA* 1985; 254:1171–1172.
76. Chodak GW, Wald V, Parmer E, Watanabe H, Ohe H, Saitoh M: Comparison of digital examination and transrectal ultrasonography for the diagnosis of prostatic cancer. *J Urol* 1986; 135:951–954.
77. Chodak GW, Smith FL, Jensen C: Clinical assessment of transrectal ultrasonography for staging and diagnosis of prostate cancer. *J Urol* 1987; 137(4 Part 2):360A.
78. Chodak GW: The changing physical examination of prostate cancer: Correlation with transrectal ultrasound. Presented at the Second International Symposium on Transrectal Ultrasound in the Diagnosis and Management of Prostate Cancer, Detroit, Michigan, September 21–22, 1987.
79. Coffey DS, Isaacs JT: Prostate tumor biology and cell kinetics—Theory. *Urology* (Suppl) 1981; 17:40–53.
80. Coffey DS, Isaacs JT: Control of prostate growth. *Urology* 1981; 17:17–24.
81. Cohen JM, Resnick MI: The use of transrectal ultrasonography in the diagnosis of stage A prostatic carcinoma. *World J Urol* 1983; 1:12–14.
82. Cooner WH, Eggers GW, Lichtenstein P: Prostate cancer: New hope for early diagnosis. *Ala Med* 1987; 56:13–16.
83. Cordes M, Tunn UW, Neidl K, Haasner E: Prostatic cancer. Staging via transrectal prostatic sonography and computed tomography with histopathological correlation. *ROFO* 1987; 146:412–414.
84. Crawford ED, Haynes AL, Story MW, Borden TA: Prevention of urinary tract infection and sepsis following transrectal prostatic biopsy. *J Urol* 1982; 127:449–451.
85. Creaven PJ, Madajewicz S, Mittelman A: New potential treatment modalities for disseminated prostatic cancer. *Urol Clin North Am* 1984; 11:343–356.
86. Cruisinberry RA, Kramolowsky EV, Loening SA: Percutaneous transperineal placement of gold 198 seeds for treatment of carcinoma of the prostate. *Prostate* 1987; 11:59–67.
87. Culp OS, Meyer JJ: Radical prostatectomy in the treatment of prostatic cancer. *Cancer* 1973; 32:1113–1118.
88. Cutler SJ, Young JL Jr: *Natl Cancer Inst Monogr* 1975; 41.
89. Dahl DS, Wilson CS, Middleton RG, Bourne HH: Pelvic lymphadenectomy for staging localized prostatic cancer. *J Urol* 1974; 112:245–246.
90. Dahnert WF, Hamper UM, Walsh PC, Eggleston JC, Sanders RC: The echogenic focus in prostatic sonograms, with xeroradiographic and histopathologic correlation. *Radiology* 1986; 159:95–100.
91. Dahnert WF, Hamper UM, Eggleston JC, Walsh PC, Sanders RC: Prostatic evaluation by transrectal sonography with histopathologic correlation: The echopenic appearance of early carcinoma. *Radiology* 1986; 158:97–102.
92. Davidson M: Problematic prostatic prediction [Letter to the Editor]. *JAMA* 1985; 254:1173.
93. Davison P, Malament M: Urinary contamination as a result of transrectal biopsy of the prostate. *J Urol* 1971; 105:545–546.

94. deKernion JB, Lindner A: Chemotherapy of hormonally unresponsive prostatic carcinoma. *Urol Clin North Am* 1984; 11:319–326.
95. Denis LJ: Computed tomography versus ultrasonotomography. In: *Diagnostic Ultrasound in Urology and Nephrology* (H Watanabe, JH Holmes, HH Holm, BB Goldberg, Editors). Igaku-Shoin, New York, 1981, pp. 186–189.
96. Denis L, Braeckman J, Keuppens F: Ultrasonography and computed tomography in the staging of bladder and prostate cancers. In: *Progress and Controversies in Oncological Urology* (KH Kurth, FMJ Gebruyne, FH Schroeder, TAW Splinter, TDJ Wagener, Editors). Alan R. Liss, New York, 1984, pp. 3–21.
97. Denkhaus H, Dierkopf W, Grabbe E, Donn F: Comparative study of suprapubic sonography and computed tomography for staging of prostatic carcinoma. *Urol Radiol* 1983; 5:1–9.
98. Denkhaus H, Dierkopf W, Grabbe E, Donn F: Comparative study of suprapubic sonography and computed tomography for staging of prostatic carcinoma. *Radiology*, 1983; 149:904.
99. deVere White R, Deitch AD, Tomashefsky P, Olsson CA: Flow cytometry in prostatic adenocarcinoma. *World J Urol* 1983; 1:55–61.
100. Devonec M, Codas H, Provensal B, Chapelon JY, Dubernard JM, Cathignol D: Evaluation of endorectal ultrasonography in the diagnosis of prostatic cancer using a high-frequency sectorial intracavitary probe. *Ann Urol* 1987; 21:17–22.
101. Dhom G, Degro S: Therapy of prostatic cancer and histopathologic follow-up. *Prostate* 1982; 3:531–542.
102. Diamond DA, Berry SJ, Jewett HJ, Eggleston JC, Coffey DS: A new method to assess metastatic potential of human prostate cancer: Relative nuclear roundness. *J Urol* 1982; 128:729–734.
103. Dobbs HJ, Husband JE: The role of CT in the staging and radiotherapy planning of prostatic tumours. *Br J Radiol* 1985; 58:429–436.
104. Donker PJ, Kakiailatu F: Preoperative evaluation of patients with bladder outlet obstruction with particular regard to excretory urography. *J Urol* 1978; 120:685–686.
105. Donohue RE, Fauver HE, Whitesel JA, Pfister RR: Staging prostatic cancer: A different distribution. *J Urol* 1979; 122:327–329.
106. Donohue RE, Mani JH, Whitesel JA, Mohr S, Scanavino D, Augspurger RR, Biber RJ, Fauver HE, Wettlaufer JN, Pfister RR: Pelvic lymph node dissection. Guide to patient management in clinically locally confined adenocarcinoma of the prostate. *Urology* 1982; 20:559–565.
107. Dowlen LW Jr, Block NL, Politano VA: Complications of transrectal biopsy of the prostate. *South Med J* 1974; 67:1453–1456.
108. Ducassou JD, Daou N, Hoarau T, Serment G, Hermanowicz M, Ducassou J: L'echographie prostatique par voie trans-rectale. Rapport preliminaire a propos de notre experience portant sur plus de 400 cas. *J Urol (Paris)* 1986; 92:249–270.
109. Dunn JE Jr: Cancer epidemiology in populations of the United States with emphasis on Hawaii and California—and Japan. *Cancer Res* 1975; 35:3240–3245.
110. Eggleston JC, Walsh PC: Radical prostatectomy with preservation of sexual function: Pathological findings in the first 100 cases. *J Urol* 1985; 134:1146–1148.
111. Elder JS, Catalona WJ: Management of newly diagnosed metastatic carcinoma of the prostate. *Urol Clin North Am* 1984; 11:283–295.
112. Elder JS, Scott WW, Nyberg LM: Overview of past and current philosophy of prostatic cancer. *Prostate* 1980; 1:287–301.
113. Elkon D, Kim JA, Constable WC: Anatomic localization of radioactive gold seeds of the prostate by computer-aided tomography. *Comput Tomogr* 1981; 5:89–93.
114. Emory TH, Reinke DB, Hill AL, Lange PH: Use of CT to reduce understaging in prostatic cancer: Comparison with conventional staging techniques. *AJR* 1983; 141:351–354.
115. Emtage JB, Perez-Marrero R: Extension of carcinoma of prostate along perineal needle biopsy tract. *Urology* 1986; 27:548–549.
116. Epstein JI, Paull G, Eggleston JC, Walsh PC: Prognosis of untreated stage A1 prostatic carcinoma: A study of 94 cases with extended followup. *J Urol* 1986; 136:837–839.
117. Epstein NA, Fatti LP: Prostatic carcinoma: Some morphological features affecting prognosis. *Cancer* 1976; 37:2455–2465.
118. Ernster VL, Winkelstein W Jr, Selvin S, Brown SM, Sacks ST, Austin DF, Mandel SA, Bertolli TA: Race, socioeconomic status, and prostatic cancers. *Cancer Treat Rep* 1977; 61:187–191.
119. Esposti PL: Cytologic malignancy grading of prostatic carcinoma by transrectal aspiration biopsy. *Scand J Urol Nephrol* 1971; 5:199–209.
120. Fair WR, Heston WDW, Kadmon D, Crane DB, Catalona WJ, Ladenson JH, McDonald JM, Noll BW, Harvey G: Prostatic cancer, acid phosphatase, creatine kinase-BB and race: A prospective study. *J Urol* 1982; 128:735–738.
121. Fair WR, Kadmon D: Carcinoma of the prostate: Diagnosis and staging. *World J Urol* 1983; 3–11.
122. Falkowski WS, O'Conner VJ Jr: Long-term survivor of prostatic carcinoma with lung metastasis. *J Urol* 1981; 125:260–262.
123. Fellows GJ, Cannell LB, Ravichandran G: Transrectal ultrasonography compared with voiding cystourethrography after spinal cord injury. *Br J Urol* 1987; 59:218–221.

124. Flanders WD: Review: Prostate cancer epidemiology. *Prostate* 1984; 5:621–629.
125. Flanigan RC, Mohler JL, King CT, Atwell JR, Umer MA, Loh FK, McRoberts JW: Preoperative lymph node evaluation in prostatic cancer patients who are surgical candidates: The role of lymphangiography and computerized tomography scanning with directed fine needle aspiration. *J Urol* 1985; 134:84–87.
126. Flocks RH, Culp D, Porto R: Lymphatic spread from prostatic cancer. *J Urol* 1959; 81:194–196.
127. Flocks RH, Culp DA, Elkins HB: Present status of radioactive gold therapy in management of prostatic cancer. *J Urol* 1959; 81:178–184.
128. Fornage BD, Touche DH, Deglaire M, Faroux MJC, Simatos A: Real-time ultrasound-guided prostatic biopsy using a new transrectal linear-array probe. *Radiology* 1983; 146:547–548.
129. Fornage BD: Normal US anatomy of the prostate. *Ultrasound Med Biol* 1986; 12:1011–1021.
130. Foti AG, Cooper JF, Herschman H, Malvaez RR: Detection of prostatic cancer by solid-phase radioimmunoassay of serum prostatic acid phosphatase. *N Engl J Med* 1977; 297:1357–1361.
131. Franks LM: Latent carcinoma of the prostate. *J Pathol Bacteriol* 1954; 68:603–616.
132. Franks LM: Etiology, epidemiology, and pathology of prostatic cancer. *Cancer* 1973; 32:1092–1095.
133. Franks LM: Benign prostatic hyperplasia: Gross and microscopic anatomy. In: *Benign Prostatic Hyperplasia* (JT Grayhack, WJD Wilson, MJ Scherbenske, Editors), NIAMDD Workshop Proceedings, February 20–21, 1975. DHEW Publication Number (NIH) 76-1113, pp. 63–89. Washington, D.C., U.S. Government Printing Office, 1976.
134. Freiha FS, Bagshaw MA: Carcinoma of the prostate: Results of post-irradiation biopsy. *Prostate* 1984; 5:19–25.
135. Frentzel-Beyme B, Ledwa D: Echomorphology of the prostate. *Ultraschall Med* 1986; 7:7–16.
136. Friedland GW, Perkash I: Neuromuscular dysfunction of the bladder and urethra. *Semin Roentgenol* 1983; 18:255–266.
137. Fritzsche PJ, Axford PD, Ching VC, Rosenquist RW, Moore RJ: Correlation of transrectal sonographic findings in patients with suspected and unsuspected prostatic disease. *J Urol* 1983; 130:272–274.
138. Fujino A, Scardino PT: Transrectal ultrasonography for prostatic cancer: Its value in staging and monitoring the response to radiotherapy and chemotherapy. *J Urol* 1985; 133:806–810.
139. Fujino A, Scardino PT: Transrectal ultrasonography for prostatic cancer. II. The response of the prostate to definitive radiotherapy. *Cancer* 1986; 57:935–940.
140. Gaeta JF, Asirwatham JE, Miller G, Murphy GP: Histologic grading of primary prostatic cancer: A new approach to an old problem. *J Urol* 1980; 123:689–693.
141. Gaeta JF: Glandular profiles and cellular patterns in prostatic cancer grading. National prostatic cancer project system. *Urology* (Suppl) 1981; 17:33–37.
142. Gammelgaard J, Holm HH: Transurethral and transrectal ultrasonic scanning in urology. *J Urol* 1980; 124:863–868.
143. Gammelgaard J, Holm HH: Transurethral scanning of the prostate. In: *Diagnostic Ultrasound in Urology and Nephrology* (H Watanabe, JH Holmes, HH Holm, BB Goldberg, Editors). Igaku-Shoin, New York, 1981, pp. 153–156.
144. Ganem EJ: The prognostic significance of an elevated serum acid phosphatase level in advanced prostatic carcinoma. *J Urol* 1956; 76:179–181.
145. Gardiner RA, Fitzpatrick JM, Constable AR, Cranage RW, O'Donoghue EPN, Wickham JEA: Improved techniques in radionuclide imaging of prostatic lymph nodes. *Br J Urol* 1979; 51:561–564.
146. Garrett PG, Herman JG, Rawlings GA, Hawkins NV, Gospodarowicz MK, Keen CW, Rider WD: Radical external beam radiation therapy for prostate carcinoma. *J Can Assoc Radiol* 1984; 35:139–143.
147. Garrett WJ: The octoson in nephrology. In: *Diagnostic Ultrasound in Urology and Nephrology* (H Watanabe, JH Holmes, HH Holm, BB Goldberg, Editors). Igaku-Shoin, New York, 1981, pp. 55–65.
148. Ghanadian R, Puah CM: The clinical significance of steroid hormone measurements in the management of patients with prostatic cancer. *World J Urol* 1983; 1:49–54.
149. Gittes RF, McCullough DL: Occult carcinoma of the prostate: An oversight of immune surveillance—A working hypothesis. *J Urol* 1974; 112:241–244.
150. Gittes RF: Prostate-specific antigen [Editorial]. *N Engl J Med* 1987; 317:954–955.
151. Gleason DF, Mellinger GT: Prediction of prognosis for prostatic adenocarcinoma by combined histological grading and clinical staging. *J Urol* 1974; 111:58–64.
152. Gleason DF and The Veterans Administration Cooperative Urological Research Group: *Histologic Grading and Clinical Staging of Prostatic Carcinoma*. Lea & Febiger, Philadelphia, 1977.
153. Goldberg BB, Pollack HM: Ultrasonic aspiration biopsy transducer. *Radiology* 1973; 108:667–671.
154. Goldberg BB, Pollack HM: Ultrasonic aspiration transducer. *Radiology* 1972; 102:187–189.
155. Goldenberg DM, DeLand FH: Clinical studies of prostatic cancer imaging with radiolabeled antibodies against prostatic acid phosphatase. *Urol Clin North Am* 1984; 11:277–281.
156. Goldsmith MF: Modifications in prostate cancer operation preserve potency. *JAMA* 1983; 250:2897–2899.
157. Goldstein A: *Quality Assurance in Diagnostic Ultrasound: A Manual for the Clinical User*. American Institute of Ultrasound in Medicine, New York, 1980.
158. Goldstein A: Pertinent physics of an optimal examination. *The Use of Transrectal Ultrasound in the Diagnosis and Management of Prostate Cancer* (F Lee, RD McLeary, Editors). Alan R. Liss, New York, 1987, pp. 31–48.

159. Golimbu M, Morales P, Al-Askari S, Shulman Y: CAT scanning in staging of prostatic cancer. *Urology* 1981; 18:305–308.
160. Graversen PH, Gasser TC, Madsen PO, Corle DK: Early prostatic cancer: Radical prostatectomy versus placebo. *J Urol* 1987; 137(4 Part 2):364A.
161. Gray JM: Prostate gland: Anatomy, hyperplasia, cytologic atypia, adenocarcinoma, and tumor markers. *The Use of Transrectal Ultrasound in the Diagnosis and Management of Prostate Cancer* (F Lee, RD McLeary, Editors). Alan R. Liss, New York, 1987, pp. 15–30.
162. Gray J, Lee F: Transrectal ultrasound examination of prostate cancer with anatomic correlation. Presented at the Second International Symposium on Transrectal Ultrasound in the Diagnosis and Management of Prostate Cancer, Detroit, Michigan, September 21–22, 1987.
163. Grayhack JT, Bockrath JM: Diagnosis of carcinoma of prostate. *Urology* (Suppl) 1981; 17:54–60.
164. Grayhack JT, Assimos DG: Prognostic significance of tumor grade and stage in the patient with carcinoma of the prostate. *Prostate* 1983; 4:13–31.
165. Green N: Value of radiotherapy for adenocarcinoma of the prostate simulating primary rectal carcinoma. *J Urol* 1974; 112:247–248.
166. Green N, Bodner H, Broth E: Prostate cancer: Experience with definitive irradiation in the aged. *Urology* 1985; 25:228–232.
167. Greenberg M, Neiman HL, Brandt TD, Falkowski W, Carter M: Ultrasound of the prostate. Analysis of tissue texture and abnormalities. *Radiology* 1981; 141:757–762.
168. Greenberg M, Neimen HL, Vogelzang R, Falkowski W: Ultrasonographic features of prostatic carcinoma. *J Clin Ultrasound* 1982; 10:307–312.
169. Greenberg RN, Reilly PM, Luppen KL, Piercy S: Chronic prostatitis: Comments on infectious etiologies and antimicrobial treatment. *Prostate* 1985; 6:445–448.
170. Greenwald P, Kirmss V, Polan AK, Dick VS: Cancer of the prostate among men with benign prostatic hyperplasia. *J Natl Cancer Inst* 1974; 53:335–340.
171. Griffiths GJ, Clements R, Jones DR, Roberts EE, Peeling WB, Evans KT: The ultrasound appearances of prostatic cancer with histological correlation. *Clin Radiol* 1987; 38:219–227.
172. Griffiths GJ, Crooks AJR, Roberts EE, Evans KT, Buck AC, Thomas PJ: Ultrasonic appearances associated with prostatic inflammation: A preliminary study. *Clin Radiol* 1984; 35:343–345.
173. Grossman HB, Batata M, Hilaris B, Whitmore, WF Jr: ^{125}I implantation for carcinoma of prostate. Further follow-up of first 100 cases. *Urology* 1982; 20:591–598.
174. Grossman IC, Carpiniello V, Greenberg SH, Malloy TR, Wein AJ: Staging pelvic lymphadenectomy for carcinoma of the prostate: Review of 91 cases. *J Urol* 1980; 124:632–634.
175. Guileyardo JM, Sarma DP, Johnson WD, Akazaki K, Correa P: Incidental prostatic carcinoma: Tumor extent versus histologic grade. *Urology* 1982; 20:40–42.
176. Guinan P, Bush I, Ray V, Vieth R, Rao R, Bhatti R: The accuracy of the rectal examination in the diagnosis of prostate carcinoma. *N Engl J Med* 1980; 303:499–503.
177. Guinan P, Bhatti R, Ray P: An evaluation of prostate specific antigen in prostatic cancer. *J Urol* 1987; 137:686–689.
178. Hallemans E, Declereq G, Denis L: Transrectal ultrasono-tomography. *Eur Urol* 1977; 3:37–40.
179. Halpert B, Schmalhorst WR: Carcinoma of the prostate in patients 70 to 79 years old. *Cancer* 1966; 19:695–698.
180. Hamilton S, Fitzpatrick JM: Ultrasound diagnosis of a prostatic cyst causing acute urinary retention. *J Ultrasound Med* 1987; 6:385–387.
181. Hamper UM, Dahnert WF, Eggelston JC, Walsh PC, Sanders RC: Ultrasonography of prostatic carcinoma employing amplitude-enveloped (AM) and frequency-demodulated (FM) imaging. *J Ultrasound Med* 1986; 5:557–562.
182. Hara S, Yamaguchi A, Miyazaki Y: Monitoring of transurethral resection of the prostate. In: *Diagnostic Ultrasound in Urology and Nephrology* (H Watanabe, JH Holmes, HH Holm, BB Goldberg, Editors). Igaku-Shoin, New York, 1981, pp. 179–182.
183. Harada M, Mostofi FK, Corle DK, Byar DP, Trump BF: Preliminary studies of histologic prognosis in cancer of the prostate. *Cancer Treat Rep* 1977: 61:223–225.
184. Harada K, Igari D, Tanahashi Y: Gray scale transrectal ultrasonography of the prostate. *J Clin Ultrasound* 1979; 7:45–49.
185. Harada K, Tanahashi Y, Igari D, Numata I, Orikasa S: Clinical evaluation of inside echo patterns in gray scale prostatic echography. *J Urol* 1980; 124:216–220.
186. Harada K: Cystitis and other diseases. In: *Diagnostic Ultrasound in Urology and Nephrology* (H Watanabe, JH Holmes, HH Holm, BB Goldberg, Editors). Igaku-Shoin, New York, 1981, pp. 104–108.
187. Harada K: Prostatic calculi. In: *Diagnostic Ultrasound in Urology and Nephrology* (H Watanabe, JH Holmes, HH Holm, BB Goldberg, Editors). Igaku-Shoin, New York, 1981, pp. 171–174.
188. Harrison GSM: The prognosis of prostatic cancer in the younger man. *Br J Urol* 1983; 55:315–320.
189. Hastak SM, Gammelgaard J, Holm HH: Ultrasonically guided transperineal biopsy in the diagnosis of prostatic carcinoma. *J Urol* 1982; 128:69–71.

190. Hastak SM, Gammelgaard J, Holm HH: Transrectal ultrasonic volume determination of the prostate—A preoperative and postoperative study. *J Urol* 1982; 127:1115–1118.
191. Haugen OA, Harbitz TB: Prostatic weight in elderly men. An analysis in an autopsy series. *Acta Pathol Microbiol Scand [A]*, 1972; 80:769–777.
192. Heaney JA, Chang HC, Daly JJ, Prout GR Jr: Prognosis of clinically undiagnosed prostatic carcinoma and the influence of endocrine therapy. *J Urol* 1977; 118:283–287.
193. Heller JE: Prostatic acid phosphatase: Its current clinical status. *J Urol* 1987; 137:1091–1103.
194. Henneberry M, Carter MF, Neiman HL: Estimation of prostatic size by suprapubic ultrasonography. *J Urol* 1979; 121:615–616.
195. Hennig RC, Wilson SR: Suprapubic sonographic detection of prostate carcinoma. *J Clin Ultrasound* 1985; 13:101–106.
196. Herman SD, Friedman AC, Radecki PD, Caroline DF: Incidental prostatic carcinoma detected by MRI and diagnosed by MRI/CT-guided biopsy. *AJR* 1986; 146:351–352.
197. Herr HW: Interstitial irradiation for localized prostate cancer. *Semin Urol* 1983; 1:222–228.
198. Hoekstra WJ, Schroeder FH: The role of lymphangiography in the staging of prostatic cancer. *Prostate* 1981; 2:433–440.
199. Holm HH: Instrumentation and techniques. In: *Diagnostic Ultrasound in Urology and Nephrology* (H Watanabe, JH Holmes, HH Holm, BB Goldberg, Editors). Igaku-Shoin, New York, 1981, pp. 25–31.
200. Holm HH, Gammelgaard J: Transurethral scanning. In: *Diagnostic Ultrasound in Urology and Nephrology* (H Watanabe, JH Holmes, HH Holm, BB Goldberg, Editors). Igaku-Shoin, New York, 1981, pp. 84–89.
201. Holm HH: Ultrasonically guided puncture. Central canal transducer. In: *Diagnostic Ultrasound in Urology and Nephrology* (H Watanabe, JH Holmes, HH Holm, BB Goldberg, Editors). Igaku-Shoin, New York, 1981, pp. 233–243.
202. Holm HH, Gammelgaard J: Ultrasonically guided precise needle placement in the prostate and the seminal vesicles. *J Urol* 1981; 125:385–387.
203. Holm HH, Juul N, Pedersen JF, Hansen H, Stroyer I: Transperineal ^{125}iodine seed implantation in prostatic cancer guided by transrectal ultrasonography. *J Urol* 1983; 130:283–286.
204. Holm HH, Juul N, Torp-Pederson S, Rasmussen F, Laursen F, Bak M: Ultrasonographic guided ^{125}I-seed in prostate cancer. Presented at the 1st Danish Symposium on Uroradiology, September 7–10, 1987, Copenhagen, Denmark.
205. Holm HH, Gammelgaard J: Ultrasonically guided precise needle placement in the prostate and seminal vesicles. *Radiology* 1981; 141:284.
206. Holmes JH: Early applications in ultrasound in study of kidney and bladder. In: *Diagnostic Ultrasound in Nephrology* (H Watanabe, JH Holmes, HH Holm, BB Goldberg, Editors). Igaku-Shoin, New York, 1981, pp. 1–10.
207. Holmes JH: Instrumentation and techniques. In: *Diagnostic Ultrasound in Urology and Nephrology* (H Watanabe, JH Holmes, HH Holm, BB Goldberg, Editors). Igaku-Shoin, New York, 1981, pp. 75–84.
208. Huben R, Natarajan N, Pontes E, Mettlin C, Smart CR, Murphy GP: Carcinoma of prostate in men less than fifty years old. Data from American College of Surgeons' National Survey. *Urology* 1982; 20:585–588.
209. Huben RP, Schellhammer PF: The role of routine followup bone scans after definitive therapy of localized prostatic cancer. *J Urol* 1982; 128:510–512.
210. Huben RP, Murphy GP: Prostate cancer: An update. *CA* 1986; 36:274–292.
211. Huben RP, Murphy GP: Transrectal ultrasonography of the prostate and prostate cancer—An update. *Appl Pathol* 1985; 3:198–205.
212. Huben RP: The U.S.A. experience: Diagnosis and follow-up of prostate malignancy by transrectal ultrasound. *The Use of Transrectal Ultrasound in the Diagnosis and Management of Prostate Cancer* (F Lee, RD McLeary, Editors). Alan R. Liss, 1987, pp. 153–160.
213. Hudson PB, Finkle AL, Hopkins JA, Sproul EE, Purdy Stout AP: Prostatic cancer. XI. Early prostatic cancer diagnosed by arbitrary open perineal biopsy among 300 unselected patients. *Cancer* 1954; 7:690–703.
214. Hussey M: *Basic Physics and Technology of Medical Diagnostic Ultrasound*. Elsevier, New York, 1985.
215. Hutchison GB: Incidence and etiology of prostate cancer. *Urology* (Suppl) 1981; 17:4–10.
216. Ishibe T, Usui T, Nihira H: Prognostic usefulness of serum acid phosphatase levels in carcinoma of the prostate. *J Urol* 1974; 112:237–240.
217. Jaeger N, Radeke HW, Adolphs HD: Die pathologische harnblase im sonographischen bild. *Ultraschall Med* 1983; 4:98–105.
218. Jakobsen H, Juul N: Influence of vasectomy on the volume of the non-hyperplastic prostate in men. *Int J Androl* 1985; 8:13–20.
219. Jensen M, Bruskewitz RC, Iversen P, Madsen PO: Significance of prostatic weight in prostatism. *Urol Int* 1983; 38:173–178.
220. Jewett HJ: The present status of radical prostatectomy for stages A and B prostatic cancer. *Urol Clin North Am* 1975; 2:105–124.
221. Johnson DE, von Eschenbach AC: Roles of lymphangiography and pelvic lymphadenectomy in staging prostate cancer. *Urology* (Suppl) 1981; 17:66–71.

222. Kadow C, Gingell JC, Penry JB: Prostatic ultrasonography: A useful technique? *Br J Urol* 1985; 57:440–443.
223. Kaplan WD, Whitmore WF, Gittes RF: Visualization of canine and human prostatic lymph nodes following intraprostatic injection of technetium-99m-antimony sulfide colloid. *Invest Radiol* 1980; 15:34–38.
224. Kaufman JJ, Rosenthal M, Goodwin WE: Methods of diagnosis of carcinoma of the prostate: A comparison of clinical impression, prostatic smear, needle biopsy, open perineal biopsy and transurethral biopsy. *J Urol* 1954; 72:450–465.
225. Kaufman JJ, Ljung BM, Walther P, Waisman J: Aspiration biopsy of prostate. *Urology* 1982; 19:587–591.
226. Killian CS, Yang N, Emrich LJ, Vargas FP, Kuriyama M, Wang MC, Slack NH, Papsidero LD, Murphy GP, Chu TM and the Investigators of the National Prostatic Cancer Project: Prognostic importance of prostate-specific antigen for monitoring patients with stages B2 to D1 prostate cancer. *Cancer Res* 1985; 45:886–891.
227. Killian CS, Emrich LJ, Vargas FP, Yang N, Wang MC, Priore RL, Murphy GP, Chu TM: Relative reliability of five serially measured markers for prognosis of progression in prostate cancer. *J Natl Cancer Inst* 1986; 76:179–185.
228. Kim RY, Brascho DJ, Wilson EE: Use of ultrasound scan in prostatic I-125 implantation. *Int J Radiat Oncol Biol Phys* 1984; 10:1971–1973.
229. Kimura A, Nakamura S, Niizuma M, Hoshino T, Niijima T, Ohashi Y, Eng D, Higuchi T: Quantitative analysis of ultrasonogram of the prostate. *J Clin Ultrasound* 1986; 14:501–507.
230. King WW, Wilkiemeyer RM, Boyce WH, McKinney WM: Current status of prostatic echography. *JAMA* 1973; 226:444–447.
231. Kirk D, Hinton CE, Shaldon C: Transitional cell carcinoma of the prostate. *Br J Urol* 1979; 51:575–578.
232. Kirk D: Trial and tribulations in prostatic cancer. *Br J Urol* 1987; 59:375–379.
233. Klein LA: Prostatic carcinoma. *N Engl J Med* 1979; 300:824–833.
234. Klimas R, Bennett B, Gardner WA Jr: Prostatic calculi: A review. *Prostate* 1985; 7:91–96.
235. Kohnen PW, Drach GW: Patterns of inflammation in prostatic hyperplasia: A histologic and bacteriologic study. *J Urol* 1979; 121:755–760.
236. Kojima M, Watanabe H, Ohe H, Miyashita H, Inaba T: Kinetic evaluation of the effect of LHRH analog on prostatic cancer using transrectal ultrasonotomography. *Prostate* 1987; 10:11–17.
237. Komine Y, Kimura A, Niizuma M, Nakamura S, Kawabe K, Niijima T: Transurethral ultrasonotomography of the prostate. *Prostate* (Suppl) 1981; 1:53–57.
238. Komine Y, Kimura A, Niizuma M: Transurethral ultrasonotomography of the prostate. *Radiology* 1982; 144:217.
239. Koss LG, Woyke S, Schreiber K, Kohlberg W, Freed SZ: Thin needle aspiration biopsy of the prostate. *Urol Clin North Am* 1984; 11:237–251.
240. Kossoff G: Technical considerations and potential developments in diagnostic ultrasound in nephrology. In: *Diagnostic Ultrasound in Urology and Nephrology* (H Watanabe, JH Holmes, HH Holm, BB Goldberg, Editors). Igaku-Shoin, New York, 1981, pp. 16–21.
241. Kratochwil A: The transplanted kidney. In: *Diagnostic Ultrasound in Urology and Nephrology* (H Watanabe, JH Holmes, HH Holm, BB Goldberg, Editors). Igaku-Shoin, New York, 1981, pp. 49–55.
242. Kratochwil A: Demonstration of the prostate by rectal and transabdominal scanning. In: *Diagnostic Ultrasound in Urology and Nephrology* (H Watanabe, JH Holmes, HH Holm, BB Goldberg, Editors). Igaku-Shoin, New York, 1981, pp. 147–153.
243. Kremkau FW: *Diagnostic Ultrasound Physical Principles and Exercises*, 2nd edition. Grune and Stratton, New York, 1984.
244. Kroes R, Beems RB, Bosland MC, Bunnik GSJ, Sinkeldam EJ: Nutritional factors in lung, colon, and prostate carcinogenesis in animal models. *Fed Proc* 1986; 45:136–141.
245. Kumasaka GH: Diagnostic considerations in transrectal ultrasonic imaging of the prostate gland. *The Use of Transrectal Ultrasound in the Diagnosis and Management of Prostate Cancer* (F Lee, RD McLeary, Editors). Alan R. Liss, New York, 1987, pp. 57–72.
246. Kumasaka GH, Lee F, McLeary RD, Borlaza GS, Littrup PJ, Gray J, Davis R: Transrectal ultrasound of normal and benign hypertrophy of the prostate and differential diagnosis of hypoechoic lesions of the prostate [Abstract]. *Radiology* 1987; 165(P):216.
247. Kuriyama M, Wang MC, Lee CL, Papsidero LD, Killian CS, Inaji H, Slack NH, Nishiura T, Murphy GP, Chu TM: Use of human prostate-specific antigen in monitoring prostate cancer. *Cancer Res* 1981; 41:3874–3876.
248. Kuriyama M, Wang MC, Lee CL, Killian CS, Papsidero LD, Inaji H, Loor RM, Lin MF, Nishiura T, Slack NH, Murphy GP, Chu TM: Multiple marker evaluation in human prostate cancer with the use of tissue-specific antigens. *J Natl Cancer Inst* 1982; 68:99–105.
249. Leach GE, Cooper JF, Kagan AR, Snyder R, Forsythe A: Radiotherapy for prostatic carcinoma: Post-irradiation prostatic biopsy and recurrence patterns with long-term followup. *J Urol* 1982; 128:505–509.
250. LeDuc IE: The anatomy of the prostate and the pathology of early benign hypertrophy. *J Urol* 1939; 42:1217–1241.

251. Lee DJ, Leibel S, Shiels R, Sanders R, Siegelman S, Order S: The value of ultrasonic imaging and CT scanning in planning the radiotherapy for prostate carcinoma. *Cancer* 1980; 45:724–727.
252. Lee F, Gray JM, McLeary RD, Meadows TR, Kumasaka GH, Borlaza GS, Straub WH, Lee F Jr, Solomon MH, McHugh TA, Wolf RM: Transrectal ultrasound in the diagnosis of prostate cancer: Location, echogenicity, histopathology, and staging. *Prostate* 1985; 7:117–129.
253. Lee F, Gray JM, McLeary RD, Lee F Jr, McHugh TA, Solomon MH, Kumasaka GH, Straub WH, Borlaza GS, Murphy GP: Prostatic evaluation by transrectal sonography: Criteria for diagnosis of early carcinoma. *Radiology* 1986; 158:91–95.
254. Lee F, Littrup PJ, McLeary RD, Kumusaka GH, Borlaza GS, McHugh TA, Soiderer MH, Roi LD: Needle aspiration and core biopsy of prostate cancer: Comparative evaluation with biplanar transrectal US guidance. *Radiology* 1987; 163:515–520.
255. Lee F, Littrup PJ, Kumasaka GH, Borlaza GS, McLeary RD: The use of transrectal ultrasound in the diagnosis, guided biopsy, staging and screening of prostate cancer. *RadioGraphics* 1987; 7:627–644.
256. Lee F, Littrup PJ, McLeary RD, Kumasaka GH, Borlaza GS, McHugh TA, Soiderer MH, Roi LD: Transrectal ultrasound: Diagnosis of prostate cancer by a new biplane ultrasound guided biopsy technique. Comparison of thin needle cytology and histology with large core biopsy. *J Urol* 1987; 137(4 Part 2):354A.
257. Lee F, McLeary RD: Ultrasound guided biopsy techniques: Transperineal and transrectal. Presented at the Second International Symposium on Transrectal Ultrasound in the Diagnosis and Management of Prostate Cancer, Detroit, Michigan, September 21–22, 1987.
258. Lee F, Meiselman L, Torp-Pedersen S: The development of ultrasound guided iodine-125 therapy—The Copenhagen–Ann Arbor Experience. Presented at the Second International Symposium on Transrectal Ultrasound in the Diagnosis and Management of Prostate Cancer, Detroit, Michigan, September 21–22, 1987.
259. Lee F: Transrectal ultrasound in the diagnosis, staging, guided needle biopsy, and screening for prostate cancer. *The Use of Transrectal Ultrasound in the Diagnosis and Management of Prostate Cancer* (F Lee, RD McLeary, Editors). Alan R. Liss, New York, 1987, pp. 73–110.
260. Lee F, Littrup P, Kumasaka GH, Borlaza GS, McLeary RD, Torp-Pedersen S: Transrectal ultrasound of prostate cancer utilizing transrectal guidance and an automatic biopsy system [Abstract]. *Radiology* 1987; 165(P):432.
261. Lee F, Littrup PJ, Torp-Pedersen S, McLeary RD, Kumasaka GH, Borlaza GS: Transrectal ultrasound of prostate cancer with use of transrectal guidance and an automatic biopsy system [Abstract]. *Radiology* 1987; 165(P):215.
262. Lee F Jr, Lee F, Solomon MH, Straub WH, McLeary RD: Sonographic demonstration of prostatic abscess. *J Ultrasound Med.* 1986; 5:101–102.
263. Lee MS, Kurup P, Chung-Bin A, Zusag T, Hendrickson FR: Treatment planning with CAT scanning for prostatic carcinoma. *Ill Med J* 1981; 160:429–431.
264. Lee SB, Lee F, Solomon MH, McLeary RD, Kumasake GH, Straub WH: Seminal vesicle abscess diagnosis by transrectal ultrasound. *J Clin Ultrasound* 1986; 14:546–549.
265. Legge DA, Good CA, Ludwig J: Roentgenologic features of pulmonary carcinomatosis from carcinoma of the prostate. *AJR* 1971; 111:360–364.
266. Leissner KH, Tisell LE The weight of the human prostate. *Scand J Urol Nephrol* 1979; 13:137–142.
267. Lepor H, Ross A, Walsh PC: The influence of hormonal therapy on survival of men with advanced prostatic cancer. *J Urol* 1982; 128:335–340.
268. Lerner RM, Rubens D: Distal ureteral calculi: Diagnosis by transrectal sonography. *AJR* 1986; 147:1189–1191.
269. Lerski RA, Barnett E, Morley P: Ultrasound equipment for intra-rectal imaging of the prostate. *Br J Radiol* 1979; 52:225–226.
270. Leung FW, Casciato DA: Carcinoma of prostate presenting as symptomatic abdominal mass. *Urology* 1982; 20:78–79.
271. Levine MS, Arger PH, Coleman BG, Mulhern CB Jr, Pollack HM, Wein AJ: Detecting lymphatic metastases from prostatic carcinoma: Superiority of CT. *AJR* 1981; 137:207–211.
272. Lidell HT, McDougal WS, Burks DD, Fleischer AC: Ultrasound versus digitally directed prostatic needle biopsy. *J Urol* 1986; 135:716–718.
273. Lieskovsky G, Skinner DG, Weisenburger T: Pelvic lymphadenectomy in the management of carcinoma of the prostate. *J Urol* 1980; 124:635–638.
274. Lilienfeld RM, Berman M, Khedkar M, Sporer A: Comparative evaluation of intravenous urogram and ultrasound in prostatism. *Urology* 1985; 26:310–312.
275. Lin BP, Davies WR, Hormata PA: Prostatic aspiration cytology. *Pathology* 1979; 11:607–614.
276. Lindell MM, Doubleday LC, von Eschenbach AC, Libshitz HI: Mediastinal metastases from prostatic carcinoma. *J Urol* 1982; 128:331–334.
277. Ling D, Lee JKT, Heiken JP, Balfe DM, Glazer HS, McClennan BL: Prostatic carcinoma and benign prostatic hyperplasia: Inability of MR imaging to distinguish between the two diseases. *Radiology* 1986; 158:103–107.
278. Liskow A: External radiotherapy for localized prostate cancer. *Semin Urol* 1983; 1:217–221.

279. Littrup PJ: The development of a three dimensional prostate model. *The Use of Transrectal Ultrasound in the Diagnosis and Management of Prostate Cancer* (F Lee, RD McLeary, Editors). Alan R. Liss, New York, 1987, pp. 213–218.
280. Littrup PJ, Lee F, Wu D, Lee A, McLeary RD, Kumasaka GH: Transrectal ultrasound of seminal vesicle and ejaculatory duct pathology: Clinical correlations [Abstract]. *Radiology* 1987; 165(P):216.
281. Ljung BM: Fine-needle aspiration biopsy of the prostate gland: Technique and review of the literature. *Semin Urol* 1985; 3:18–26.
282. Ljung BM, Cherrie R, Kaufman JJ: Fine needle aspiration biopsy of the prostate gland: A study of 103 cases with histologic followup. *J Urol* 1986; 135:955–958.
283. Loening S, Lubaroff D: Cryosurgery and immunotherapy for prostatic cancer. *Urol Clin North Am* 1984; 11:327–336.
284. Loening SA, Rosenberg SJ: Percutaneous placement of radioactive gold seeds in localized prostatic carcinoma. *Urology* 1987; 29:250–252.
285. Loprinzi CL: Prostatic cancer. *South Med J* 1982; 75:193–196.
286. Luciani L, Piscioli F: Accuracy of transcutaneous aspiration biopsy in the definitive assessment of nodal involvement in prostatic carcinoma. *Br J Urol* 1983; 55:321–325.
287. MacIntyre RC, Peron SE, Madrazo B, Cerny JC: Ultrasound guided needle biopsy of the prostate gland. *J Urol* 1987; 137(4 Part 2);242A.
288. Martin DS: Prostatic ultrasonography: Applicability in a small hospital. *South Med J* 1986; 79:1261–1263.
289. Maier U, Czerwenka K, Neuhold N: The accuracy of transrectal aspiration biopsy of the prostate: An analysis of 452 cases. *Prostate* 1984; 5:147–151.
290. McDicken WN: *Diagnostic Ultrasonic Principles and Use of Instruments*, 2nd edition. John Wiley & Sons, New York, 1981.
291. McHugh T: The value of transrectal ultrasound for the urologist. Presented at the Second International Symposium on Transrectal Ultrasound in the Management of Prostate Cancer, Detroit, Michigan, September 21–22, 1987.
292. McLaughlin AP, Saltzstein SL, McCullough DL, Gittes RF: Prostatic carcinoma: Incidence and location of unsuspected lymphatic metastasis. *J Urol* 1976; 115:89–93.
293. McLeary RD: The performance of an optimal transrectal examination of the prostate. *The Use of Transrectal Ultrasound in the Diagnosis and Management of Prostate Cancer* (F Lee, RD McLeary, Editors). Alan R. Liss, New York, 1987, pp. 49–56.
294. McLeary RD: Future developments in ultrasonic imaging of the prostate. *The Use of Transrectal Ultrasound in the Diagnosis and Management of Prostate Cancer* (F Lee, RD McLeary, Editors). Alan R. Liss, New York, 1987, pp. 209–212.
295. McMillen SM, Wettlaufer JN: The role of repeat transurethral biopsy in stage A carcinoma of the prostate. *J Urol* 1976; 116:759–760.
296. McNeal JE: Morphogenesis of prostatic carcinoma. *Cancer* 1965; 18:1659–1666.
297. McNeal JE: Regional morphology and pathology of the prostate. *Am J Clin Pathol* 1968; 49:347–357.
298. McNeal JE: Origin and development of carcinoma in the prostate. *Cancer* 1969; 23:24–34.
299. McNeal JE: The prostate and prostatic urethra: A morphologic synthesis. *J Urol* 1972; 107:1008–1016.
300. McNeal JE: Origin and evolution of benign prostatic enlargement. *Invest Urol* 1978; 15:340–345.
301. McNeal JE: Anatomy of the prostate: An historical survey of divergent views. *Prostate* 1980; 1:3–13.
302. McNeal JE: The zonal anatomy of the prostate. *Prostate* 1981; 2:35–49.
303. McNeal JE: Normal and pathologic anatomy of prostate. *Urology* (Suppl) 1981; 17:11–16.
304. McNeal JE: The prostate gland. *1983 Monogr Urol* 1983; 4:3–33.
305. McNeal JE, Bostwick DG: Anatomy of the prostatic urethra. *JAMA* 1984; 251:890–891.
306. McNeal JE: Anatomy of the prostate and morphogenesis of BPH. *Prog Clin Biol Res* 1984; 145:27–53.
307. McNeal JE, Kindrachuk RA, Freiha FS, Bostwick DG, Redwine EA, Stamey TA: Patterns of progression in prostate cancer. *Lancet* 1986, 1:60–63.
308. McNeal JE: The window of curability. Presented at the Second International Symposium on Transurethral Ultrasound in the Diagnosis and Management of Prostate Cancer, Detroit, Michigan, September 21–22, 1987.
309. Meares ME: Prostatitis and related disorders. In: *Campbell's Urology*, 5th edition (PC Walsh, RF Gittes, AD Perlmutter, TA Stamey, Editors). W. B. Saunders, Philadelphia, 1986, pp. 868–887.
310. Melchoir J, Valk WL, Foret JD, Mebust WK: Transurethral prostatectomy: Computerized analysis of 2,223 consecutive cases. *J Urol* 1974; 112:634–642.
311. Melograna F, Oertel YC, Kwart AM: Prospective controlled assessment of fine needle prostatic aspiration. *Urology* 1982; 19:47–51.
312. Miller SS, Garvie WHH: The evaluation of prostate size by ultrasonic scanning: A preliminary report. *Br J Urol* 1973; 45:187–191.
313. Miyashita H, Watanabe H, Ohe H, Saitoh M, Oogama Y, Iijima S: Transrectal ultrasonotomography of the canine prostate. *Prostate* 1984; 5:453–457.
314. Miyazaki Y, Yamaguchi A, Hara S: The value of transrectal ultrasonography in preoperative assessment for transurethral prostatectomy. *J Urol* 1983; 129:48–50.

315. Mobley TL, Frank IN: Influence of tumor grade on survival and on serum acid phosphatase levels in metastatic carcinoma of the prostate. *J Urol* 1968; 99:321–323.
316. Moore GH, Lawshe B, Murphy J: Diagnosis of adenocarcinoma in transurethral resectates of the prostate gland. *Am J Surg Pathol* 1986; 10:165–169.
317. Moore RA: The evolution and involution of the prostate gland. *Am J Pathol* 1936; 12:599–624.
318. Moore RA: Benign hypertrophy and carcinoma of the prostate. *Surgery* 1944; 16:152–167.
319. Morgan CL, Calkins RF, Cavalcanti EJ: Computed tomography in the evaluation, staging, and therapy of carcinoma of the bladder and prostate. *Radiology* 1981; 140:751–761.
320. Mostofi FK: Grading of prostatic carcinoma. *Cancer Chemother Rep Part 1* 1975; 59:111–117.
321. Mostofi FK: Problems of grading carcinoma of prostate. *Semin Oncol* 1976; 3:161–169.
322. Mugharbil ZH, Childs C, Tannenbaum M, Schapira H: Carcinoma of prostate metastatic to penis. *Urology* 1985; 25:314–315.
323. Mukamel E, Hanna J, deKernion JB: Pitfalls in preoperative staging in prostate cancer. *Urology* 1987; 30:318–321.
324. Mundy AR: Urinary hydroxyproline excretion in carcinoma of the prostate. A comparison of 4 different modes of assessment and its role as a marker. *Br J Urol* 1979; 51:570–574.
325. Murnaghan GF, Tynan AP, Farnsworth RH, Harvey K: Chronic prostatitis—An Australian view. *Br J Urol* 1973; 45:55–59.
326. Murphy GP: Cancer of the prostate. *Cancer* 1973; 32:1089–1091.
327. Murphy GP: The diagnosis of prostatic cancer. *Cancer* 1976; 37:589–596.
328. Murphy GP, Gaeta JF: Tumors of the seminal vesicles. In: *Campbell's Urology* 5th edition (PC Walsh, RF Gittes, AD Perlmutter, TA Stamey, Editors), W. B. Saunders, Philadelphia, 1986, pp. 1612–1614.
329. Murphy GP, Natarajan N, Pontes JE, Schmitz RL, Smart CR, Schmidt JD, Mettlin C: The national survey of prostate cancer in the United States by the American College of Surgeons. *J Urol* 1982; 127:928–934.
330. Murphy GP, Gaeta J, Priore R: Pattern of care and follow-up of stages A1, B1 prostatic cancers from multicenter group, The National Prostatic Cancer Treatment Group (NPCTG). *Urology* 1987; 29:258–261.
331. Myrtle JF: Clinical utility of PSA in the management of prostate cancer. Presented at the Second International Symposium on Transrectal Ultrasound in the Diagnosis and Management of Prostate Cancer, Detroit, Michigan, September 21–22, 1987.
332. Nadji M, Tabei SZ, Castro A, Chu TM, Murphy GP, Wang MC, Morales AR: Prostatic-specific antigen: An immunohistologic marker for prostatic neoplasms. *Cancer* 1981; 48:1229–1232.
333. Naidich DP, Freedman MT, Bowerman JW, Siegelman SS: Ten section approach to computed tomography of the pelvis. *Skeletal Radiol* 1980; 5:213–217.
334. NCRP Report No. 74: Biological Effects of Ultrasound: Mechanisms and Clinical Implications. National Council on Radiation Protection and Measurements, 7910 Woodmont Ave., Bethesda, MD 20814, December 30, 1983.
335. Nemoto R, Harada M, Uchida K, Koiso K: Incidental carcinoma of the prostate in Japan: Histological characteristics and tumor size. *Appl. Pathol* 1985; 3:215–220.
336. Newman AJ Jr, Graham MA, Carlton CE Jr, Lieman S: Incidental carcinoma of the prostate at the time of transurethral resection: Importance of evaluating every chip. *J Urol* 1982; 128:948–950.
337. Niijima T, Nakamura S, Shiraishi T: Transurethral scanning and scanning via abdominal wall. In: *Diagnostic Ultrasound in Urology and Nephrology* (H Watanabe, JH Holmes, HH Holm, BB Goldberg, Editors). Igaku-Shoin, New York, 1981, pp. 96–104.
338. Obrant KO: Transurethral electroresection of prostatic adenoma. *Scan J Urol Nephrol* 1976; 10:26–32.
339. O'Flynn JD: The management of simple prostatic hyperplasia. *Br J Hosp Med* 1969; February:562–574.
340. Ohe H: Benign prostatic hypertrophy. Ultrasonic diagnosis of benign prostatic hypertrophy by means of transrectal ultrasonotomography. In: *Diagnostic Ultrasound in Urology and Nephrology* (H Watanabe, JH Holmes, HH Holm, BB Goldberg, Editors). Igaku-Shoin, New York, 1981, pp. 123–129.
341. Ohe H, Watanabe H, Saitoh M, Pontes JE, Murphy GP: Evaluation of effect of treatment for primary lesions of stage D2 prostatic cancer by means of transrectal ultrasonotomography. *Tohoku J Exp Med* 1986; 149:307–316.
342. Ohlsen H, Ekman P, Ringertz H: Assessment of prostatic size with computed tomography. *Acta Radiol Diagn (Stockh)* 1982; 23:219–223.
343. Ohnishi K, Watanabe H, Ohe H: Development of benign prostatic hypertrophy estimated from ultrasonic measurement with long-term follow up. *Tohoku J Exp Med* 1987; 151:51–56.
344. Onik G, Cobb C, Cohen J, Porterfield B: Ultrasound correlation of prostate cryosurgery [Abstract]. *Radiology* 1987; 165(P):216.
345. Osterling JE, Brendler CB, Epstein JI, Kimball AW Jr, Walsh PC: Correlation of clinical stage, serum prostatic acid phosphatase and preoperative gleason grade with final pathological stage in 275 patients with clinically localized adenocarcinoma of the prostate. *J Urol* 1987; 138:92–98.
346. Otto RJ, Klein BD, Bradley WG: Transrectal surface coil imaging of the prostate [Abstract]. *Radiology* 165(P):236, 1987.
347. Pang SMW, Keresteci AG, Rankin JT, Jewett MAS: Role of preoperative urography in benign prostatic hyperplasia. *Urology* 1979; 14:292–294.

348. Parfitt HE Jr, Smith JA Jr, Gliedman JB, Middleton RG: Accuracy of staging in A1 carcinoma of the prostate. *Cancer* 1983; 51:2346–2350.
349. Parra RO, Wolf RM, Huben RP: Echogenic patterns of local pelvis recurrences following radical pelvic surgery as evaluated by transrectal ultrasonography. *J Urol* 1987; 137(4 Part 2):243A.
350. Paul DB, Loening SA, Narayana AS, Culp DA: Morbidity from pelvic lymphadenectomy in staging carcinoma of the prostate. *J Urol* 1983; 129:1141–1144.
351. Paulson DF and the Uro-Oncology Research Group: Radical surgery for the management of prostatic carcinoma. *World J Urol* 1983; 1:29–35.
352. Paulson DF, Lin GH, Hinshaw W, Stephani S: Radical surgery versus radiotherapy for adenocarcinoma of the prostate. *J Urol* 1982; 128:502–504.
353. Paulson DF, Stone AR, Walther PJ, Tucker JA, Cox EB: Radical prostatectomy: Anatomical predictors of success or failure. *J Urol* 1986; 136:1041–1043.
354. Paulson DF, Cox EB: Does transurethral resection of the prostate promote metastatic disease? *J Urol* 1987; 138:90–91.
355. Peeling WB, Griffiths GJ, Evans KT, Roberts EE: Diagnosis and staging of prostatic cancer by transrectal ultrasonography. A preliminary study. *Br J Urol* 1979; 51:565–569.
356. Peeling WB, Griffiths GJ: Imaging of the prostate by ultrasound. *J Urol* 1984; 132:217–224.
357. Peeling WB, Griffiths GJ, Jones DR, Ryan PG, Roberts EE, Evans KT: The United Kingdom experience: Clinical trials for carcinoma of the prostate monitored by ultrasound. In: *The Use of Transrectal Ultrasound in the Diagnosis and Management of Prostate Cancer* (F Lee, RD McLeary, Editors). Alan R. Liss, New York, 1987, pp. 161–176.
358. Peneau M, Arbeille P, Pourcelot L, Pourcelot D, Plais JF, Fetissof F, Lanson Y: Tentative de classification de la semiologie echographique de la prostate par confrontation anatomo-ultrasonique de trente-quatre cas. *Ann Urol* 1985; 19:19–25.
359. Penkert A, Ristau U: Vergleich von prostatasonogrammen und den dazugehorigen histologischen grobflachenschnitten. *Ultraschall Med* 1986; 7:17–20.
360. Penkert A: Ultraschallgesteuerte biopsieverfahren der prostata. *Ultraschall Med* 1986; 7:21–24.
361. Perkash I, Friedland GW: Real-time gray-scale transrectal linear array ultrasonography in urodynamic evaluation. *Semin Urol* 1985; 3:49–59.
362. Pfau A: Prostatitis: A continuing enigma. *Urol Clin North Am* 1986; 13:695–715.
363. Pfitzenmaier, Malzacher F: A special device for the objective size measurement of the prostata via transrectal sonography. *Ultraschall Med* 1983; 4:13–14.
364. Pilepich MV, Perez CA, Prasad S: Computed tomography in definitive radiotherapy of prostatic carcinoma. *Int J Radiat Oncol Biol Phys* 1980; 6:923–926.
365. Pilepich MV, Perez CA, Bauer W: Prognostic parameters in radiotherapeutic management of localized carcinoma of the prostate. *J Urol* 1980; 124:485–487.
366. Pilepich MV, Bagshaw MA, Asbell SO, Hanks GE, Krall JM, Emami BN, Bard RH: Radical prostatectomy or radiotherapy in carcinoma of prostate. The dilemma continues. *Urology* 1987; 30:18–21.
367. Pinck BD, Corrigan MJ, Jasper P: Pre-prostatectomy excretory urography: Does it merit the expense? *J Urol* 1980; 123:390–391.
368. Pollen JJ: The role of radiography, computed tomography and bone scanning in prostatic cancer. *Prostate* 1980; 1:251–258.
369. Pollen JJ: Bone scanning in prostatic cancer. *Urology* (Suppl) 1981; 17:31–32.
370. Pontes JE: New assays for prostatic acid phosphatase and alkaline phosphatase isoenzymes. *Urology* (Suppl) 1981; 17:38–39.
371. Pontes JE, Chu TM, Slack N, Karr J, Murphy GP: Serum prostatic antigen measurement in localized prostatic cancer: Correlation with clinical course. *J Urol* 1982; 128:1216–1218.
372. Pontes JE, Eisenkraft S, Watanabe H, Ohe H, Saitoh M, Murphy GP: Preoperative evaluation of localized prostatic carcinoma by transrectal ultrasonography. *J Urol* 1985; 134:289–291.
373. Poon PY, McCallum RW, Henkelman MM, Bronskill MJ, Sutcliffe SB, Jewett MAS, Rider WD, Bruce AW: Magnetic resonance imaging of the prostate. *Radiology* 1985; 154:143–149.
374. Porena M, Vespasiani G, Virgili G, Lombi R, Mearini E, Rosi P, Micali F: Real-time transrectal sonographic voiding cystourethrography. *Urology* 1987; 30:171–175.
375. Powis RL, Powis WJ: *A Thinker's Guide to Ultrasonic Imaging*, Urban & Schwarzenberg, Baltimore, 1984.
376. Pradhan BK, Chandra K: Morphogenesis of nodular hyperplasia-prostate. *J Urol* 1975; 113:210–213.
377. Prout GR Jr: Diagnosis and staging of prostatic carcinoma. *Cancer* 1973; 32:1096–1103.
378. Prout GR Jr, Griffin PP, Daly JJ, Shipley WU: Nodal involvement as prognostic indicator in prostatic carcinoma. *Urology* (Suppl) 1981; 17:72–79.
379. Ragde H: Prostate cancer screening by digital and transrectal ultrasound. Presented at the Second International Symposium on Transrectal Ultrasound in the Diagnosis and Management of Prostate Cancer, Detroit, Michigan, September 21–22, 1987.
380. Raghavaiah NV, Jordan WP Jr: Prostatic lymphography. *J Urol* 1979; 121:178–181.

381. Ray P: Techniques in the fine needle aspiration biopsy of the prostate. In: *The Use of Transrectal Ultrasound in the Diagnosis and Management of Prostate Cancer* (F Lee, RD McLeary, Editors). Alan R. Liss, New York, 1987, pp. 111–124.
382. Reindl P: Darstellung der prostata mittels transrektaler sonographie. *Morphol Med* 1982; 2:75–80.
383. Reindl P: *Die Transrektale Transversale Sonographie der Prostata*. Springer-Verlag, Berlin, 1984.
384. Resnick MI, Willard JW, Boyce WH: Recent progress in ultrasonography of the bladder and prostate. *J Urol* 1977; 117:444–446.
385. Resnick MI, Willard JW, Boyce WH: Ultrasonic evaluation of the prostatic nodule. *J Urol* 1978; 120:86–89.
386. Resnick MI: Evaluation of prostatic carcinoma: Noninvasive and preoperative techniques. *Prostate* 1980; 1:311–320.
387. Resnick MI: Noninvasive techniques in evaluating patients with carcinoma of prostate. *Urology* (Suppl) 1981; 17:25–30.
388. Resnick MI: Gray scale and high frequency transrectal scanning. In: *Diagnostic Ultrasound in Urology and Nephrology* (H Watanabe, JH Holmes, HH Holm, BB Goldberg, Editors). Igaku-Shoin, New York, 1981, pp. 156–161.
389. Resnick MI: Detection of early prostatic cancer. In: *Diagnostic Ultrasound in Urology and Nephrology* (H Watanabe, JH Holmes, HH Holm, BB Goldberg, Editors). Igaku-Shoin, New York, 1981, pp. 166–170.
390. Resnick MI: Use of transrectal ultrasound in evaluating prostatic cancer. *J Urol* 1985; 134:314.
391. Resnick MI: Transrectal ultrasound guided versus digitally directed prostate biopsy. *J Urol* 1987; 137(4 Part 2):241A.
392. Riccabona M, Hammer J, Schorn A: Percutaneous, perineal, ultrasound-controlled implantation of ^{125}iodine in prostatic cancer: Tecnnics, report of initial experiences and comparison with the retropubic method of implantation. *Urolge* 1987; 26:15–21.
393. Rifkin MD: Diagnostic imaging of the lower genitourinary tract. Raven Press, New York, 1985.
394. Rifkin MD, Kurtz AB: Ultrasound of the prostate. *Ultrasound Annual 1983* (RC Sanders, Editor). Raven Press, New York, 1983, pp. 95–132.
395. Rifkin MD, Kurtz AB, Goldberg BB: Prostate biopsy utilizing transrectal ultrasound guidance: Diagnosis of nonpalpable cancers. *J Ultrasound Med* 1983; 2:165–167.
396. Rifkin MD, Kurtz AB, Goldberg BB: Sonographically guided transperineal prostatic biopsy: Preliminary experience with a longitudinal linear-array transducer. *AJR* 1983; 140:745–747.
397. Rifkin MD, Kurtz AB, Choi HY, Goldberg BB: Endoscopic ultrasonic evaluation of the prostate using a transrectal probe: Prospective evaluation and acoustic characterization. *Radiology* 1983; 149:265–271.
398. Rifkin MD: Sonourethrography: Technique for evaluation of prostatic urethra. *Radiology* 1984; 153:791–792.
399. Rifkin MD, Goldberg BB: Lower urinary tract and testes. *Abdominal Ultrasonography*, 2nd edition (BB Goldberg, Editor). John Wiley & Sons, New York, 1984, pp. 425–480.
400. Rifkin MD: Intraoperative and endoscopic ultrasound. *Radiological Society of North America Categorical Course Syllabus* (BB Goldberg, Editor). American College of Radiology, Washington, D.C., 1984, pp. 201–213.
401. Rifkin MD: Transrectal prostatic ultrasonography: Comparison of linear array and radial scanners. *J Ultrasound Med* 1985; 4:1–5.
402. Rifkin MD: Ultrasonography of the lower genitourinary tract. *Urol Clin of North Am* 1985; 12:645–656.
403. Rifkin MD, Kurtz AB: Prostate ultrasound. *Clin Diag Ultrasound* 1986; 18:195–227.
404. Rifkin MD, Friedland GW, Shortliffe L: Prostatic evaluation of transrectal endosonography: Detection of carcinoma. *Radiology* 1986; 158:85–90.
405. Rifkin MD: Endorectal prostate ultrasound. Clinical implications. *AJR* 1987; 148:1137–1142.
406. Rifkin MD: Intraoperative and endoscopic ultrasound of the genitourinary system. *Clin Diagn Ultrasound* 1987; 22:191–217.
407. Rifkin MD: Transrectal ultrasound in America. Presented at the Second International Symposium on Transrectal Ultrasound in the Diagnosis and Management of Prostate Cancer, Detroit, Michigan, September 21–22, 1987.
408. Rifkin MD: Prostatic ultrasound [Abstract]. *Radiology* 1987; 165(P):257.
409. Rifkin MD: Prostate imaging [Abstract]. *Radiology* 1987; 165(P):220.
410. Rifkin MD: Endorectal prostatic ultrasound: Significance of nonpalpable lesions [Abstract]. *Radiology* 1987; 165(P):215.
411. Rifkin MD, Choi H: Endorectal prostate ultrasound: Implications of the small peripheral lesions in hypoechoic endorectal US of the prostate. *Radiology* 1988; 106:619–622.
412. Rifkin MD, Kurtz AB: Bladder, seminal vesicles and prostate. In: *An Atlas of Genitourinary Sonography* (BG Coleman, Editor). Igaku-Shoin, Tokyo 1988; 363–405.
413. Rifkin MD: Inflammation of the prostate, seminal vesicles and scrotum. In: *Emmets Clinical Urology*, 5th edition (H Pollack, Editor). W.B. Saunders, Philadelphia (*in press*).

414. Roehrborn CG, Chinn HKW, Fulgham PF, Simpkins KL, Peters PC: The role of transabdominal ultrasound in the preoperative evaluation of patients with benign prostatic hypertrophy. *J Urol* 1986; 135:1190–1193.
415. Rohr HP, Bartsch G: Human benign prostatic hyperplasia: A stromal disease? *Urology* 1980; 16:625–626.
416. Romero Aguirre C, Tallada MB, Mayayo TD, Perales LC, Romero JM: Evaluation comparative du volume prostatique par l'echographie transabdominale, le profil uretral et la radiologie. *J d'Urologie* 1980; 86:675–679.
417. Ronnberg L, Ylostalo P, Jouppila P: Estimation of the size of the seminal vesicles by means of ultrasonic B-scanning: A preliminary report. *Fertil Steril* 1978; 30:474–475.
418. Rosenberg S, Sogani PC, Parmer EA, Miller DG: Screening of ambulatory patients for prostate cancer by transrectal ultrasonography. *J Urol* 1987; 137(4 Part 2):241A.
419. Ross RK, Deapen DM, Casagrande JT, Paganini-Hill A, Hendersen BE: A cohort study of mortality from cancer of the prostate in Catholic priests. *Br J Cancer* 1981; 43:233–235.
420. Rotkin ID: Studies in the epidemiology of prostate cancer: Expanded sampling. *Cancer Treat Rep* 1977; 61:173–180.
421. Rous SN, Mallouh C: Prostatic carcinoma: The relationship between histologic grade and incidence of early metastases. *J Urol* 1972; 108:905–907.
422. Rullis I, Shaeffer JA, Lilien OM: Incidence of prostatic carcinoma in the elderly. *Urology* 1975; 6:295–297.
423. Saitoh M: Bladder calculi. In: *Diagnostic Ultrasound in Urology and Nephrology* (H Watanabe, JH Holmes, HH Holm, BB Goldberg, Editors). Igaku-Shoin, New York, 1981, pp. 109–110.
434. Saitoh M: Testicular vessels. In: *Diagnostic Ultrasound in Urology and Nephrology* (H Watanabe, JH Holmes, HH Holm, BB Goldberg, Editors). Igaku-Shoin, New York, 1981, pp. 227–231.
425. Saitoh M: Needle placement with real-time guidance. In: *Diagnostic Ultrasound in Urology and Nephrology* (H Wantanabe, JH Holmes, HH Holm, BB Goldberg, Editors). Igaku-Shoin, New York, 1981, pp. 243–249.
426. Saitoh M, Watanabe H, Ohe H: Ultrasonically guided puncture for the prostate and seminal vesicles with transrectal real-time linear scanner. *J Kyoto Pref Univ Med* 1981; 90:47–53.
427. Saitoh N, Okui K, Sarashina H, Suzuki M, Arai T, Nunomura M: Evaluation of echographic diagnosis of rectal cancer using intrarectal ultrasonic examination. *Dis Colon Rectum* 1986; 29:234–242.
428. Salo JO, Kivisaari L, Rannikko S, Lehtonen T: Computerized tomography and transrectal ultrasound in the assessment of local extension of prostate cancer before radical retropubic prostatectomy. *J Urol* 1987; 137:435–438.
429. Salo JO, Rannikko S, Makinen J, Lehtonen T: Echogenic structure of prostatic cancer imaged on radical prostatectomy specimens. *Prostate* 1987; 10:1–9.
430. Sanders RC, Hamper UM, Dahnert WF: Update on prostatic ultrasound. *Urol Radiol* 1987; 9:110–118.
431. Sause WT, Richards RS, Plenk HP: Prostatic carcinoma: 5-year followup of patients with surgically staged disease undergoing extended field radiation. *J Urol* 1986; 135:517–519.
432. Scardino PT: The prognostic significance of biopsies after radiotherapy for prostatic cancer. *Semin Urol* 1983; 1:243–251.
433. Schacht MJ, Garnett JE, Grayhack JT: Biochemical markers in prostatic cancer. *Urol Clin North Am* 1984; 11:253–267.
434. Schapira HE: Prostatic needle biopsy in patients after abdominoperineal resection. *Urology* 1982; 20:76–77.
435. Schiebler ML, Pollack HM, Tomaszewski JE, Kressel HY, Altman H, Cohen EK, Wein AJ, Axel L: High-resolution MR imaging of prostatic carcinoma and benign prostatic hypertrophy with histopathological correlation [Abstract]. *Radiology* 165(P):235, 1987.
436. Schiebler ML, Cohen EK, Allen KS, Glickstein MF, Axel L, Kressel HY, Pollack, HM: Staging of prostatic adenocarcinoma with MR imaging at 1.5T [Abstract]. *Radiology* 165(P):235, 1987.
437. Schmidt JD: Prostate cancer: Confirming the diagnosis evaluating the extent of disease. *Your Patient & Cancer* 1984; 4:41–50.
438. Schmidt JD: Treatment of localized prostatic carcinoma. *Urol Clin North Am* 1984; 11:305–309.
439. Schroeder FH, Blom JHM, Hop WCJ, Mostofi FK: Incidental carcinoma of the prostate treated by total prostatectomy. The prognostic impact of microscopic tumor extension and grade. *World J Urol* 1983; 15–23.
440. Schuller J, Walther V: Transrectal ultrasound tomography by electronic linear scanner. *Ultraschall Med* 1983; 4:7–12.
441. Schuman LM, Mandel J, Blackard C, Bauer H, Scarlett J, McHugh R: Epidemiologic study of prostatic cancer: Preliminary report. *Cancer Treat Rep* 1977; 61:181–186.
442. Scott R Jr, Mutchnik DL, Laskowski TZ, Schmalhorst WR: Carcinoma of the prostate in elderly men: Incidence, growth characteristics and clinical significance. *J Urol* 1969; 101:602–607.
443. Scully RE, Galdabini JJ, McNeely BU: Presentation of a case. *N Engl J Med* 1980; 302:1246–1251.
444. Sekine H, Oka K, Takehara Y: Transrectal longitudinal ultrasonotomography of the prostate by electronic linear scanning. *J Urol* 1982; 127:62–65.
445. Shapeero LG, Friedland GW, Perkash I: Transrectal sonographic voiding cystourethrography: Studies in neuromuscular bladder dysfunction. *AJR* 1983; 141:83–90.

446. Sheldon CA, Williams RD, Fraley EE: Incidental carcinoma of the prostate: A review of the literature and critical reappraisal of classification. *J Urol* 1980; 124:626–631.
447. Shinohara K, Wheller TM: Ultrasonic determination of extracapsular extension: A clinicopathologic study. *J Urol* 1987; 137(4 Part 2):242A.
448. Shipley WU, Kopelson G, Novack DH, Ling CC, Dretler SP, Prout GR Jr: Preoperative irradiation, lymphadenectomy and ^{125}iodine implant for patients with localized prostatic carcinoma: A correlation of implant dosimetry with clinical results. *J Urol* 1980; 124:639–642.
449. Sieber PR, Rohner TJ Jr: Importance of acid phosphatase in response criteria for prostate cancer. *Urology* 1987; 30:316–317.
450. Siegel AL, Tomaszewski JE, Wein AJ, Hanno PM: Invasive carcinoma of prostate presenting as rectal carcinoma. *Urology* 1986; 27:162–164.
451. Silverberg E, Holleb AI: Cancer statistics, 1972. *CA* 1972; 22:2–20.
452. Silverberg E: Cancer statistics, 1977. *CA* 1977; 27:26–41.
453. Silverberg E: Cancer statistics, 1979. *CA* 1979; 29:6–21.
454. Silverberg E: Cancer statistics, 1980. *CA* 1980; 30:23–38.
455. Silverberg E: Cancer statistics, 1981. *CA* 1981; 31:13–28.
456. Silverberg E: Cancer statistics, 1982. *CA* 1982; 32:15–31.
457. Silverberg E: Cancer statistics, 1983. *CA* 1983; 33:9–25.
458. Silverberg E: Cancer statistics, 1984. *CA* 1984; 34:7–23.
459. Silverberg E: Cancer statistics, 1985. *CA* 1985; 35:19–35.
460. Silverberg E, Lubera J: Cancer statistics, 1986. *CA* 1986; 36:9–25.
461. Silverberg E, Lubera J: Cancer statistics, 1987. *CA* 1987; 37:2–19.
462. Slack NH, Murphy CP: A decade of experience with chemotherapy for prostate cancer. *Urology* 1983; 22:1–7.
463. Slack NH, Murphy GP: Criteria for evaluating patient responses to treatment modalities for prostatic cancer. *Urol Clin North Am* 1984; 11:337–341.
464. Slack NH, Lane WW, Priore RL, Murphy GP: Prostatic cancer. Treated at a categorical center, 1980–1983. *Urology* 1986; 27:205–213.
465. Soiderer MH: Histologic and cytologic diagnosis of prostate carcinoma by ultrasound-guided needle biopsy. In: *The Use of Transrectal Ultrasound in the Diagnosis and Management of Prostate Cancer* (F Lee, RD McLeary, Editors). Alan R. Liss, New York, 1987, pp. 125–132.
466. Spaulding J: Carcinoma of the prostate in the elderly. *Front Radiat Ther Oncol* 1986; 20:133–138.
467. Spigelman SS, McNeal JE, Freiha FS, Stamey TA: Rectal examination in volume determination of carcinoma of the prostate: Clinical and anatomical correlations. *J Urol* 1986; 136:1228–1230.
468. Spirnak, JP, Resnick MI: Clinical staging of prostatic cancer: New modalities. *Urol Clin North Am* 1984; 11:221–235.
469. Spirnak JP, Resnick MI: Transrectal ultrasonography. *Urology* 1984; 23:461–467.
470. Sridhar KN, Woodhouse CRJ: Prostatic infiltration in leukaemia and lymphoma. *Eur Urol* 1983; 9:153–156.
471. Stamey TA: Cancer of the prostate. An analysis of some important contributions and dilemmas. *1983 Monogr Urol* 1983; 4:68–92.
472. Stamey TA, Hay A, Constantinou CE, McNeal J, Freiha FS: The role of transrectal ultrasound (TRUS) in the diagnosis and management of prostate cancer. *J Urol* 1987; 137(4 Part 2):242A.
473. Stamey TA, Yang N, Hay AR, McNeal JE, Freiha FS, Redwine E: Prostate-specific antigen as a serum marker for adenocarcinoma of the prostate. *N Engl J Med* 1987; 317:909–916.
474. Stassi J, Rifkin MD: Correlative imaging of the lower genitourinary tract. *Urologic Imaging and Interventional Techniques* (WH Bush, Editor). Urban & Schwarzenberg, New York (*in press*).
475. Staszewski J, Haenszel W: Cancer mortality among the Polish-born in the United States. *J Natl Cancer Inst* 1965; 35:291–297.
476. Steele R, Lees REM, Kraus A, Rao C: Sexual factors in the epidemiology of cancer of the prostate. *J Chronic Dis* 1971; 24:29–37.
477. Steyn JH, Smith FW: Nuclear magnetic resonance (NMR) imaging of the prostate. *Br J Urol* 1984; 56:679–681.
478. Stone AR, Merrick MV, Chisholm GD: Prostatic lymphoscintigraphy. *Br J Urol* 1979; 51:556–560.
479. Sugao H, Takiuchi H, Sakura T: Transrectal longitudinal ultrasonography of prostatic abscess. *J Urol* 1986; 136:1316–1317.
480. Sugiura H, Hasegawa S: Transrectal prostatography: Its use in prostatic hypertrophy. *Am J Roentgenol Radium Ther Nucl Med* 1969; 107:796–802.
481. Sukov RJ, Scardino PT, Sample WF, Winter J, Confer DJ: Computed tomography and transabdominal ultrasound in the evaluation of the prostate. *J Comput Assist Tomogr* 1977; 1:281–289.
482. Swank-Bordewijk SCG, van Kleffens HJ: Investigation of changes in CT-number in the prostate after radiotherapy. *Int J Radiat Oncol Biol Phys* 1984; 10:659–664.
483. Swee DE: Problematic prostatic prediction [Letter to the Editor]. *JAMA* 1985; 254:1172.
484. Swyer GIM: Post-natal growth changes in the human prostate. *J Anat* 1944; 78:130.

485. Takahashi H: Biological effects of ultrasound in urology and nephrology. In: *Diagnostic Ultrasound in Urology and Nephrology* (H Watanabe, JH Holmes, HH Holm, BB Goldberg, Editors). Igaku-Shoin, New York, 1981, pp. 21–24.
486. Tanahashi Y, Watanabe H, Igari D, Harada K, Saitoh M: Volume estimation of the seminal vesicles by means of transrectal ultrasonotomography: A preliminary report. *Br J Urol* 1975; 47:695–702.
487. Tanahashi Y: Seminal vesicles. In: *Diagnostic Ultrasound in Urology and Nephrology* (H Watanabe, JH Holmes, HH Holm, BB Goldberg, Editors). Igaku-Shoin, New York, 1981, pp. 162–165.
488. Tanahashi Y: Visualization of internal glands. In: *Diagnostic Ultrasound in Urology and Nephrology* (H Watanabe, JH Holmes, HH Holm, BB Goldberg, Editors). Igaku-Shoin, New York, 1981, pp. 141–147.
489. Tanahashi Y: Monitoring of cryosurgery. In: *Diagnostic Ultrasound in Urology and Nephrology* (H Watanabe, JH Holmes, HH Holm, BB Goldberg, Editors). Igaku-Shoin, New York, 1981, pp. 183–186.
490. Tanaka S: Prostatitis. In: *Diagnostic Ultrasound in Urology and Nephrology* (H Watanabe, JH Holmes, HH Holm, BB Goldberg, Editors). Igaku-Shoin, New York, 1981, pp. 136–141.
491. Taylor WB, Hunt JW, Foster FS, Blend R, Worthington A: A high-resolution transrectal ultrasonographic system. *Ultrasound Med Biol* 1979; 5:129–138.
492. Thomas R, Lewis RW, Sarma DP, Coker GB, Rao MK, Roberts JA: Aid to accurate clinical staging—Histopathologic grading in prostatic cancer. *J Urol* 1982; 128:726–728.
493. Thompson IM, Ernst JJ, Gangai MP, Spence CR: Adenocarcinoma of the prostate: Results of routine urological screening. *J Urol* 1984; 132:690–692.
494. Thornhill BA, Morehouse HT, Coleman P, Hoffman-Tretin JC: Prostatic abscess: CT and sonographic findings. *AJR* 1987; 148:899–900.
495. Tisnado J, Amendola MA, Walsh JW, Jordan RL, Turner MA, Krempa J: Computed tomography of the perineum. *AJR* 1981; 136:475–481.
496. Tolis G, Koutsilieris M, Fazekas ATA, Patton R: Transabdominal ultrasonography in the evaluation of patients with advanced prostatic carcinoma: Effects of castration and of chronic administration of a gonadotropin releasing hormone agonistic analogue. *Prostate* 1983; 4:595–600.
497. Torp-Pedersen S, Holm HH, Littrup PJ: Transperineal I-125 seed implantation in prostate cancer guided by transrectal ultrasound. *The Use of Transrectal Ultrasound in the Diagnosis and Mangement of Prostate Cancer* (F Lee, RD McLeary, Editors). Alan R. Liss, New York, 1987, pp. 143–152.
498. Totterman S, Spataro R, Rubens D, Szumowski J, Weiss SL, Katzberg RW, Lerner RM: Fat suppression technique in detection and staging of cervical, bladder and prostate carcinoma [Abstract]. *Radiology* 1987; 165(P):235.
499. Tsuchida S, Yamaguchi O: Urodynamics. In: *Diagnostic Ultrasound in Urology and Nephrology* (H Watanabe, JH Holmes, HH Holm, BB Goldberg, Editors). Igaku-Shoin, New York, 1981, pp. 221–227.
500. Utz DC, Farrow GM: Pathologic differentiation and prognosis of prostatic carcinoma. *JAMA* 1969; 209:1701–1705.
501. Van Engelshoven JMA, Kreel L: Computed tomography of the prostate. *J Comput Assist Tomogr* 1979; 3:45–51.
502. Vardi Y, Ginesin Y, Levin DR: Preoperative evaluation of prostatic size by urethral pressure profilometry. *Eur Urol* 1985; 11:257–259.
503. Veterans Administration Co-Operative Urological Research Group: Treatment and survival of patients with cancer of the prostate. *Surg Gynecol Obstet* 1967; May:1011–1017.
504. Vihko P, Kontturi M, Lukkarinen O, Vihko R: Radioimmunoassayable prostate-specific acid phosphatase in peripheral and bone marrow sera compared in diagnosis of prostatic cancer patients. *J Urol* 1982; 128:739–741.
505. Vihko P, Kontturi M, Lukkarinen O, Ervasti J, Vihko R: Screening for carcinoma of the prostate. Rectal examination, and enzymatic and radioimmunologic measurements of serum acid phosphatase compared. *Cancer* 1985; 56:173–177.
506. Vilmann P, Hancke S, Strange-Vognsen HH, Nielsen K, Sorensen SM: The reliability of transabdominal ultrasound scanning in the determination of prostatic volume. An autopsy study. *Scand J Urol Nephrol* 1987; 21:5–7.
507. Vijverberg PLM, Dabhoiwala NF, deReijke TM: Transrectal ultrasonographically guided implantation of transperineal I-125 seeds for prostatic cancer. *J Urol* 1987; 137(4 Part 2):367A.
508. Vollmer RT: Prostate cancer and chip specimens: Complete versus partial sampling. *Hum Pathol* 1986; 17:285–290.
509. Wajsman Z: Lymph node evaluation in prostatic cancer: Is pelvic lymph node dissection necessary? *Urology* (Suppl) 1981; 17:80–82.
510. Wallace DM, Chisholm GD, Hendry WF: T.N.M. classification for urological tumours (U.I.C.C.)—1974. *Br J Urol* 1975; 47:1–12.
511. Walls WJ, Lin F: Ultrasonic diagnosis of seminal vesicle cyst. *Radiology* 1975; 114:693–694.
512. Walker ARP: Prostate cancer—Some aspects of epidemiology risk factors, treatment and survival. *Afr Med J* 1986; 69:44–47.
513. Walker WC, Bowles WT: Transvesical seminal vesiculostomy in treatment of congenital obstruction of seminal vesicles: Case report. *J Urol* 1968;99:324–326.

514. Walsh JW, Amendola MA, Konerding KF, Tisnado J, Hazra TA: Computed tomographic detection of pelvic and inguinal lymph-node metastases from primary and recurrent pelvic malignant disease. *Radiology* 1980; 137:157–166.
515. Walsh PC, Donker PJ: Impotence following radical prostatectomy: Insight into etiology and prevention. *J Urol* 1982; 128:492–497.
516. Walsh PC: Benign prostatic hyperplasia. *Campbell's Urology*, 5th edition (PC Walsh, RF Gittes, AD Perlmutter, TA Stamey, Editors). W.B. Saunders, Philadelphia, 1986, pp. 1248–1267.
517. Walsh PC: Personal communication, 1987.
518. Walz PH, Wenderoth U, Jacobi GH: Suprapubic transvesical sonography of the prostate: Determination of prostate size. *Eur Urol* 1983; 9:148–152.
519. Wang MC, Valenzuela LA, Murphy GP, Chu TM: Purification of a human prostate specific antigen. *Invest Urol* 1979; 17:159–163.
520. Watanabe H: Preventive oncology project for prostatic cancer. Personal communication.
521. Watanabe H, Kaiho H, Tanaka M, Terasawa Y: Diagnostic application of ultrasonotomography to the prostate. *Invest Urol* 1971; 8:548–559.
522. Watanabe H, Igari D, Tanahashi Y, Harada K, Saitoh M: Transrectal ultrasonotomography of the prostate. *J Urol* 1975; 114:734–740.
523. Watanabe H, Saitoh M, Mishina T, Igari D, Tanahashi Y, Harada K, Hisamichi S: Mass screening program for prostatic diseases with transrectal ultrasonotomography. *J Urol* 1977; 117:746–748.
524. Watanabe H, Date S, Ohe H, Saitoh M, Tanaka S: A survey of 3,000 examinations by transrectal ultrasonotomography. *Prostate* 1980; 1:271–278.
525. Watanabe H, Ohe H, Ando K, Sawamura Y, Niijima T, Nakamura S, Orikasa S, Tanahashi Y, Imamura K, Yoshida H: The effect of estramustine phosphate on prostatic cancer estimated by transrectal ultrasonotomography. *Prostate* 1981; 2:155–161.
526. Watanabe H: General review of diagnostic ultrasound in urology and nephrology. In: *Diagnostic Ultrasound in Urology and Nephrology* (H Watanabe, JH Holmes, HH Holm, BB Goldberg, Editors). Igaku-Shoin, New York, 1981, pp. 10–16.
527. Watanabe H: Instrumentation and techniques. In: *Diagnostic Ultrasound in Urology and Nephrology* (H Watanabe, JH Holmes, HH Holm, BB Goldberg, Editors). Igaku-Shoin, New York, 1981, pp. 119–123.
528. Watanabe H: Prostatic cancer. Diagnosis. In: *Diagnostic Ultrasound in Urology and Nephrology* (H Watanabe, JH Holmes, HH Holm, BB Goldberg, Editors). Igaku-Shoin, New York, 1981, pp. 130–135.
529. Watanabe H, Mishina T: Mass screening program for prostatic disease. In: *Diagnostic Ultrasound in Urology and Nephrology* (H Watanabe, JH Holmes, HH Holm, BB Goldberg, Editors). Igaku-Shoin, New York, 1981, pp. 174–179.
530. Watanabe H: Natural history of benign prostatic hypertrophy. *Ultrasound Med Biol* 1986; 12:567–571.
531. Watanabe H: Historical perspectives on the use of transrectal sonography of the prostate. *The Use of Transrectal Ultrasound in the Diagnosis and Management of Prostate Cancer* (F Lee, RD McLeary, Editors). Alan R. Liss, New York, 1987, pp. 5–14.
532. Watanabe H: Preventive oncology project for prostatic cancer. *The Use of Transrectal Ultrasound in the Diagnosis and Management of Prostate Cancer* (F Lee, RD McLeary, Editors). Alan R. Liss, New York, 1987, pp. 133–142.
533. Watanabe H: The Japanese experience: Use of transrectal ultrasound in the evaluation of tumor response to various treatment modalities. *The Use of Transrectal Ultrasound in the Diagnosis and Management of Prostatic Cancer* (F Lee, RD McLeary, Editors). Alan R. Liss, New York, 1987, pp. 195–208.
534. Weinberger, Pitlik SD, Rabinovitz M, Morduchowicz, Rosenfeld JB, Cytron S, Servadio C: Per-rectal ultrasonography for diagnosis of and guide to drainage of prostatic abscess. *Lancet* 1985; 2:772.
535. Weinerman PM, Arger PH, Pollack HM: CT evaluation of bladder and prostate neoplasms. *Urol Radiol* 1982; 4:105–114.
536. Weinerman PM, Arger PH, Coleman BG, Pollack HM, Banner MP, Wein AJ: Pelvic adenopathy from bladder and prostate carcinoma: Detection by rapid-sequence computed tomography. *AJR* 1983; 140:95–99.
537. Wenderoth UK, Jacobi GH: Gonadotropin-releasing hormone analogues for palliation of carcinoma of the prostate. *World J Urol* 1983; 1:40–48.
538. Weyrauch HM, Nesbet JD: Use of triethylene thio-phosphoramide (thio-TEPA) in treatment of advanced carcinoma of prostate. *J Urol* 1959; 81:185–193.
539. Whelan JP, Chin JL, Shapre JR, Davis IR: Transrectal needle aspiration versus transperineal needle biopsy in diagnosis of carcinoma of prostate. *Urology* 1986; 27:410–414.
540. Whitmore WF Jr: The natural history of prostatic cancer. *Cancer* 1973; 32:1104–1112.
541. Whitmore WF Jr: Natural history and staging of prostate cancer. *Urol Clin North Am* 1984; 11:205–220.
542. Whitmore WF Jr: Stage A prostatic cancer. *J Urol* 1986; 136:883.
543. Whittingham TA: Ultrasonic estimation of the volume of the enlarged prostate. *Br J Radiol* 1973; 46:68–70.
544. Wild SR, McDicken WN, Anderson T: Evaluation of a new type of rotating ultrasound transducer for examination of the prostate gland. *Br J Radiol* 1983; 56:483–484.

545. Willems JS, Lowhagen T: Transrectal fine-needle aspiration biopsy for cytologic diagnostic and grading of prostatic carcinoma. *Prostate* 1981; 2:381–395.
546. Williams G, Wallace DM, Bloom HJG: A reconsideration of the biology of carcinoma of the prostate. *Br J Urol* 1974; 46:61–64.
547. Wilson JM, Kemp IW, Stein GJ: Cancer of the prostate. Do younger men have a poorer survival rate? *Br J Urol* 1984; 56:391–396.
548. Winklestein W Jr, Ernster VL: Epidemiology and etiology in: *Prostatic Cancer* (GP Murphy, Editor). PSG Publishing Company, Littleton, Mass., 1979, pp. 1–17.
549. Wolf RM, Dragone N: Monitoring the effect of external beam radiation on localized prostate cancer with transrectal ultrasound. *J Urol* 1987; 137(4 Part 2):242A.
550. Wong W, Saito T, Ogawa H: Radiologic detection of prostatic carcinoma by double contrast retrograde urethrocystography. *J Urol* 1975; 114:746–751.
551. Wynder EL, Mabuchi K, Whitmore WF Jr: Epidemiology of cancer of the prostate. *Cancer* 1971; 28:344–360.
552. Wynder EL, Laakso K, Sotarauta, Rose DP: Metabolic epidemiology of prostatic cancer. *Prostate* 1984; 5:47–53.
553. Yatani R, Chigusa I, Akazaki K, Stemmermann GN, Welsh RA, Correa P: Geographic pathology of latent prostatic carcinoma. *Int J Cancer* 1982; 29:611–616.
554. Young JL Jr, Percy CL, Asire AJ, et al: Cancer incidence and mortality in the United States 1973–77. *Natl Cancer Inst Monogr* 1981; 57:1–9.
555. Zagoria RJ, Papanicolaou N, Pfister RC, Stafford SA, Young HH: Seminal vesicle abscess after vasectomy: Evaluation of transrectal sonography and CT. *AJR* 1987; 149:137–138.
556. Zaridze DG, Boyle P: Cancer of the prostate: Epidemiology and aetiology. *Br J Urol* 1987; 59:493–502.
557. Zincke H, Campbell JT, Utz DC, Farrow GM, Anderson MJ Jr: Confidence in the negative transrectal needle biopsy. *Surg Gynecol Obstet* 1973; 136:78–80.
558. Zincke H, Farrow GM, Myers RP, Benson RC Jr, Furlow WL, Utz DC: Relationship between grade and stage of adenocarcinoma of the prostate and regional pelvic lymph node metastasis. *J Urol* 1982; 128:498–501.
559. Zincke H, Utz DC, Thule PM, Taylor WF: Treatment options for patients with stage D1 (T0/3, N1/2, M0) adenocarcinoma of prostate. *Urol* 1987; 30:307–315.

Subject Index

A

Abdominal (transabdominal) approach for prostate ultrasound, 31–33
  acute prostatitis demonstrated with, 222
  benign prostatic hypertrophy demonstrated with, 193–195
  normal sonographic anatomy demonstrated with, 51–56
    echogenic appearances of prostate and, 51, 54
    on sagittal scans, 51, 53, 55
    of seminal vesicles, 51, 53
    on transverse (axial) scans, 51–53
  patient position for, 51
  prostate size determined with, 94–95
  seminal vesicle abscess demonstrated with, 228
  seminal vesicle cysts demonstrated with, 235, 236
  seminal vesicle neoplasms demonstrated with, 238
  seminal vesicle size determined with, 98–100
  voiding abnormalities evaluated with, 245
Abscesses
  prostatic, 224, 225
  seminal vesicle, 226–228
Acetylcholine, detrusor affected by, 243
Acoustic widows, as solution to imaging problems, 26
Adenomas
  cystic, infertility caused by, 235
  hyperplastic, on axial endorectal sonogram, 203, 204
α-Adrenergic drugs
  bladder neck affected by, 243
  urethra affected by, 243
Aging, prostate cancer pathogenesis and, 144
Air, ultrasound images affected by, 26
Alpha-blockers
  bladder neck affected by, 244
  urethra affected by, 244
Androgen, and prostate cancer pathogenesis, 145
Anechoic lesions, in sonographic approach to prostatic disease, 104, 105
Anterior fibromuscular stroma, normal sonographic anatomy and
  on axial endorectal sonogram, 68–72
  on sagittal endorectal sonogram, 74, 75
Anterior fibromuscular zone, normal sonographic anatomy and, on axial endorectal sonogram, 72
Anterior prostatic fat and fascia, 5, 6

normal sonographic anatomy and
  on axial endorectal sonogram, 67
  on sagittal endorectal sonogram, 76
Anticholinergics, bladder contractility affected by, 244
Antihistamines, bladder contractility affected by, 244
Aspiration biopsy, for prostate cancer grading, 147
Autonomic nervous system, abnormalities of, voiding abnormalities caused by, 241–243
Axial scanning, technique for, 45

B

Bacteroides fragilis, prostatitis caused by, 221
Benign prostatic hypertrophy (benign prostatic hyperplasia), 191–220
  bladder neck obstruction and, 245
  clinical manifestations of, 193
  diffuse, on axial endorectal sonogram, 204
  general considerations of, 191–192
  imaging of, 193
  incidence of, 192
  nodules impinging on urethra or bladder neck caused by, 255–257
  pathogenesis of, 192–193
    microscopic classification and, 192–193
    transitional zone and, 192
  post-transurethral resection
    endorectal ultrasound of, 200, 209, 210–213
    ultrasound monitoring of, 209, 214–215
  prostate cancer pathogenesis and, 145
  prostatic calculi and, 216–219
    endorectal sonograms of, 217–219
    endourethral sonogram of, 216
  prostatic cysts and, 219, 220
  sonographic characteristics of, 193–200
    using endorectal approach, 196–200, 201–208
    using endourethral approach, 195–196, 197
    using transabdominal approach, 193–195, 196
    using transperineal approach, 195
Beta-blockers, urethra affected by, 243
Beta-stimulants, urethra affected by, 244
Bethanecol, detrusor affected by, 243
Biopsy. *See also* Transperineal biopsy; Transrectal biopsy; Ultrasound guided biopsy
  complications of, 116–117
  conventional, 114–116

Biopsy (contd.)
  core-needle, 113
    for prostate cancer grading, 147
  cytologic aspiration, 114
    for prostate cancer grading, 148
  techniques for, 113–139
  transperineal, 114–116, 118–130
  transrectal, 114–116, 117, 130–139
  ultrasounded-guided, 117–139
    as clinical indication for endorectal sonography, 265
    sagittally oriented scanners for, 90, 91
    transperineal, 118–130
    transrectal, 130–139
Biopty needle, for core needle biopsy, 113, 114
  gun or trigger for, 115
Biplane probes, 35–37, 38, 39
  with guides for biopsies, 120
Blacks, prostate cancer in, 141, 144, 145
Bladder, urinary. See Urinary bladder
Bladder neck nodules, imaging of, 255–256
Bladder neck obstruction
  etiology of, 245
  imaging of, 250, 254
Blastomycosis, prostatitis caused by, 221
Bones, ultrasound images affected by, 25–26
Bowel movement, blood in
  as complication of transperineal biopsy, 139
  as complication of transrectal biopsy, 139
  as complication of ultrasound guided transrectal biopsy, 130
BPH. See Benign prostatic hypertrophy

C
Calculi
  axial versus sagittal orientation in evaluation of, 91
  in benign prostatic hypertrophy, 216–219
  echogenicity of, 216
    carcinomas and, 219
  endorectal sonograms showing, 217–219
  endourethral sonogram showing, 216
  prostate cancer pathogenesis and, 146
  in sonographic approach to prostatic disease, 102
Cancer. See also Neoplasms
  of prostate. See also Prostate cancer
    general considerations of, 141–155
    percutaneous radiation treatment for, 185–190
    sonographic characteristics of, 157–184
Central zone
  anatomy of, 12
  cancer originating in, 146
  normal sonographic anatomy and
    on axial endorectal sonogram, 67, 68, 69
    on sagittal endorectal sonogram, 74, 75
  in sonographic approach to prostatic disease, 102
Chiba needle, for core needle biopsy, 114
Cholinergic drugs, detrusor affected by, 243
Clostridium perfringens, prostatitis caused by, 221
Coccydioidomycosis, prostatitis caused by, 221
Computed tomography, in prostate imaging, 1
Contact scanning, 18
Core needle biopsy, 113, 114, 115
  for prostate cancer grading, 147

Corpora amylacea, prostatic calculi and, 216, 217
Cryptococcus, prostatitis caused by, 221
Curability, window of, in prostate cancer, 155
Cystography, prostate size determined by, 93
Cystometrogram, bladder pressure studied with, 244
Cysts
  axial versus sagittal orientation in evaluation of, 91
  in benign prostatic hypertrophy, 219–220
    endorectal sonograms demonstrating, 220
  endorectal sonograms demonstrating, 207
  in seminal vesicle, infertility caused by, 235, 236–237
Cytologic aspiration, for prostate biopsy, 114

D
Denovilliers' fascia, 5
Detrusor muscle, drugs affecting, 243, 244
Detrusor muscle-bladder neck dyssynergia
  bladder neck obstruction and, 245
  voiding abnormalities and, 241, 242
Detrusor muscle hyperreflexic abnormalities, voiding abnormalities and, 241, 242
Detrusor muscle-sphincter dyssynergia, voiding abnormalities and, 241, 242
Diabetes mellitus, hypotonic areflexic bladder caused by, 241, 242
Diamond system, for prostate cancer grading, 147
Drugs, voiding abnormalities caused by, 243, 244
Dysreflexia, autonomic, 241–243

E
Echogenicity, in sonographic approach to prostatic disease, 102
  focal disease and, 102
Ejaculatory ducts
  embryologic development of, 5
  normal sonographic anatomy and
    on axial endorectal sonogram, 68, 69
    on sagittal endorectal sonogram, 74, 75, 79
  obstruction and dilatation of causing infertility, 229–232
    longitudinal scanner for evaluation of, 231
    sonogram findings in, 230
Electromyogram, voiding abnormalities studied with, 244
Endorectal approach for prostate ultrasound, 34–44. See also Endorectal probe; Endorectal prostate scanners
  acute prostatitis demonstrated with, 222, 223
  benign prostatic hypertrophy demonstrated with, 196–200, 201–208
  biopsy guided with, 118–139. See also Endorectal ultrasound guided biopsy
  chronic prostatitis demonstrated with, 222
  clinical implications of, 259–266
  clinical indications for, 264–265
    algorithm for, 261
    biopsy guidance, 265
    future potential, 266
    inflammatory disease, 265
    normal prostate, 265
    palpable mass, 264–265

screening, 265
sonourethrography, 265
differential diagnoses using, 259–266
  benign disease, 260
  peripherally oriented hypoechoic lesion, 260, 262
  prostate cancer, 259–260
equipment for, 35–37, 38
normal sonographic anatomy demonstrated with, 57–91
  in axial orientation, 62–74
  comparison of axial and sagittal images with, 76–91
  in sagittal orientation, 74–76
patient preparation for, 42–44
probe insertion for, 44
prostate cancer demonstrated with, 259–260
prostate size determined with, 95, 96–97
  planimetric calculation for, 96
prostatic abscess demonstrated with, 224, 225
prostatic calculi demonstrated with, 217–219
prostatic cysts demonstrated with, 220
as screening modality, 184, 260–264, 265
seminal vesicle abscess demonstrated with, 227
seminal vesicle cysts demonstrated with, 235, 237
seminal vesicle neoplasms demonstrated with, 239
seminal vesiculitis demonstrated with, 226
transducer preparation for, 38–42
transurethral resection studied with, 200, 209, 210–213
Endorectal probe
  biplane, 35–37, 38, 39
  insertion of, 44
  preparation of, 38–42
    double cover technique for, 42, 43
    single-sheath (cover) technique, 38–42
Endorectal prostate scanners, 27–30, 34–44
  biplane probes for, 35–36, 38, 39
  chair for, 35
  longitudinally oriented, 35, 37
  patient positioning for, 43, 44
  patient preparation and, 42–44
  probe insertion and, 44
  probe positioning and, 27–30
  radial scanners, 35, 36
  scan-plane thickness and, 30
  sector scanners, 35, 37
  transducers for, 38–42
    double-cover technique for, 42, 43
    single-sheath (cover) technique for, 38–42
Endorectal ultrasound guided biopsy
  anesthesia for, 117
  as clinical indication for endorectal sonography, 265
  freehand guidance for, 118
  general considerations for, 117
  guidance systems for, 118, 119, 120, 121
  patient position for, 117
  sterile precautions for, 117
  transperineal, 118–130
    axial orientation, 119–122
    sagittal orientation, 122–130
  transperineal versus transrectal, 130, 139
    accuracy of, 130
    benefits of, 139
    complications of, 139
    patient positioning for, 130
  transrectal, 130–139
    curvable needle for, 137–138
    guidance systems for, 131, 132, 133, 134
Endourethral approach for prostate ultrasound, 33–34
  benign prostatic hypertrophy demonstrated with, 195–196
  normal sonographic anatomy demonstrated with, 56–67
  prostate enlargement and, 56
  of prostatic urethra, 56
  prostate size determined with, 95
  prostatic calculi demonstrated with, 216
  transurethral resection monitored with, 209, 214–215
Environment, prostate cancer pathogenesis and, 145
Ephedrine
  bladder neck affected by, 243
  urethra affected by, 243
Escherichia coli, prostatitis caused by, 221
Estrogen, and prostate cancer pathogenesis, 145
External sphincter, and anatomy of the prostate, 6

F
Fat, ultrasound images affected by, 25
Fibromas, of seminal vesicle, infertility caused by, 235
Fibromuscular nodules, in benign prostatic hypertrophy, 192
Fibromyoadenomatous nodules, in benign prostatic hypertrophy, 193
Fibrovascular nodules, in benign prostatic hypertrophy, 192
Focus characteristics, ultrasound images affected by, 23

G
Gaeta system, for prostate cancer grading, 147
Genetics, prostate cancer pathogenesis and, 144
Gleason system, for prostate cancer grading, 146–147
Gray scale images, 16–17
Guanethidine, bladder contractlity affected by, 244

H
Hair, body, ultrasound images affected by, 26
Halo sign
  on axial endorectal sonogram, 203
  in sonographic approach to prostatic disease, 102
Hematospermia
  as complication of transperineal biopsy, 139
  as complication of transrectal biopsy, 130, 139
Hematuria
  as complication of percutaneous radiation treatment of prostate cancer, 190
  as complication of transperineal biopsy, 139
  as complication of transrectal biopsy, 130, 139
Hormones, prostate cancer pathogenesis and, 145

Hyperadenomatous nodules, in benign prostatic hypertrophy, 193
Hyperechoic lesions
  in prostate cancer, 169, 176–177
  in sonographic approach to prostatic disease, 107, 109–110, 111
Hyperplasia, benign prostatic, 191–220. See also Benign prostatic hypertrophy
Hyperplastic nodules, impingement of on bladder base, longitudinal orientation for evaluation of, 90, 91
Hypertrophy, benign prostatic, 191–220. See also Benign prostatic hypertrophy
Hypoechoic lesions
  in prostate cancer, 163–165, 166–168, 169, 170–171
  in sonographic approach to prostatic disease, 104–107

I
Image preservation, 46
Imipramine
  bladder neck affected by, 243
  urethra affected by, 243
Immersion scanning, 18
Impotence, as complication of percutaneous radiation treatment of prostate cancer, 190
Infection
  as complication of percutaneous radiation treatment of prostate cancer, 190
  prostate cancer pathogenesis and, 145–146
Infertility, male
  ejaculatory duct obstruction and dilatation causing, 229–232
  and seminal vesicle disease, 229–239
    absence of causing, 232–234
    congenital abnormalities causing, 232
    cysts causing, 235, 236–237
    postsurgical acquired disease causing, 235
    primary neoplasms causing, 235, 238–239
Inflammation
  endorectal ultrasound in evaluation of, 265
  of prostate, 221–224, 225. See also Abscesses, prostatic; Prostatitis
  of seminal vesicle, 225–228. See also Abscesses, seminal vesicle; Seminal vesiculitis
Internal sphincter, normal sonographic anatomy and, 6
  on axial endorectal sonogram, 68
  on sagittal endorectal sonogram, 74
Iodine-125, for percutaneous radiation treatment of prostate cancer, 185–190
  half life and, 185–186
  half value layer and, 185–186
Isoechoic lesions
  in prostate cancer, 165–169, 172–173
  in sonographic approach to prostatic disease, 107, 108, 109
Isoproterenol, urethra affected by, 244

L
Levator ani muscles, normal sonographic anatomy and, on axial endorectal sonogram, 67

Line array, 19
Line density, ultrasound images affected by, 21–22
Longitudinally oriented endorectal scanners, 35, 37
Lymph nodes, in sonographic approach to prostatic disease, 103

M
Magnetic resonance imaging (MRI)
  dilated urethra demonstrated with, 245
  in prostate imaging, 1–2
Malignant seeding, as complication of prostate biopsy, 117
Mayo Clinic system, for prostate cancer grading, 147
MD Anderson (MDA) Hospital system, for prostate cancer grading, 147
Mechanical sector scanner, 18–19
Median furrow (median sulcus)
  and anatomy of prostate, 6
  appearance of on endourethral sonograms, 56
Median hypertrophy, 193. See also Benign prostatic hypertrophy
Mesonephros, in embryogenesis of urogenital system, 3–4
Methacholine, detrusor affected by, 243
Micturition, 241
Middle lobe hypertrophy, 193. See also Benign prostatic hypertrophy
Mixed echogenicity
  in prostate cancer, 169, 174
  in sonographic approach to prostatic disease, 107, 112
Mostofi system, for prostate cancer grading, 147
Muscular nodules, in benign prostatic hypertrophy, 192
Myomas, of seminal vesicle, infertility caused by, 235

N
Neoplasms. See also Cancer
  of seminal vesicle, infertility caused by, 235, 238–239
Nicotine, detrusor affected by, 243
Nipple sign
  normal sonographic anatomy and, on sagittal endorectal sonogram, 74–76, 90
  prostate cancer and, 179
  in sonographic approach to prostatic disease, 103

O
Obturator internus muscles, normal sonographic anatomy and, on axial endorectal sonogram, 67
Orientals, prostate cancer in, 144

P
Pain, as complication of percutaneous radiation treatment of prostate cancer, 190
Pelvis, male, and anatomy of the prostate
  axial diagrams of, 9, 10

coronal diagrams of, 7, 8
sagittal diagram of, 6
Perineal approach for prostate ultrasound. *See* Transperineal approach for prostate ultrasound
Peripheral zone
  anatomy of, 11–12
  cancer originating in, 146
  normal sonographic anatomy and
    on axial endorectal sonogram, 67, 68–73
    laterally placed longitudinally oriented sonogram of, 80, 81
    on sagittal endorectal sonogram, 74, 75
  in sonographic approach to prostatic disease, 102
Periurethral glandular tissue, normal sonographic anatomy and
  on axial endorectal sonogram, 68, 69
  on sagittal endorectal sonogram, 75
Periurethral glandular zone, 12–14
Phased array. *See* Sector array
Phenothiazine, bladder contractility affected by, 244
Phenoxybenzamine
  bladder neck affected by, 244
  urethra affected by, 244
Phentolamine
  bladder neck affected by, 244
  urethra affected by, 244
Phenylephrine
  bladder neck affected by, 243
  urethra affected by, 243
Piezoelectric transducers, in pulse-echo ultrasound scanning, 17–18
Preservation of images, 46
Progesterone, urethra affected by, 244
Pronephros, in embryogenesis of urogenital system, 3
Propantheline, bladder contractility affected by, 244
Propranalol, urethra affected by, 243
Prostadynia, 221
Prostate gland
  abdominal approach in ultrasound study of, 31–33. *See also* Abdominal approach for prostate ultrasound
  apex of, longitudinal orientation for evaluation of, 90, 91
  atrophy of, prostatic cancer and, 145
  axial scanning of, 45
  base of, longitudinal orientation for evaluation of, 90, 91
  benign hypertrophy of, 191–220. *See also* Benign prostatic hypertrophy
  calculi in. *See* Calculi
  cancer of, 141–184. *See also* Prostate cancer
    general considerations of, 141–155
    percutaneous radiation treatment for, 185–190
    sonographic characteristics of, 157–184
  central zone of. *See* Central zone
  cysts of. *See* Cysts
  embryology of, 3–5
    and ejaculatory ducts, 5
    and seminal vesicles, 5
    and sex determination, 4
    and urinary bladder, 3–4
    and vas deferens, 4
  endorectal approach in ultrasound study of, 34–44. *See also* Endorectal approach for prostate ultrasound
  endourethral approach in ultrasound study of, 33–34. *See also* Endourethral approach for prostate ultrasound
  glandular, zones of, 11–12
  gross anatomy of, 5–11
    axial diagrams of, 9, 10
    coronal diagrams of, 7, 8, 12
    lobar, 6–8
    sagittal diagram of, 6
    specimen showing, 11
  histologic anatomy of, 11–14
    in curved coronal section, 12
  inflammation of, 221–224, 225. *See also* Abscesses, prostatic; Prostatitis
  lateral margins of, axial orientation for evaluation of, 90, 91
  normal, endorectal ultrasound in evaluation of, 265
  normal sonographic anatomy of, 51–91
    abdominal approach demonstrating, 51–55
    with axial endorectal scanners, 57, 58–59
    on axial endorectal sonograms, 57–74, 64–67, 68–73
    axial image characteristics, 90–91
    comparison of on axial and sagittal endorectal sonograms, 76–91
    echogenic appearances of, 51, 54
    endorectal approach demonstrating, 57–91
    endourethral approach demonstrating, 56–57
    laterally placed longitudinally oriented sonogram of, 80, 81
    longitudinal orientation of to seminal vesicle and vas deferens, 77–78
    perineal approach demonstrating, 56
    and relationship to seminal vesicles, 82–83, 83–84, 88–89
    with sagittal endorectal scanners, 60–61, 62
    on sagittal endorectal sonograms, 74–76
    sagittal image characteristics, 90–91
    and sequential appearance on transaxial approach, 62
    on transverse transabdominal scans, 52, 53
  peripheral zone of. *See* Peripheral zone
  periurethral, 12–14. *See also* Periurethral glandular zone
  sagittal scanning of, 45–46, 47–48, 49
  size determination of, 93–97
    cystography for, 93
    digital rectal examination for, 93
    endorectal examination for, 95, 96–97
    endourethral examination for, 95
    formulas for, 94–95
    intravenous pyelography for, 93
    planimetric calculation of, 96, 98
    tables for, 95, 96
    techniques for, 93
    transabdominal transverse and longitudinal orientations for, 94, 95
    ultrasound for, 93, 94–96, 97, 98
  sonographic approach to evaluation of, 101–112
    anechoic lesions in, 104, 105
    echogenicity in, 103–112

Prostate gland (contd)
    focus or area of abnormality in, 101–103
    hyperechoic lesions in, 107, 109–111
    hypoechoic lesions in, 104–107
    isoechoic lesions in, 107, 108, 109
    mixed echogenicity in, 107, 112
    periprostatic space in, 103
    symmetrical versus asymmetrical internal architecture of, axial orientation for evaulation of, 90, 91
    transition zone of. See Transition zone
    transperineal approach for ultrasound study of, 33. See also Transperineal approach for prostate ultrasound
    tumors of, axial versus sagittal images for evaluation of, 91. See also Prostate cancer
    ultrasound guided biopsies of, 117–139. See Ultrasound guided biopsy
    weight of. See Prostate, size determination of
    zonal anatomy of, 11–14
        pathologic processes and, 14
Prostate cancer
    atrophy of prostate and, 145
    benign prostatic hypertrophy and, 184
    biopsy for. See Biopsy; Transperineal biopsy; Transrectal biopsy
    capsular invasion and, 179
    classification of, 146, 147
    death rate from, 141, 142, 143
    detection of
        accuracy of sonography in, 184
        and screening with endorectal sonography, 260–264, 265
    differential diagnoses and, endorectal sonography in, 259–260
    dissemination patterns of, 154–155
    endorectal approach in evaluation of, 259–260
    general considerations of, 141–155
        anatomy of development of, 146
        classification of, 146, 147
        dissemination patterns of, 154–155
        grading systems for, 146–148
        metastatic potential of, 155
        pathogenesis of, 144–146
        significant versus insignificant (incidental), 155
        staging of, 148–154
    grading systems for, 146–148
        aspiration biopsy and, 148
        core biopsy and, 147
        cytology and, 148
        Diamond system for, 147
        Gaeta system for, 147
        Gleason system for, 146–147, 148
        limitations of, 147–148
        Mayo Clinic system for, 147
        MD Anderson (MDA) Hospital system for, 147
        Mostofi system for, 147
    incidence of, 142
    metastatic potential of, 155
    mortality rate from, 144
    newly diagnosed cases of, 141, 143
    pathogenesis of, 144–146
        age in, 144
        benign prostatic hyperplasia in, 145
        environmental factors in, 145
        genetics in, 144
        hormonal influence in, 145
        infectious agents in, 145–146
        national predisposition in, 144
        race in, 144–145
    percutaneous placement of radioactive seeds for, 185–190
        ancillary treatment and, 188
        complications of, 188–190
        follow-up studies of, 188
        general considerations for, 185–186
        planning for, 186
        procedure for, 186–188, 189, 190
        success of, 188
    prevalence of, 142
    racial predilection of, 141, 144
    significant versus insignificant (incidental), 155
    site of development of, 146
    sonographic characteristics of, 157–184
        historical perspective of, 157–163
        hyperechoic lesions, 169, 176–177
        hypoechoic lesions, 163–165, 166–168, 169, 170–171
        isoechoic lesions, 165, 168–169, 172–173
        mixed echogenic lesions, 169, 174–175
    staging of, with ultrasound, 181–182, 183
    staging systems for, 148–154
        comparison of, 153
        revised TNM, 153–154
        TNM, 150
        updated TNM, 150, 152–153
        Whitmore Jewett, 148–150, 151
    transitional zone cancer, 177
    tumor extension and, 177–178
Prostate-seminal vesicle angle
    normal sonographic anatomy of
        longitudinal image of in midline, 85, 86–87
        longitudinal image of laterally, 85, 86–87
        on sagittal endorectal sonogram, 74, 90
    prostate cancer and, 181, 182, 183
    in sonographic approach to prostatic disease, 103
Prostatic capsule
    lateral bulges of, axial orientation for evaluation of, 90, 91
    normal sonographic anatomy and
        on axial endorectal sonogram, 67, 74
        on sagittal endorectal sonogram, 76
    in sonographic approach to prostatic disease, 102
    periprostatic tissues and, 103
    tumor extension to, 177–178
    tumor invasion of, 178, 179–181
Prostatic nodules, imaging of, 255–257
Prostatitis, 221–223
    acute, imaging studies of, 222, 223
    bacterial
        classification of, 221
        organisms causing, 221
    chronic, imaging studies of, 222
    general considerations of, 221–222
    histologic study of, 222
    nonbacterial, classification of, 221
    prostate cancer pathogenesis and, 146

P

Prozacin HCl
  bladder neck affected by, 244
  urethra affected by, 244
Pulse echo principle, in ultrasound imaging, 16–17
Pyelogram, intravenous, in benign prostatic hypertrophy, 193

R

Race, prostate cancer affected by
  incidence and, 141, 144
  pathogenesis and, 144, 145
Radial scanners, 35, 36
Radioactive seed implantation, ultrasound guided, 185–190
  ancillary treatment and, 188
  complications of, 188–190
  follow-up studies of, 188
  general considerations in, 185–186
  planning for, 186
  procedure for, 186–188, 189, 190
  success of, 188
Radiography, in prostate imaging, 1
Radionuclide studies, in prostate imaging, 1
Real time ultrasound, 18–19, 20, 21
Rectal examination, prostate size determined by, 93
Rectal ulcer, as complication of percutaneous radiation treatment of prostate cancer, 190
Rectum, normal sonographic anatomy and
  on axial endorectal sonogram, 64, 67
  with perineal approach, 56
Renal obstruction, as complication of percutaneous radiation treatment of prostate cancer, 190
Reserpine, bladder contractility affected by, 244
Resolution, spatial. *See* Spatial resolution

S

Sagittal scanning, technique for, 45–46, 47–48, 49
Sampling volume, ultrasound images affected by, 22
Santorini's plexus, and anatomy of prostate, 5
Scan plane thickness, ultrasound images affected by, 24
Scar tissue, ultrasound images affected by, 26
Sclerotic prostatic atrophy, prostatic cancer and, 145
Screening, for prostate cancer
  and accuracy of sonography in detection, 184
  endorectal ultrasound for, 260–264, 265
Sector (phased) array, 19, 20
Sector scanner, 35, 37
Seminal vesicle
  abdominal approach in ultrasound study of, 31–32
  anatomy and, 5, 6
  asymmetric enlargement of, abscesses and, 226
  diseases of causing infertility, 229–239
    absence of, 232–234
    congenital abnormalities, 232
    cysts, 235, 236–237
    postsurgical acquired disease, 235
    primary neoplasms, 235, 238–239
  embryologic development of, 5
  inflammation of, 225–228. *See also* Abscesses, seminal vesicle; Seminal vesiculitis

  normal sonographic anatomy and
    abdominal approach demonstrating, 51, 53, 55
    on axial endorectal sonogram, 62, 63, 64, 65–66, 67
    laterally placed longitudinally oriented sonogram of, 80, 81
    longitudinal orientation of to prostate, 77–78
    perineal approach demonstrating, 56
    and relationship to prostate, 82–83, 83–84, 88–89
    on sagittal endorectal sonogram, 74, 75, 76
    and sequential appearance on transaxial approach, 62
    on transverse transabdominal scans, 53
  size determination of, 98–100
    abdominal approach for, 99
    normal range for, 100
    symmetry and, 100
  in sonographic approach to prostatic disease, 103
  symmetry of
    axial versus sagittal orientation in evaluation of, 91
    size and, 100
Seminal vesicle angle. *See* Prostate-seminal vesicle angle
Seminal vesiculitis, 225, 226
Sepsis, as complication of prostate biopsy, 116
  transperineal biopsy, 139
  transrectal biopsy, 139
Sex determination, 4
Sexual activity, prostate cancer pathogenesis and, 145
Side lobes, ultrasound images affected by, 23–24
Small parts scanners, 26–27
Sonourethrography
  endorectal approach for, 265
  voiding abnormalities studied with, 245–250, 251
Spatial resolution, ultrasound images affected by, 21–22
Sphincter
  external. *See* External sphincter
  internal. *See* Internal sphincter
Spinal cord injury, voiding abnormalities caused by, 243
Spinal needle, for core needle biopsy, 114
Static scanners, 18
Stroma, anterior fibromuscular. *See* Anterior fibromuscular stroma
Suprapubic approach for prostate ultrasound. *See* Abdominal approach for prostate ultrasound

T

Time-gain compensation (TGC) curves, for normal sonographic anatomy, 51, 54
Tissue attenuation, ultrasound images affected by, 24–25
TNM staging system, for prostate cancer, 150–154
  comparison of with other systems, 153
  correlation of with Whitmore-Jewett system, 151
  revised, 153–154
  updated, 150, 152–153

Transabdominal approach to prostate ultrasound. *See* Abdominal approach to prostate ultrasound
Transition zone
 anatomy of, 14
 benign prostatic hyperplasia in, 192
 cancer originating in, 146, 177
 normal sonographic anatomy and
  on axial endorectal sonogram, 69
  on sagittal endorectal sonogram, 75
Transperineal approach for prostate ultrasound, 33
 benign prostatic hypertrophy demonstrated with, 195
 normal sonographic anatomy demonstrated with, 56
Transperineal biopsy, 114–116
 complications of, 116–117
 ultrasound guided, 118–130
  accuracy of, 130
  accuracy of sagittal orientation, 122
  axial orientation, 119–122
  benefits of, 130, 139
  biplane probe for, 127, 128–129
  comparison of with transrectal biopsy, 130, 139
  complications of, 139
  and echogenically inhomogeneous lesion in sagittal orientation, 123
  freehand, 118
  general considerations of, 118
  guides for, 120, 121
  and limitations of axial orientation, 119–122
  patient position for, 122, 130
  with probe guide, 119, 120
  for prostate cancer, 124–125, 126
  and sagittal orientation, 122–130
  technique for in sagittal orientation, 127–130
Transrectal biopsy, 116, 117
 complications of, 116–117
 ultrasound guided, 130–139, 131
  accuracy of, 130
  benefits of, 139
  comparison of with transperineal biopsy, 130, 139
  complications of, 130, 139
  curvable needle for, 137–138
  guide system for, 132–134
  longitudinally oriented, 135, 136, 137–138
  patient discomfort and, 130
  patient positioning for, 130
  technique for, 130, 135–138
Transurethral approach for prostate ultrasound. *See* Endourethral approach for prostate ultrasound
Transurethral resection (TUR)
 defect from. *See* TUR defect
 endorectal ultrasound after, 200, 209–213
 infertility caused by, 235
 ultrasound monitoring of, 209, 214–215
Tru Cut needle, for core needle biopsy, 113, 114
Tuberculosis, prostatitis caused by, 221
α-Tubocarine, bladder contractility affected by, 244
TUR. *See* Transurethral resection
TUR defect, 209
 on axial endorectal sonogram, 203, 212
 endorectal sonograms of, 210–213

U

Ultrasound
 approaches for, 31–44. *See also specific approach, e.g.,* Abdominal approach for prostate ultrasound; Endorectal approach for prostate ultrasound
  abdominal, 31–33
  endorectal, 34–44
  endourethral, 33–34
  transperineal, 33
 image generation and, 16–19
  equipment design and, 17–18
  pulse-echo principle in, 16–17
  real-time scanners and, 18–19
 image generation difficulties and, 19–26
  acoustic windows and, 26
  air and, 26
  body hair and, 26
  bones and, 25–26
  fat and, 25
  focus characteristics and, 23
  scan plane thickness and, 24
  scar tissue and, 26
  side lobes and, 23–24
  spatial resolution and, 21–22
  tissue attenuation and, 24–25
 and new high-quality images, 26–30
  endorectal prostate scanners for, 27–30
  small-parts scanners for, 26–27
 physical principles of, 15–30
  image generation and, 16–19
  image generation difficulties and, 19–26
  new high-quality images and, 26–30
 in prostate imaging, 2
 techniques for, 45–46
  axial scanning, 45
  image preservation and, 46
  sagittal scanning, 45–46, 47–48, 49
Ultrasound guided biopsy, 117–139. *See also* Endorectal ultrasound guided biopsy; Transperineal biopsy; Transrectal biopsy
 general considerations of, 117
  sterile precautions in technique for, 117–118
 sagittally oriented scanners for, 90, 91
 transperineal, 118–130
  in axial orientation, 119–122
  comparison of with transrectal, 130, 139
  in sagittal orientation, 122–130
 transrectal, 130–139
  comparison of with transperineal, 130, 139
Ureterocele, infertility caused by, 232
Urethra, prostatic, 241–258
 abdominal approach in ultrasound study of, 32–33
 appearance of with abdominal approach, 55
 appearance of with endourethral approach, 56
 autonomic nervous system abnormalities and, 241–243
 on axial endorectal sonogram, 70, 71, 72, 73
 bladder hyperreflexia and, 255
 bladder neck obstruction and, 245, 250–254
 cystometrogram in evaluation of, 244
 drug-induced disorders and, 243
 electromyogram in evaluation of, 244

imaging techniques and, 245–250, 251
longitudinal orientation for evaluation of, 90, 91
neuromuscular disorders of, 241, 242
prostatic nodules and, 255–257
on sagittal endorectal sonogram, 74, 75, 76, 77
in sonographic approach to prostatic disease, 102
spinal cord injury and, 243
urethrometrogram in evaluation of, 244
and urodynamic studies for evaluation of voiding difficulties, 243–244
Urethrometrogram, urethral pressures measured with, 244
Urinary bladder
abdominal approach in ultrasound study of, 32–33
and anatomy of prostate, 5
contracted, 241, 242
drugs contracting, 243
drugs relaxing, 244
embryologic development of, 3–4
hyperreflexia of, imaging of, 255
impingement of disease on, longitudinal orientation for evaluation of, 90, 91
neck of, obstruction of. See Bladder neck obstruction
noncontracted, 241, 242
normal sonographic anatomy and
on axial endorectal sonogram, 64, 67
with perineal approach, 56
on sagittal endorectal sonogram, 76
on transverse transabdominal scans, 52, 53
Urogenital diaphragm, normal sonographic anatomy and, on sagittal endorectal sonogram, 76
Urogram, intravenous, in benign prostatic hypertrophy, 193

V

Vas deferens
and anatomy of prostate, 5
embryologic development of, 4
normal sonographic anatomy and
abdominal approach demonstrating, 55
on axial endorectal sonogram, 62, 63, 64
longitudinal orientation of to prostate, 77–78
on sagittal endorectal sonogram, 74
Vasovagal reaction
as complication of transperineal biopsy, 139
as complication of transrectal biopsy, 139
VCU. See Voiding cystourethrogram
Venereal disease, prostate cancer pathogenesis and, 145
Verumontanum, normal sonographic anatomy and
on axial endorectal sonogram, 67, 70, 71
on sagittal endorectal sonogram, 75
Vim Silverman needle, for core needle biopsy, 113
Voiding abnormalities
and autonomic nervous system disorders, 241–243
bladder hyperreflexia and, 255
bladder neck obstruction and, 245
imaging of, 250–254
cystometrogram in study of, 244
drug induced disorders and, 243, 244
electromyogram in study of, 244
imaging techniques in evaluation of, 245–249, 250, 251
neuromuscular disorders causing, 241, 242
prostatic nodules and, 255–258
spinal cord injury and, 243
urethrometrogram in study of, 244
urodynamic studies of, 243–244
Voiding cystourethrogram (VCU), voiding abnormalities studied with, 245
Voiding sonourethrography, 245–250, 251

W

Westcott needle, for core needle biopsy, 114
Whitmore Jewett staging system, for prostate cancer, 148–150
comparison of with other systems, 153
correlation of with TNM system, 151
Window of curability, in prostate cancer, 155
Wolffian duct, in embryogenesis of urogenital system, 3–5